Falls in Epileptic and Non-epileptic Seizures During Childhood

Fondazione Pierfranco e Luisa Mariani
viale Bianca Maria 28
20129 Milan, Italy

Falls in Epileptic and Non-epileptic Seizures During Childhood

International Colloquium of the Pierfranco e Luisa Mariani Foundation
Milan State University, 12–14 October 1995

Edited by
A. Beaumanoir, F. Andermann,
G. Avanzini and L. Mira

Mariani Foundation Paediatric Neurology Series: 6
Series Editor: Maria Majno

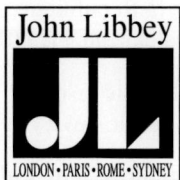

British Library Cataloguing in Publication Data

Falls in epileptic and non-epileptic seizures during childhood
  Mariani Foundation paediatric neurology series: vol. 6
  1. Epilepsy in children
  I. Beaumanoir, A. II. Fondazione Pierfranco e Luisa Mariani
  616.9'2'853

ISSN: 0969-0301
ISBN: 0 86196 540 X

Published by

**John Libbey & Company Ltd, 13 Smiths Yard, Summerley Street,
London SW18 4HR, England.** Telephone: 0181-947 2777: Fax 0181-947 2664
John Libbey and Company Pty Ltd, Level 10, 15–17 Young Street, Sydney, 2000, Australia.
John Libbey Eurotext Ltd, 127 Avenue de la République, 92120 Montrouge, France.
John Libbey - C.I.C. s.r.l., via Lazzaro Spallanzani 11, 00161 Rome, Italy.

© 1997 John Libbey & Company Ltd. All rights reserved.
Unauthorised duplication contravenes applicable laws.

Printed in Hong Kong by Dah Hua Printing Press Co., Ltd.

Contents

	A tribute to Henri Gastaut *Anne Beaumanoir*	vii
Chapter 1	The problem of falls in the symptomatology of epileptic and non-epileptic seizures during childhood in Gastaut's works and today *Anne Beaumanoir and Jean-Louis Gastaut*	1

PART I

Chapter 2	Physiological mechanisms involved in falling *Jean Massion*	11
Chapter 3	Epilepsy and the development of cortical connectivity *Giorgio M. Innocenti*	19
Chapter 4	Cortical maturation and electroclinical epxression of epileptic falls *Giuliano Avanzini, Flavio Villani, Laura Canafoglia and Tiziana Granata*	29
Chapter 5	Muscular silent period following transcranial magnetic stimulation: contribution of peripheral and central mechanisms *Paolo M. Rossini and Simone Rossi*	45
Chapter 6	Clinical and neurophysiological features of different forms of epileptic falls *Guido Rubboli, Roberto Michelucci, Franco Valzania, Lucio Parmeggiani, Stefano Meletti, Elena Gardella, Romana Rizzi, Anna Zaniboni and Carlo Alberto Tassinari*	53

PART II

Chapter 7	Study of epileptic falls: methodologies and polygraphies *Michelle Bureau and Henri Régis*	65
Chapter 8	Infantile spasms and tonic seizures *Silvana Franceschetti, Tiziana Granata, Simona Binelli, Laura Canafoglia and Giuliano Avanzini*	75
Chapter 9	Semeiological features of non-epileptic falls *Giuseppe Gobbi and Antonella Pini*	83

PART III

Chapter 10	Epileptic syndromes with drop seizures in children *Charlotte Dravet, Renzo Guerrini and Michelle Bureau*	95
Chapter 11	Falls in epileptic syndromes of adolescence *Pierre Thomas and Karine Ostrowsky*	113
Chapter 12	Falls in epileptic seizures with partial onset *Arnaud Biraben and Patrick Chauvel*	125
Chapter 13	Outcome of children's epileptic falls *Pierre Loiseau, Pierre Jallon and Jean-Michel Pédespan*	137

PART IV

Chapter 14	The pharmacological treatment of epileptic falls *Francesco Viani, Antonino Romeo, Maurizio Viri and Elda Fabiola Gonano*	147
Chapter 15	Indications and results of surgical treatment (excluding callosotomy) in children with epileptic falls *Claudio Munari, Lorella Minotti, Giorgio Lo Russo, Philippe Kahane, Filippo Leocata, Stefano Francione, Laura Tassi, Matilde Di Leo, Pier Paolo Quarato, Dominique Hoffmann and Alim Louis Benabid*	159
Chapter 16	Corpus callosum section for the treatment of epileptic falls or drop attacks: an effective palliative approach *Mario A. Alonso-Vanegas, Frederick Andermann and André Olivier*	175
Chapter 17	Seizures and the risk of injury in four different clinical severity populations *Giorgio Capizzi, Piernanda Vigliano, Maresa Perenchio and Giovanni Asteggiano*	193
Chapter 18	The social life of the epileptic child presenting falls *Laura Mira, Bona Oxilia and Carlo Zerbi*	199
Chapter 19	The fall in epileptic children: psychopathological and humanistic aspects *René Soulayrol*	207
	Synopsis *Giuliano Avanzini*	213
	Index	219

A tribute to Henri Gastaut

Anne Beaumanoir

Henri Gastaut, a master of epileptology, died on 14 July 1995. The Fondazione Pierfranco e Luisa Mariani wished to devote the Colloquium entitled 'Epileptic and non-epileptic falls in childhood' in honour of his memory.

Henri Gastaut's contribution to the understanding of seizures and of epilepsies is impressive for it includes the identification of several epileptic syndromes such as reflex photogenic epilepsy, startle epilepsy, the HHE syndrome, West syndrome and the Lennox–Gastaut syndrome. Unilateral seizures have been described in his clinical laboratory, where research was also carried out on diagnostic procedures to differentiate epileptic seizures from anoxo-ischaemic attacks. The results of research in his laboratory at the Faculty of Medicine in Marseille contributed to the fractionation of the so-called psychomotor epilepsy.

An admirer as well as a friend of William Lennox, he discussed with him astatic seizures, which have been the main topic of debate in this Colloquium. Henri Gastaut was a passionate pioneer of epileptology development. An exceptional educator, he always gave the best of himself as a teacher especially in the occasion of the 25 'Colloques de Marseilles' which he organized and animated from 1951 to 1975. Their success is witnessed by the increasing number of participants: 34 in the first, about 100 in the second, and then 200 to 300 in the following ones. About half of the physicians who regularly attended his didactic meetings were Italian.

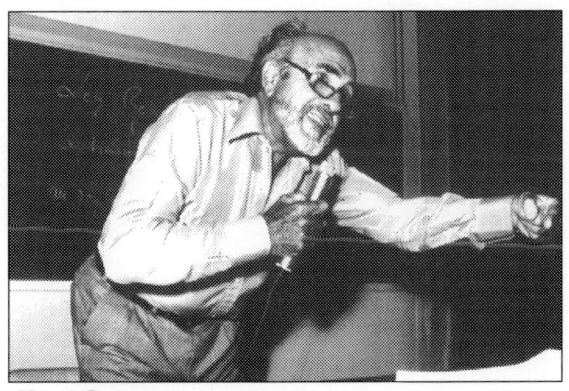
Henri Gastaut

During this Colloquium, relevant studies by Henri Gastaut as well as others have been discussed by some of those who had the privilege to follow his teachings over several months or years. Among the 33 authors who are included in this book, eleven have been his pupils or his collaborators.

Chapter 1

The problem of falls in the symptomatology of epileptic and non-epileptic seizures during childhood in Gastaut's works and today

Anne Beaumanoir and Jean-Louis Gastaut[*]

Fondazione Pierfranco e Luisa Mariani, Neurologia infantile, viale Bianca Maria 28, 20129 Milan, Italy
[*]*Service de Neurologie, Hôpital Ste Marguerite, Boulevard Ste Marguerite, 13009 Marseille, France*

Until the last century, the fall characterized epilepsy and marked the epileptic patient. Since the Assyrians, epilepsy – the *morbus caducum* of Paracelsus – has knocked man down. Today the terms 'fall' and 'drop attack' still have a negative meaning for epileptologists who observed that falls are an ominous sign in the evolution of generalized and partial epilepsies.

The advent of the EEG permitted the distinction between falls accompanied by epileptic EEG paroxysms and falls without EEG modification or without an epileptic EEG abnormality. The contribution of polygraphy and cinematography (and later of video recordings) to the identification of falls was soon acknowledged. Therefore, since the 1960s, thanks mainly to the works of Gastaut and his group, 'static seizures', as Hunt (1922) called them, have been classified in different electroclinical types: myoclonias, tonic seizures, atonic seizures, partial seizures and non-epileptic attacks with falls. Gastaut's works led in 1969 to the first proposal of a classification of the epileptic seizures, which as far as epileptic falls are concerned has been since then very little modified (Classification of 1981). His works also led to the book on *Epileptic seizures* by Gastaut & Broughton (1972) and to the *Dictionnaire de l'Épilepsie* by Gastaut, edited by WHO in 1973, which is the source of the definitions of the first part of this chapter. This part, meant as an homage to Henri Gastaut, remembers his work in the field of seizures with falls. The second part is a brief introduction which takes into account data acquired in the years preceding the Colloquium of which this book represents the outcome.

Part I

Myoclonias

Myoclonia is a 'brief and involuntary contraction of one or more muscles, without body displacement if a small muscle acts on a big part, with displacement in the opposite case. The muscular potentials accompanying the myoclonia are followed by a muscular activity of interferential type prolonging the contraction or, on the contrary, by an inhibition. The myoclonia is caused by a dysfunction of the structure involved in motor activity, from the cerebral cortex to the spinal motor neuron (*Dictionnaire de l'Épilepsie*). Epileptic myoclonias leading to a fall correspond to massive epileptic myoclonias of very short duration. They involve 'simultaneously agonist and antagonist muscles (if they do not have reciprocal innervation) of several symmetrical segments (usually head, neck, upper limbs) or of the whole body' (Gastaut, 1968). When the myoclonia is global, causing flexion of the legs, fall is possible as in Janz's Impulsive PM (Janz & Christian, 1957, 1994). This is a propulsive fall. Gastaut & Broughton (1972) emphasize the accompanying signs: the patient widens his fingers, any object held in the hand is thrown forwards, and the fall usually occurs in flexion though sometimes in extension. The EEG accompaniment of epileptic myoclonias is a generalized spike, polyspike or polyspike-wave. The spike predominates in the central regions of the scalp, the slow wave is more anterior. During the slow wave following the spike, inhibition may occur, usually associated with post myoclonic inhibition of the muscle tone. Falling may result either from myoclonus of flexor muscles of the legs or from the post myoclonic hypotonia, or even from both in succession (Gastaut & Broughton, 1972).

The definition of myoclonia, and specifically of epileptic myoclonia, given by Gastaut in 1968 does not differ from the more recent definition by Fahn *et al.* (1986) which is usually referred to as a landmark: 'The epileptic myoclonia is a sudden, brief, brisk and involuntary movement due to a massive muscular contraction (positive myoclonia) or to a muscular inhibition (negative myoclonia) originating in the CNS.'

Tonic seizures

Gastaut *et al.* (1965) described three types of tonic seizures according to the muscles which become hypertonic. 'The axial tonic seizures, the axorhyzomelic tonic seizures, the global tonic seizures' which can cause a fall in the standing subject, as pointed out by Chatrian *et al.* (1982). There is a semeiological continuum among these three types of seizures. The global tonic seizure is the most complete one. In fact, every axial tonic seizure begins with a contraction of the neck muscles followed by those of the face 'which usually fixates the head rigidly in line with the body axis, or may displace it somewhat forwards or backwards, depending upon whether flexor or extensor groups predominate. The axorhyzomelic tonic seizure begins as an axial tonic seizure, but the attack is more extensive owing to added participation of the arms and sometimes leg girdle muscles. In the global tonic seizure these changes are associated with contraction to the very periphery of the limbs. The arms are flung upwards and are semi-flexed in front of the head with clenching of the fists. The lower limbs are in triple flexion or, less often, in forced extension.' If the subject is standing, a fall is possible. The duration of the spasm depends on its extension, ranging from 2–3 s up to 10–12 s. The stiffening of the extremities, sometimes the cry caused by forced expiration, and mostly the accompanying autonomic signs permit the differential diagnosis with other postural tonic epileptic or non-epileptic seizures, such as the 'convulsive syncopal attacks', the 'tetanic attack' or the 'hysterical attack'. Gastaut

& Broughton (1972) stressed the absence of opisthotonic posturing in epileptic tonic seizures. Since epileptic tonic seizures do not entail decerebration, they do not show opisthotonic posturing, at variance with convulsive syncopal attacks in which such a mechanism may be at play. According to Gastaut & Broughton, infantile spasms consist 'of a more or less generalized contraction, often of such a brief duration that it appears clinically as a form of myoclonus' (Gastaut & Broughton, 1972). Infantile spasms occurring before the age of the upright position do not cause fall; however 'the spasm confined to the axial muscles of the head, neck and sometimes trunk causes head nodding'.

Tonic seizures are exaggerated by slow sleep, as it is usually the case in the Lennox–Gastaut syndrome, of which they are the hallmark (Gastaut, 1982; Beaumanoir & Dravet, 1992).

Infantile spasms, though not pathognomonic of West syndrome, are nonetheless its most obvious clinical sign.

EEG and polygraphy recordings play a role in the diagnosis of tonic seizures and infantile spasms. On an EEG tonic seizures are represented by discharges of low amplitude spikes, beginning as fast spikes and slowing down to about 10 Hz while their amplitude increases. The duration of the discharge ranges from a few seconds to 10 s; when it is long it usually ends with a burst of diffuse slow waves. Tonic spasms may also present these same EEG patterns, but more often they present only a decreased amplitude of the rhythms, usually preceded by a hypersynchronous slow wave which in the case of West syndrome stands out on the hypsarrhythmic tracing.

Atonic seizures

Gastaut & Régis (1961) make a distinction between atonic absences and atonic seizures, which they called epileptic drop attacks to emphasize their short duration. They define this type of seizure as a reduction or elimination of the postural tone of very short duration which can involve all the postural muscles (with the patient falling to the ground) or only those of the head (the head falls on the chest: epilepsy 'nutans').

Epileptic drop attacks, called 'astatic seizures' by Lennox, are the only epileptic seizures which always cause a fall.

Gastaut with Tassinari & Bureau-Paillas (1966) studied the atonic seizures from the electroclinical and cinematographical point of view. They confirmed the usual association of atonic and myoclono-atonic seizures in the same patient.

As Dravet et al. (1988) point out in the wake of the studies on drop attacks by Gastaut and his school, only myoclonias can be identified by a characteristic EEG pattern. On an EEG, atonic seizures may be accompanied by a burst of polyspike wave followed by generalized spikes and slow waves, or else by discharges of slow spike-waves followed (or not) by fast rhythms. Whichever is the case, the loss of tone accompanies the slow waves.

As far as the pathogenesis of the epileptic atonic fall is concerned, in 1968 Tassinari, Régis & Gastaut excluded a mechanism such as 'spinal silent period' because of the duration of atonia. Furthermore, Gastaut & Broughton (1972), observed that during an atonic seizure, whether cephalic, global or focal, the slow waves always predominate in the central regions (C3–C4) of one or both of the two hemiscalps. This led them to postulate a role of the motor cortex in the genesis of epileptic atonia. Moreover, Tassinari & Gastaut (1969) described a peculiar kind of muscular inhibition in the epileptic subject: the 'related epileptic silent period', which they showed to be present in generalized as well as focal atonic seizures.

In their work of 1972 Gastaut & Broughton make a distinction among brief, prolonged and focal atonic seizures. Prolonged seizures, up to 10 min in duration, are most often 'akinetic' seizures: the child is motionless, sometimes on the ground, and the spikes and waves are slow, diffuse and rhythmical. On the contrary, when the atonic seizure is brief, the slow spikes and waves are diffuse and less rhythmical.

In the epileptic unilateral drop attack the hypotonia may be consistently asymmetrical, the child always falling on one side. Most striking of all are the unilateral atonic epileptic seizures giving rise to transient ictal hemiplegia, to be thoroughly distinguished from the postictal Todd paralysis (Gastaut & Broughton, 1972).

Part II

Recent advances, mainly due to the new techniques of neurophysiological investigation of the motor loops in man – for instance, magnetic transcranial stimulation, the diffusion of the back averaging method of Ugawa et al. (1989), the better understanding of the mechanisms of anti-epileptic drugs, the improvement of neurosurgical techniques and the growing interest for the psychological and social aspects of epilepsy – should allow a better medical, surgical and pedagogical treatment of the epileptic child, whose epileptic falls are a major handicap.

The availability of polygraphy and video EEG allowed a better understanding of the clinical and electrophysiological features which distinguish the different types of seizures sharing the fall as their most important sign.

Ikeno et al. (1985) analysed the results of simultaneous EEG and EMG recordings and tracking videotapes of 48 epileptic falls in 15 children with Lennox–Gastaut syndrome. They described four types of seizures with falls, and stated, as already observed by Egli et al. (1985), that the most distinguishable falls are the tonic seizures. They observed that the hypertonic state continued unchanged even after the patient has fallen down. They used the term 'flexor spasms' for short-duration tonic seizures limited to the neck, the truncal muscles and the upper limbs. They described the myoclonia of the myoclono-atonic seizure, confirmed by the EMG. They observed a brief vocalization, a brief jerk of the trunk and of the upper limbs with throwing forward of any object held in the hand. However, the cause of the fall may be the subsequent global atonia. The atonic seizure is characterized by an abrupt loss of tone in antigravity muscles. The subject looks like a puppet whose strings have all been cut.

Oguni et al. (1992a) studied 36 drop seizures: 17 exhibited only deep head nodding. They distinguished two groups of atonic seizures: those characterized by abrupt falls and those in which the fall is preceded by other symptoms, most often minimal myoclonic contractions of the facial muscles and twitching of the extremities. They showed that such subtle myoclonic movements produce a post myoclonic inhibition. These transient preceding signs correspond to the length of the spike and the atonia to the ascendant phase of the slow wave of the generalized bilateral synchronous polyspike wave.

A post myoclonic inhibition is also likely in the nine observations of status epilepticus by Kanazawa & Kawai (1990), characterized by repetitive asymmetrical atonia in which the loss of tone corresponds to the slow wave of the spike and wave complex. An epileptic negative myoclonus (ENM) might also be present, as in several cases of partial epilepsy (Cirignotta & Lugaresi, 1991; Oguni et al., 1992b; Guerrini et al., 1993). The first description of this disorder was made by Tassinari in 1981. In the same year Cirignotta et al. (1981) studied the role of posture in the muscular activities which accompany the spike-wave discharge. The fall of an arm may be the effect of a phasic inhibition resulting in the silence of agonist and antagonist muscles while maintaining a posture. The ENM always manifests itself as 'a brief postural lapse of a segment without evidence of myoclonia' (Ford et al., 1995). An ENM may involve the facial muscles as well as the limb muscles. It may be unilateral or bilateral according to the motor areas involved. According to Tassinari et al. (1995) it corresponds to 'a paroxysmal event involving primarily or secondarily the centro-parietal and frontal supplementary motor areas'.

Oguni et al. (1994), in their study of the myoclonias of the juvenile myoclonic epilepsy, think that the fall could be caused, at least in part, by a loss of balance when the upper trunk suffers a propulsive contraction leading to a sudden shift of the centre of gravity.

The fall is always the result of a sudden loss of muscle tone, or, rather, of postural control, and/or of a disruption of balance. When a sudden movement displaces the sustaining polygon, a fall occurs if the physiological adjusting reactions cannot be brought into action. The fall may also result from a defective cortical control on the lower structures involved in maintaining tone, mainly in the brainstem. The reduction or suppression, during an episode of altered consciousness, of the multisensorial information involved in maintaining the species normal posture may also facilitate the fall.

When the fall occurs during an epileptic discharge, the sensorimotor and/or pre-motor areas, either unilaterally or bilaterally, are usually primarily or secondarily involved. Drop attacks occurring in a subject with an epileptic frontal focus are very frequent, as shown by Geier, Bancaud et al. (1977) and many others. They often occur when the EEG shows bilateral bursts of spikes and waves, which correspond to the secondary bisynchronia of the electroencephalograph. Thus, a transcallosal transmission may be inferred with the ensuing consequences on the therapeutical decision.

The functional systems allowing man the erect posture, the ability to straighten up, to maintain equilibrium and to walk without support are gradually acquired. Therefore the semeiology of the fall evolves with the maturation of the feedback control of posture and equilibrium. The basic mechanisms of partial or global falls are similar whatever is the cause, epileptic or not, of the seizure provoking them, but they differ according to the abnormal movement (myoclonia, spasm, atonia) which is its consequence. The level of the discharge, the age of the patient, the posture of the patient at the time of the attack and other factors, such as the state of consciousness, interact to determine the semeiology of the fall.

As was observed by the older authors, ictal symptoms preceding, following and accompanying the fall are critical for the diagnosis of the aetiology and of the seizure, as already stated by Amboise Paré in the sixteenth century, when he wrote in his eighth book: 'Epilepsie, mot grec qui signifie surprise, ou rétention de tous les sentiments dont ils aduient que le malade chet en terre s'il n'est soutenu ... comme par une syncope ou une apoplexie. Mais il y a différence car en l'apoplexie et la syncope il n'y a nul mouvement ou sentiment'. (Epilepsy, a Greek word meaning surprise, or retention of all senses causing the fall of the patient if he is not supported ... as with syncopal attacks or apoplexia. But there is a difference because in apoplexia and syncopal attacks there are neither movements nor senses.)

Acknowledgement
The authors wish to thank Dr A. van Lierde for her help with the English text.

References

Beaumanoir, A. & Dravet, Ch. (1992): The Lennox–Gastaut syndrome. In: *Epileptic syndromes in infancy, childhood and adolescence*, eds. J. Roger, M. Bureau, Ch. Dravet, A. Perret & P. Wolf, pp. 115–132. London: John Libbey.

Chatrian, G.E., Lettich, E., Wilkus, R.G. & Vallaria, J. (1982): Polygraphic and clinical observations on tonic-autonomic seizures. In: Henri Gastaut and the Marseille School's Contribution to the Neurosciences. *EEG Clin. Neurophysiol.* **suppl. 35,** 101–124.

Cirignotta, F., Montagna, P. & Lugaresi, E. (1981): Muscular inhibitory and excitatory phenomena during spike-and-wave discharges: effects of posture. *J. Neurol. Neurosurg. Psychiatry* **44,** 1172–1173.

Cirignotta, F. & Lugaresi, E. (1991): Partial motor epilepsy with 'negative myoclonus'. *Epilepsia* **32,** 54–58.

Commission on Classification and Terminology of the International League Against Epilepsy (1981): Proposal for revised clinical and electroencephalographic classification of epileptic seizures. *Epilepsia* **30,** 389–399.

Dravet, C., Bureau, M., Tassinari, C.A., Régis, H., Salamon, G.& Chiarelli, D. (1988): Different types of epileptic drop seizures in children. *Neurologia et Psychiatria* **11 (suppl. 1),** 7–16.

Egli, M., Mothersill, J., O'Kane, M. & O'Kane, F. (1985): The axial spasm. The predominant type of drop seizure in patients with secondary generalized epilepsy. *Epilepsia* **26,** 401–415.

Fahn, S., Marsden, C.D. & van Woert, M.H. (1986): Definition and classification of myoclonus. In: *Advances in epileptology,* eds. S. Fahn, C.D. Marsden & M.H. van Woert, vol. 43, pp. 1–5. New York: Raven Press.

Ford, B., Fahn, S. & Pullman, S.L. (1995): Peripherally induced electromyographic silent periods: normal physiology and disorders of motor control. In: *Negative motor phenomena*, eds. S. Fahn, M. Hallett, H.O. Luders & C.D. Marsden. *Advances in neurology*, vol. 67, pp. 321–328. Philadelphia: Lippincott-Raven.

Gastaut, H. & Régis, H. (1961): On the subject of Lennox's 'akinetic' Petit Mal. *Epilepsia* **2,** 298–305.

Gastaut, H., Roger, J., Ouahchi, S., Timsit, M. & Broughton, R. (1965): An electroclinical study of generalized seizures of tonic espression. *Epilepsia* **4,** 15–44.

Gastaut, H., Tassinari, C.A. & Bureau-Paillas, M. (1966): Etude polygraphique et clinique des effondrements atoniques épileptiques. *Rev. Neurol.* **36,** 5–21.

Gastaut, H. (1968): Séméiologie des myoclonies et nosologie analytique des syndromes myocloniques. *Rev. Neurol..* **119,** 1–30.

Gastaut, H. & Broughton, R. (1972): *Epileptic seizures. Clinical and electrographic features, diagnosis and treatment,* pp. 12–16. Springfield, IL: Charles C. Thomas.

Gastaut, H. (1973): *Dictionnaire de l'épilepsie*. Genève: Organisation Mondiale de la Santé.

Gastaut, H. (1982): The Lennox–Gastaut syndrome: Comments on the syndrome's terminology and nosological position among at the secondary generalized epilepsies of childhood. In: Henri Gastaut and the Marseille School's Contribution to the Neurosciences. *EEG Clin. Neurophysiol.* **35 (suppl.),** 35–40.

Geier, S., Bancaud, J., Tailerach, J. *et al.* (1977): The seizures of frontal lobe epilepsy. A study of clinical manifestations. *Neurology* **27,** 951–958.

Guerrini, R., Dravet, C., Genton, P. Bureau, M.,Roger, J., Rubboli, G. & Tassinari, C.A. (1993): Epileptic negative myoclonus. *Neurology* **43,** 1078–1083.

Hunt, J.R. (1922): On the occurrence of static seizures in epilepsy. *J. Nerv. Ment. Dis.* **56,** 351–356.

Ikeno, T., Shigematsu, H., Miyakoshi, M., Ohba, A., Yagi, K. & Seino, M. (1985): An analytic study of epileptic falls. *Epilepsia* **26,** 612–621.

Janz, D. & Christian, W. (1957): Impulsiv petit mal. *Dtsch. Z. Nervenheilk.* **176,** 346–386.

Janz, D. & Christian, W. (1994): Impulsive petit mal (translated into English by P. Genton). In: *Idiopathic generalized epilepsies: clinical, experimental and genetic aspects*, eds. A. Malafosse, P. Genton, E. Hirsch, C. Marescaux, D. Broglin & R. Bernasconi, pp. 229–251. London: John Libbey.

Kanazawa, O. & Kawai, I. (1990): Status epilepticus characterized by repetitive asymmetrical atonia: two cases accompanied by partial seizures. *Epilepsia* **31,** 536–543.

Oguni, H., Fukuyama, Y., Imazumi, Y. & Wehara, T.B. (1992a): Video-EEG analysis of drops seizures in myoclonic-astatic epilepsy in early childhood (Doose syndrome). *Epilepsia* **33,** 805–813.

Oguni, H.O., Sato, F., Hayashi, K., Wang, P.J. & Fukuyama, Y. (1992b): A study of unilateral brief focal atonia in childhood partial epilepsy. *Epilepsia* **33,** 75–83.

Oguni, H., Mukahira, K., Oguni, M., Uehara, T., Su, Y.H., Izumi, T. & Fukuyama, Y. (1994): Video-polygraphic analysis of myoclonic seizures in juvenile myoclonic epilepsy. *Epilepsia* **35,** 307–316.

Oeuvres complètes de Amboise Paré (1957): In: *Des monstres et des prodiges*, VIII livre, p. 80. Genève: Slatkine Editeur.

Tassinari, C.A., Régis, H. & Gastaut, H. (1968): A particular form of muscular inhibition in epilepsy: the related epileptic silent period (RESP). *Proc. Aust. Assoc. Neurol.* **5,** 595–602.

Tassinari, C.A. & Gastaut, H. (1969): A particular form of muscular inhibition in epilepsy: the related epileptic silent period. *Topical Problems Psychiatry Neurol.* **10,** 178–186.

Tassinari, C. A. (1981): New perspectives in epileptology. In: *Trends in modern epileptology*, eds. Japanese Epilepsy Association. Proceedings of the International Public Seminar on Epileptology, pp. 42–59. Tokyo: Japanese Epilepsy Association.

Tassinari, C.A., Rubboli, G., Parmeggiani, L., Valzania, F., Plasmati, R., Riguzzi, P., Michelucci, R., Volpi, L., Passarelli, D., Meletti, S., Fontana, E. & Dalla Bernardina, B. (1995): Epileptic negative myoclonus. In: *Negative motor phenomena*, eds. S. Fahn, M. Hallett, H.O. Luders & C.D. Marsden. *Advances in neurology*, vol. 67, pp. 181–198. Philadelphia: Lippincott-Raven.

Ugawa, Y., Shimpo, T. & Mannen, T. (1989): Physiological asterixis: silent period locked averaging. *J. Neurol. Neurosurg. Psychiatry* **52,** 89–92.

Chapter 2

Physiological mechanisms involved in falling

Jean Massion

Laboratoire de Neurobiologie et Mouvements, CNRS 31, chemin Joseph Aiguier, 13402 Marseille Cédex 20, France

Summary

Falling during epileptic seizures in children can be explained on the basis of a large variety of factors. In order to better understand which factors are involved and how they will intervene in balance control, a short survey on the organization of posture and balance control is presented here, which also deals with how this control is co-ordinated with that of movement. The main putative reasons for balance disturbance will be discussed, along with the role of several central structures, the functional impairment of which might result in falling.

Introduction

Fallings and balance disturbances can result from the functional impairment of a large number of brain structures. These can either intervene directly in postural or equilibrium control or be only indirectly involved.

One of the main sources of equilibrium problems is of a sensory nature. Balance is based on multisensory control. The dysfunctioning of vestibular afferents is, in fact, the most common cause of disequilibrium, which can also result however from a functional disorder at the level of the proprioceptive or visual afferents involved in balance.

A lesion of the central vestibular pathways is another frequent source of balance deficiency (Dieterich & Brandt, 1994) (Fig. 1). It can be localized at the level either of the brainstem or the cerebellum, where the head and eye position with respect to the vertical are controlled. There also exist one or several cortical vestibular areas, including the infratemporal vestibular area, where the vestibular afferent messages converge with the visual and somaesthetic inputs and are used to build up spatial maps, in which not only the respective positions of body segments are accounted for, but also their position with respect to external space (Grüsser *et al.*, 1990; Karnath, 1994; Mennemeier *et al.*, 1994). These maps also define the body's midline position. A dysfunctioning of these spatial maps is liable to result in vertical perception errors and therefore in mis-judging the body's position with respect to the external world.

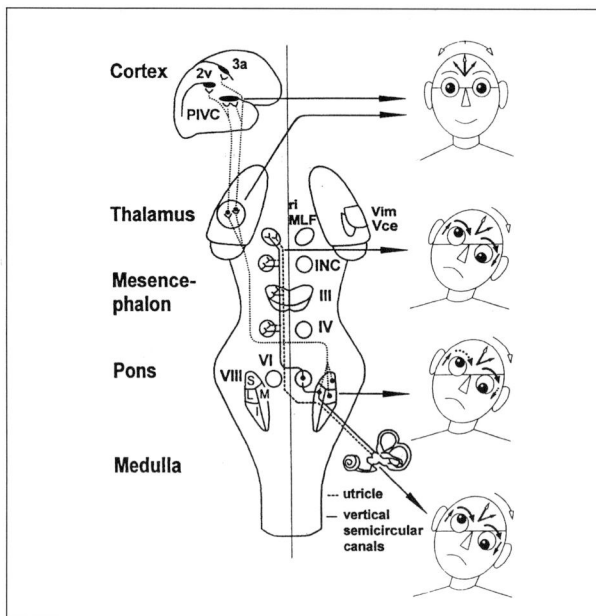

Fig. 1. *Graviceptive pathways from the otoliths and vertical semicircular canals mediating the vestibular reaction in the roll plane. They cross at pontine level. On the right, ocular tilt reaction (OTR) in relation to the level of the lesion: ipsiversive with the peripheral and pontomedullary lesions; contraversive with pontomesencephalic lesions. In the case of vestibular thalamus lesions, the tilting of the subjective vertical can be either contraversive or ipsiversive, whereas in that of vestibular cortex lesions, they tend to be preferably contraversive. OTR is not induced by supratentorial lesions above the level of the nucleus of Cajal (INC) (from Dieterich & Brandt, 1994).*

A third source of disequilibrium consists of brisk changes occurring in the muscle tone, particularly in the antigravity tone. Two sets of descending pathways acting on the segmental myotatic loop and on the segmental output stage have been identified by Mori (1987), the one excitatory and the other inhibitory, both originating from the pontine area. When the inhibitory system is excited, the standing cat stops walking and starts lying down. The reverse occurs when the excitatory system is excited, and a spastic gait is seen to emerge.

These few preliminary remarks show the wide variety of factors liable to intervene in the control of stance and balance. An attempt to sum up the present state of the art in this field should help to understand better the possible causes of falling.

Definition and function of posture

How might posture be defined? One might adopt a purely descriptive approach, and like André Thomas (1940), define posture or attitude as the positioning of the various body segments at a given time. One might also consider the neural control which is responsible for maintaining the usual posture, which is standing. This approach was adopted by Sherrington (1906), Magnus (1924) and Rademaker (1931) and then by many other authors, and resulted in the description of the whole set of postural and righting reflexes. This method of defining posture in terms of the underlying neural control is still sound in itself, but it now needs to be set in a wider framework by asking a more general question: what is the goal of a given postural control in the sensorimotor activity of living beings?

Posture can be said to serve two main functions: an antigravity function and a function consisting of acting as an interface with the external world.

(1) The antigravity function consists of resisting the force of gravity in order to build up the 'configuration' of segments which will constitute the actual posture. Postural tone is the main source on which this function depends. It also involves equilibrium control, since

under static conditions, the centre of gravity (CG) projection on to the ground has to remain inside the supporting area.

(2) The function consisting of acting as an interface with the external world for perception and action means that the position and orientation of body segments are used as reference values to compute the body's position with respect to the external world, or the position of objects in the external world with respect to the body. The posture of given segments such as the head or the trunk is also used to compute movement trajectories in external space, as in the case of hand trajectories performed towards a target.

Both of the above functions of posture are carried out not only during quiet stance but also while performing movements. As any movement *per se* is a source of postural and balance disturbance, co-ordination is needed between posture and movement. Defective co-ordination can give rise to equilibrium disturbances.

Modular versus antigravity organization of posture

In humans, erect posture raises specific control problems, due to the fact that the human stance is bipedal and the support area narrow. In addition, the CG position is quite high with respect to the supporting surface. Human stance has often been compared with an inverted pendulum oscillating around the ankle joint axis (Nashner & McCollum, 1985; Gurfinkel, 1973). Although in some situations the whole body can actually behave like an inverted pendulum, it more commonly behaves like an assembly of superimposed modules, the head, the trunk and the legs. Each module is connected to the one below by a set of muscles which undergo a specific central and peripheral control depending on the modular reference position according to the behavioural context. As first illustrated by Martin (1967), some post-encephalitic patients permanently hold their head flexed downward on to their trunk. These patients are nevertheless able to place their head at the vertical when performing a voluntary movement. This dissociation between an automatic postural head control and a voluntary control confirms the existence of automatic postural controls which are specific to each module. The example of the head is interesting because the head is equipped with three categories of receptors, visual, labyrinthine and muscle proprioceptive. The head's position can be stabilized on the basis of each category of sensors as a function of the task requirements and the context. Head posture can be stabilized for example on the basis of either the gaze direction (vision), the vertical gravity vector (otoliths) or the trunk axis (neck muscle proprioceptors) as illustrated by Berthoz & Pozzo (1988) and by Assaiante & Amblard (1993). The ability to stabilize the head on the basis of the vertical gravity vector may be used to control the posture of the other body segments in a 'top down' mode.

Besides the modular postural control, there also exists a global antigravity postural control, which is based on the brain stem excitatory and inhibitory centres (Mori, 1987) responsible for adjusting the postural tone.

What is the difference between posture and balance? Keeping balance is a constraint which affects the posture and depends on the gravity constraints. The various body segments can adopt a large variety of positions, within the limits of the joints' mechanical characteristics. There exists, however, a rule whereby the distribution of the body mass is such that the centre of gravity (CG) projection remains inside the supporting base, i.e. the area between the feet. This

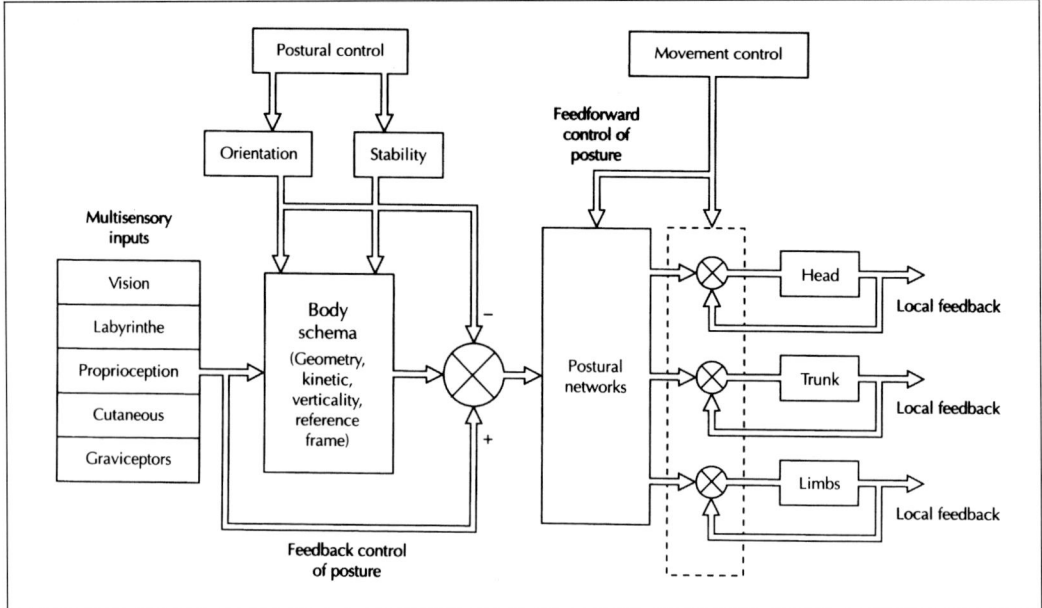

Fig. 2. This diagram summarizes the main components involved in the central organization of postural control. There are two sets of reference values, the one relating to body segment orientation and the other to whole body stability (equilibrium control). These references values, and their maintenance despite external or internal disturbances, are based on a body scheme or internal representation of the body, which includes several components, namely, body geometry and kinetics, representation of verticality and reference frame. In addition, postural networks contribute to the execution of the postural tasks. Multisensory inputs are used to build up the body scheme. These inputs also act as error-detecting sensors to evaluate the mismatch between the prescribed orientation and stability, and the actual posture. The postural reactions which occur in the presence of an error message, as well as the anticipatory postural adjustments associated with voluntary movements, are mediated via the postural networks to one or several segments. The execution of the postural reactions or anticipations is controlled on line on the basis of local feedback (from Massion, 1994).
[© 1994 Current Opinion in Neurobiology]

reference value is tightly regulated. Babinski (1899) has shown, for example, that during upper trunk forward and backward bending, movements of the hip and knee occur in opposite directions, which serve to minimize the anteroposterior CG shift resulting from the trunk movement.

Equilibrium control involves four basic items (which may also be basic to 'modular' postural control (see Massion, 1992; and Fig. 2).

(1) The *reference value* to be regulated: this value is centrally determined and as far as balance in concerned, the relevant value is the CG projection within the supporting area.

(2) The *multisensory inputs* which are used to monitor the errors between the required and actual body segment distribution. These sensory inputs are somaesthetic (proprioceptive and cutaneous), visual and labyrinthine.

(3) The *postural body scheme* is a concept which was put forward by Clement et al. (1984) and Gurfinkel (1994). It is based on the idea that there exists an internal representation of

the body segments' geometry, which is mainly based on the proprioceptive muscle afferent signals, a representation of the body segments' mass and inertia and a representation of the relationships between the body segments and the external world. Evaluating the body segments position with respect to the vertical axis is based on the use of visual, labyrinthine and body 'graviceptor' cues. Evaluating the contact forces with the ground by the hands and feet is another way of assessing the body segments' position with respect to space.

(4) The *postural reactions* are organized on the basis of sensory information associated with postural disturbance. These reactions are either slow, and under a closed loop feedback control when the disturbances encountered are slow, or consist in fast, phasic postural reactions when the disturbances are fast.

The postural reactions are flexible and depend on the selected reference value and on the postural body scheme. The reference value for balance control is not always the CG position. If, for example, someone is pushed when holding a glass of water in their hands, the postural reactions produced will be those which prevent the water from spilling and will thus give stabilizing the hand position in space priority over restoring balance (Marsden *et al.*, 1981; Droulez, 1988). The role of the support conditions is illustrated by the following example. When a standing subject is subjected to an anteroposterior acceleration, the postural reactions are organized starting with the leg muscles. If at the same time, the subjects are holding on to a firm support, the postural reactions are then seen to begin in the arm muscles (Nashner & McCollum, 1985).

This rather complex organization of posture and equilibrium control gives a good idea of the multiple causes possibly involved in falling: lesion of sensory pathways, lesion of the circuits involved in the internal representation of posture, lesion of the postural command pathways.

The anticipatory postural adjustments

Voluntary movements themselves tend to perturb posture and balance. First, they change the body's geometry, and as a result they shift the CG projection on to the ground; this is liable to cause imbalance. In addition, these movements result from internal muscular forces which are exerted along a vector corresponding to the movement direction. Reaction forces in the opposite direction are exerted on the supporting segments, on the trunk for example in the case of an arm raising movement, and their position will tend to change. In the absence of a parallel control on the supporting postural segments, which would reduce the effect of the reaction forces, the reference position of these segments will change and the movement will miss its target.

The postural disturbances due to movement performance can be minimized in two ways (see Fig. 3). First, the sensory messages signalling the postural disturbance trigger a postural reaction which will correct the change of position made by the postural segment because of the voluntary movement. This mode of correction is efficient, but it acts only after a delay, because its onset is triggered by the sensory inputs relating to the disturbance and, as a result, the correction will miss the first part of the disturbance. Secondly, anticipatory postural adjustments are controlled by the central nervous system starting before the postural and equilibrium disturbance onset, so that even its onset is minimized. This type of adjustment results from a learning process, acting on adaptive networks. Due to these anticipatory postural adjustments, the postural segments will be able to maintain their initial position during the whole movement trajectory.

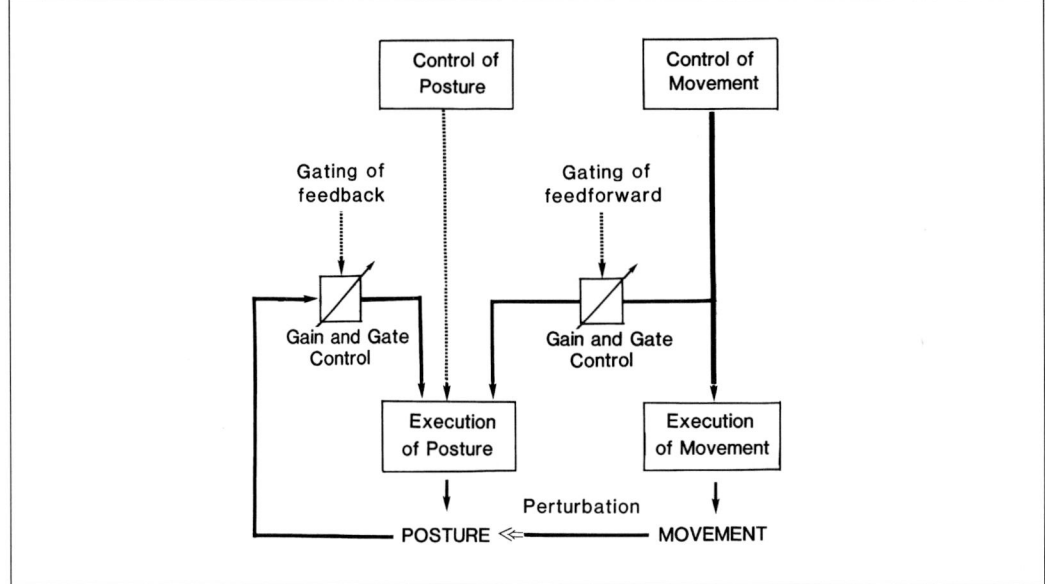

Fig. 3. Feedforward and feedback adjustment of posture. Diagram showing the two mechanisms involved in compensating for a postural disturbance. In this diagram, the central control of posture is indicated by a striped line. Two phasic mechanisms minimize the postural disturbance: they operate through a feedback loop and a feedforward control. The feedforward control acts via internal collaterals from the movement control pathways on an adaptive network involved in postural control. Both mechanisms operate under an adaptive gain and gate control [from Dufossé et al., 1988].

Anticipatory postural adjustments were first described by Belenkiy *et al.* (1967), and since then have been found to occur in many posturo-kinetic activities (Massion, 1992). They subserve three main goals:

(1) Stabilizing the orientation or the position of the postural segments which serve as an egocentric reference frame for a given segment.

(2) Controlling balance during the performance of movements, by stabilizing the CG projection onto the ground.

(3) Contributing to the movement itself, by ensuring the postural fixation of the moving segments or by using the inertia of the axial segments to increase the force of the movement.

A loss of ability to make anticipatory postural adjustments can easily lead to disequilibrium or falling.

When anticipatory postural adjustments are required in order to maintain balance during movements, their dysfunction can be directly responsible for falling. Babinski (1899) pointed out that during upper trunk bending, the axial kinematic synergies, which preserve balance by triggering opposite upper and lower segment shifts, are lost in cerebellar patients: their leg axis remains vertical when their trunk moves and falling therefore occurs. This lack of balance control seems to be attributable to a lack of appropriate thigh and hip muscle control (Viallet *et al.*, 1994).

When anticipatory postural adjustments are required in order to control the orientation of body segments such as the axis of the head or that of the trunk, their absence can also give rise to imbalance. For example, when a fast arm movement is performed in the absence of anticipatory postural adjustments, the reaction forces exerted on the trunk are no longer compensated for and the trunk position is perturbed, albeit moderately. Deficits affecting these postural adjustments will have consequences in the accuracy of the movement trajectory rather than on balance control during movement. The cortical areas which are most strongly involved in these anticipatory postural adjustments are the motor, pre-motor and supplementary motor areas and the basal ganglia.

Conclusions

The above picture outlining the present state of knowledge in the field of postural and equilibrium control shows that falling can occur for a large number of reasons. Defective peripheral and central sensory pathways, impairment of the control exerted by the brain stem and cerebellar circuits responsible for orienting eye and head position in space, hyper- or hypofunctioning of the postural tone distributing pathways, a lack of proper co-ordination between posture, equilibrium and movement are just some of the main possibilities worth considering. In order to reach a better understanding of the pathology of the falling which occurs during epileptic seizures, one should keep in mind these multiple possibilities as well as the specific brain structures which are involved in each case.

References

Assaiante, C. & Amblard, B. (1993): Ontogenesis of head stabilization in space during locomotion in children: influence of visual cues. *Exp. Brain Res.* **93,** 499–515.

Babinski, J. (1899): De l'asynergie cérébelleuse. *Rev. Neurol.* **7,** 806–816.

Belenkiy, V.E., Gurfinkel, V.S. & Paltsev, E.I. (1967): On elements of control of voluntary movements. *Biofizica* **12,** 135–141 (in Russian).

Berthoz, A. & Pozzo, T. (1988): Intermittent head stabilization during postural and locomotory tasks in humans. In: *Posture and gait: Development, adaptation and modulation,* eds. B. Amblard, A. Berthoz & F. Clarac, pp. 189–198. Amsterdam: Elsevier.

Clément, G., Gurfinkel, V.S., Lestienne, F., Lipshits, M.I. & Popov, K.E. (1984): Adaptation of postural control to weightlessness. *Exp. Brain Res.* **57,** 61–72.

Dieterich, M. & Brandt, T. (1994): Vestibular syndromes in the roll plane: topographic diagnosis from brainstem to cortex. In: *Vestibular and neural front,* eds. K. Taguchi, M. Igarashi & S. Mori, pp. 559–568. Amsterdam: Elsevier Science.

Droulez, J. (1988): Topological aspects of sensorimotor control. In: *Stance and motion: facts and concepts,* eds. V.S. Gurfinkel, M.E. Ioffé, J. Massion & J.-P. Roll, pp. 251–259. New York: Plenum Press.

Dufossé, M., Hugon, M., Massion, J. & Paulignan, Y. (1988): Two modes of adaptative change to perturbations of forearm posture. In: *Posture and gait: Development, adaptation and modulation,* eds. B. Amblard, A. Berthoz & F. Clarac, pp. 217–225. Amsterdam: Excerpta Medica.

Grüsser, O.-J., Pause, M. & Schreiter, U. (1990): Vestibular neurones in the parieto-insular cortex of monkeys (*Macaca fascicularis*) visual and neck receptor. *J. Physiol.* **430,** 559–583.

Gurfinkel E.V. (1973): Physical foundations of stabilography. *Agressologie* **14 (suppl. C),** 9–13.

Gurfinkel, V.S. (1994): The mechanisms of postural regulation in man. *Soviet Scientific Reviews F. Phys. Gen. Biol.* **7,** 59–89.

Karnath, H.-O. (1994): Subjective body orientation in neglect and the interactive contribution of neck muscle proprioception and vestibular stimulation. *Brain* **117,** 1001–1012.

Magnus, R. (1924): *Der Körperstellung.* Springer: Berlin.

Marsden, C.D., Merton, P.A. & Morton, H.P. (1981): Human postural responses. *Brain* **104,** 513–534.

Martin, J.P. (1967): *The basal ganglia and posture.* London: Pitman.

Massion, J. (1992): Movement, posture and equilibrium: interaction and coordination. *Progress in Neurobiology* **38,** 35–56.

Massion J. (1994): Postural control system. *Current Opinion in Neurobiology* **4,** 877–887.

Mennemeier, M., Chatterjee, A. & Heilman, K.M. (1994): A comparison of the influences of body and environment centred reference frames on neglect. *Brain* **117,** 1013–1021.

Mori, S. (1987): Integration of posture and locomotion in acute decerebrate cats in awake, freely moving cats. *Progress in Neurobiology* **28,** 161–195.

Nashner, L.M. & McCollum, G. (1985): The organization of human postural movements: a formal basis and experimental synthesis. *Behav. Brain Sci.* **8,** 135–172.

Rademaker, G.G.J. (1931): *Das stehen: Statische Reactionen, Gleichwichtsreaktionen und Muskeltonus unter besondere Berücksichtung ihres Verhaltens bei kleinhirnlosen Tieren.* Berlin: Springer.

Sherrington, C.S. (1906): *The integrative action of the nervous system.* London: Constable.

Thomas, A. (1940): *Equilibre et équilibration.* Masson: Paris.

Viallet, F., Massion, J., Bonnefoi-Kyriacou, B., Aurenty, R., Obadia, A. & Khalil, R. (1994): Approche quantitative de l'asynergie posturale en pathologie cérébelleuse. *Rev. Neurol.* **150,** 55–60.

Chapter 3

Epilepsy and the development of cortical connectivity

Giorgio M. Innocenti

Institut d'Anatomie, 9 rue du Bugnon, 1005, Lausanne, Switzerland

Summary

The formation of connections among cortical neurones is one of the key events in brain development. New techniques allow the visualization, reconstruction and analysis of cortical axons in experimental animal models. Here, the results obtained in the analysis of callosal axons interconnecting the primary visual areas are summarized. Several of the concepts could be generalized to other cortical axons. The geometry of callosal axons is probably responsible for a number of operations essential for cortical function. These include the establishment of precise connectional maps, synaptic weights between the axon and its targets, and timing of target activation. Abnormal axonal geometry might result in altered axonal operations with potential consequences for cortical electrogenesis. Callosal axons differentiate through several stages of exuberant growth. These lead to the formation of axons, axonal branches and synaptic boutons in excess, but progressively restricted to their sites of adult distribution. The successive growth stages and the subsequent elimination of the supernumerary axonal structures achieve different aspects of cortical connections. Synaptogenesis and synaptic elimination might be crucially involved in establishing synaptic weights between the callosal axons and their targets, with relevance for the excitatory–inhibitory balance in the developing cortex.

Introduction

Cortical neurones are heavily interconnected by axons of different lengths, using the excitatory neurotransmitters glutamate or aspartate. The efficiency of synaptic transmission across chains of cortical neurones is supposed to increase with synchronous firing (Abeles, 1991). These two characteristics suggest that epilepsy might be the state in which cerebral cortex functions, in a sense, at the best of its excitatory connectivity, unhindered by the inhibitory cortical circuitry.

The finely graded interplay between excitatory and inhibitory cortical circuits, necessary for normal cortical function, is established in development, in parallel with the formation of cortico-cortical connections. Some aspects of this process are known from studies of the callosal connections, particularly those between visual areas in the cat. Two aspects will be considered here, the differentiation of callosal axons and the role of activity, including epileptic activity on the differentiation. It may be worth noting that callosal axons are not unique in the cerebral cortex. On the contrary, there is consensus that they are representative of cortico-cortical axons in general (Hubel & Wiesel, 1967; Innocenti, 1986; Kennedy et al., 1991). Thus, most of the concepts which came into focus in the studies summarized below can probably be generalized to other cortical connections.

The corpus callosum is by far the largest fibre tract in the brain. It consists of about 23 million axons in the cat (Koppel & Innocenti, 1983) and about 56 millions in the rhesus monkey (LaMantia & Rakic, 1990a). In all species, the majority of callosal axons originate from pyramidal neurones in layer III. The infragranular layers V and VI contribute fewer axons to the corpus callosum. These are typically involved in feed-back projections from 'higher-order' to 'lower-order' areas (reviewed in Innocenti, 1986; Kennedy et al., 1991). The available electrophysiological and neurochemical information unequivocally established that these connections are mainly or exclusively excitatory in nature, although some of them terminate on inhibitory neurones and therefore have inhibitory effects on the target sites (reviewed in Innocenti, 1986; Conti & Manzoni, 1994). Each area receives afferents through the corpus callosum from the corresponding contralateral area (homotopic callosal connections) and from several other areas in the contralateral hemisphere (heterotopic callosal connections).

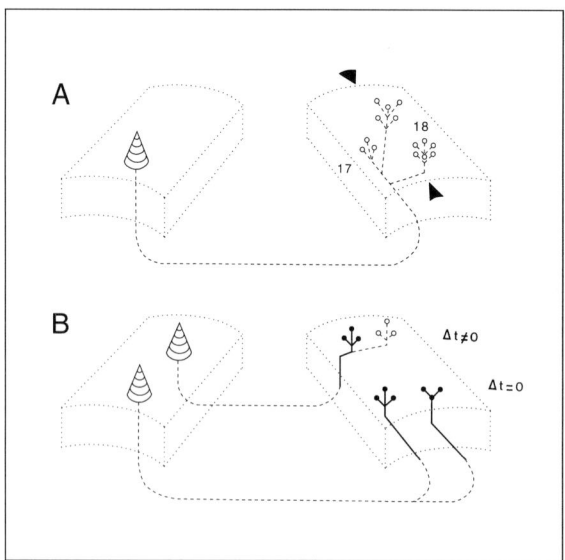

Fig. 1. Operations performed, by virtue of their geometry, by callosal axons which interconnect areas 17 and 18 of the cat. (A) illustrates mapping and differential amplification. A point in one hemisphere, corresponding to the location of the cell body, is mapped into clusters of boutons (terminal columns) that are distributed in the contralateral cortex along the border between areas 17 and 18 (filled triangles). Notice that the terminal columns contain different number of boutons, suggesting that the axon does not drive all the terminal columns with equal strength. (B) illustrates temporal transformations performed by axonal geometry. One of the two axons activates terminal columns simultaneously (the delay between the activations, $\Delta t = 0$), the other with a delay due to axonal conduction ($\Delta t \neq 0$). The active part of the axon is in full black. [Modified from Innocenti (1995).]

In addition, each area receives afferents from areas in the same hemisphere, as well as from subcortical structures. Callosal connections are often restricted to part of an area. In particular, in the primary visual areas, callosal connections are restricted to near the border between areas 17 and 18, where the vertical meridian of the visual field is represented. In addition, the neurones of origin of callosal projections (to the contralateral hemisphere) and the callosal terminal axons (from the contralateral hemisphere) were sometimes found to be distributed in discrete 'columnar' patches (reviewed in Innocenti, 1986).

New anterograde axonal tracers, and computer methods for three-dimensional reconstruction and analysis, have allowed the study of the morphology of individual callosal axons interconnecting the primary visual areas of the cat. At this new level of resolution, it became apparent that, by virtue of their geometry, individual callosal axons perform operations in the spatial, intensity and temporal domains (Fig. 1). These operations can be viewed as 'mapping', 'amplification' and 'synchronization or desynchronization' of the output signals of individual neurones. A short account of the morphology of callosal axons and their implications for cortical function is given below.

Functional implications of axonal geometry

Individual callosal axons map the three-dimensional location of their cell body of origin into that of their terminal boutons. This mapping involves topographical transformations within the cortical volume at different levels of topographical organization.

Callosal connections have thus far been considered to perform point-to-point mapping between the hemispheres. Indeed, usually, a cortical site projects to (and receives from) a roughly corresponding site in the contralateral hemisphere. This view, however, is no longer sufficiently precise. The tangential distribution of the terminal arbor of a single callosal axon greatly exceeds the territory occupied by the cell body of its parent neurone, dendrites included. Therefore, individual callosal axons diverge to their sites of termination. However, since the tangential extent of the callosal efferent zone (the volume containing callosally projecting neurones in one area) is not smaller, and if anything is larger than that of the callosal terminal territory (the volume containing the terminals of callosal axons), this implies convergence of callosal axons as well. Indeed, individual callosal axons have been seen to converge on to partially overlapping terminal territories (Houzel et al., 1994; Bressoud & Innocenti, unpublished). The values of divergence of callosal axons are known, to some extent. In the 17/18 region of the cat, individual axons can span tangentially between one hundred and several thousands square millimetres (Houzel et al., 1994). The degree of convergence (Kennedy et al., 1991), however, might be relevant to the issue of epilepsy since one would expect this parameter to be one of those which determine the strength of excitatory connections among cortical neurones.

Individual callosal axons to the primary visual areas, area 19, and to the visual areas in the suprasylvian sulcus of the cat terminate with clusters of boutons 300–600 μm across, and separated by spaces 120 to 2770 μm wide (Houzel et al., 1994). The volumes containing the clusters of callosal boutons are called *terminal columns*. The visual areas, as most other areas, are organized in 'columns' of neurones with similar functional properties, stretching from pia to white matter. In particular, the visual areas are organized in 'orientation columns', i.e. columns of neurones which detect different orientations of an elongated visual stimulus (Hubel & Wiesel, 1963). For reasons discussed elsewhere (Houzel et al., 1994), it is believed that the terminal columns of callosal axons correspond to orientation columns recognizing the same stimulus orientation as the column where the cell body lies.

Callosal axons do not usually distribute to all layers in their site of termination, although in some cases they do. Most frequently, only the supragranular and, to a lesser extent, the infragranular layers receive boutons, not layer IV. It is not known whether the callosal axons synapse specifically on one or another cell type. However, they appear to selectively contact dendritic spines rather than shafts (reviewed in Innocenti, 1986).

Callosal axons do not impinge with equal strength on all their sites of termination. Usually one or two of the terminal columns receive many more boutons than the others. The maximal ratio in the number of boutons found thus far across columns is about 1 to 50. One to 10 or 1 to 20 ratios are common (Houzel et al., 1994). Furthermore, the layers within one column usually receive different numbers of boutons. The density of boutons might be relevant to the issue of cortical epilepsy since it presumably reflects the excitatory strength (synaptic weight) of the axon at a specific terminal site. Unfortunately, nothing is known about the size of the callosal terminal boutons, their synaptic protein composition and their quantal properties of transmitter release, all of which could also contribute to the synaptic weight of the axon at its sites of termination.

Callosal axons might be critically involved in temporal transformations of spike trains originating at the cell body. Attention to this possibility was raised by the observation that the geometry callosal axons seems, occasionally, unnecessarily uneconomical in terms of axoplasmic production and maintenance (Innocenti, 1994). In particular, callosal axons often possess branches which run in parallel to their targets for several millimetres, or else exchange branches between termination columns several hundred microns apart (Houzel et al., 1994; Innocenti et al., 1994). On the whole, three kinds of axonal geometry were identified: parallel, serial and mixed (see Houzel et al., 1994).

In an attempt to clarify the possible consequences of the above mentioned geometries, we ran simulations of action potential propagation along serially reconstructed visual callosal axons, based on the well-established relationship between conduction velocity and axon diameter (Tettoni et al., 1996). The precision of the simulation is limited by a number of factors, including the accuracy of axon diameter measurement, the possibility that delays or accelerations of action potential propagation occur at the sites of axonal bifurcation, as discussed elsewhere (Innocenti et al., 1994; Tettoni et al., 1996). Nevertheless, in spite of the mentioned intractable uncertainties, the simulation of spike propagation in visual callosal axons of the cat returned interhemispheric conduction delays in the range of those measured electrophysiologically (Innocenti et al., 1994).

In callosal axons analysed to this date, we found a tendency for the geometry of the axon to achieve synchronous activation of spatially separate terminal columns with precision below the ms. The simulation also demonstrated the role of the apparently wasteful geometry mentioned above in generating the synchronous activations.

The importance of temporal factors for cortical function is highlighted by recent literature on the so called 'binding by synchrony' in the visual system and elsewhere (reviewed in Singer, 1995a) and by discussions on whether or not cerebral cortex might function at temporal precision in the ms range (Sofky & Koch, 1993; Sofky, 1994). Timing is presumably relevant to the issue of cortical epilepsy, particularly since theoretical studies stress the fact that transmission across chains of cortical neurones is most effective when neurones fire synchronously (Abeles, 1991).

The differentiation of callosal axons

Studies using retrogradely transported axonal tracers have demonstrated that callosal connections develop through a phase of exuberance in which axons are produced in excess compared to the adult. In the cat, the transient axons were found to originate from parts of the cortex which are no longer projecting into the corpus callosum in the adult, such as most of area 17, and parts of the primary somatosensory areas. Transient callosal projections were also found from the primary auditory to the visual areas (reviewed in Innocenti, 1991).

The elimination of the transitory projections is due to selective axonal deletion, rather than neuronal death (Innocenti, 1981; O'Leary et al., 1981). For the whole corpus callosum, the loss was estimated to be in the order of 70 per cent or more of the axons produced, from electron microscopic counts in both cat (Berbel & Innocenti, 1988) and monkey (La Mantia & Rakic, 1990b).

The findings mentioned above bear on one of the fundamental processes in the developing brain, the formation of connectional maps. They are not restricted to callosal connections but apply more broadly to intra-areal, inter-areal and cortico-subcortical connections (reviewed in Innocenti, 1991; see also Assal & Innocenti, 1993). The introduction of the new anterograde axonal tracers, coupled with methods for the three-dimensional reconstruction of axons and their analysis, already mentioned for the adult, significantly clarified the nature of the process. The overall conclusion is that the formation of callosal connections includes a process of axonal differentiation. In this process, several growth stages can be identified. At each stage the axon grows exuberantly but the growth is progressively constrained within the territories of adult termination.

Five stages of axonal differentiation were identified for callosal axons interconnecting the primary visual areas of the cat (Fig. 2).

The first stage identified so far, consists of the formation of the long, interhemispheric axon. It occurs mainly prenatally in the visual areas of the cat although, during the first postnatal week, axons from the primary visual areas continue to be added to the corpus callosum (Aggoun & Innocenti, 1994).

As mentioned above, many of the callosal axons formed at this stage are transient (reviewed in

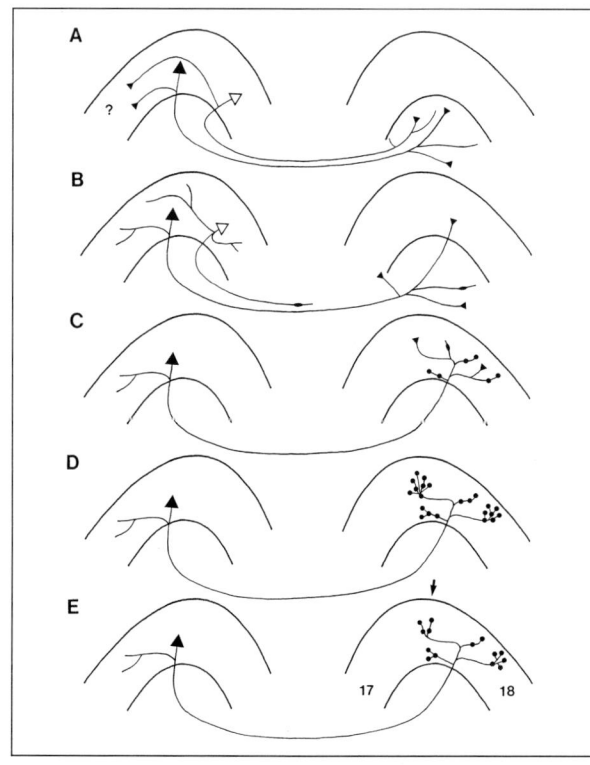

Fig. 2. Schematic representation of stages in the differentiation of callosal terminal arbours in areas 17 and 18 of the cat. (A) illustrates the stage of subcortical branching. (B) illustrates the growth into the grey matter. (C) illustrates the branching in the grey matter and the onset of synaptogenesis. (D) illustrates the peak in synaptogenesis. Notice that each stage is followed by partially regressive events, i.e. elimination of long callosal axons between (A) and (B), of subcortical branches between (B) and (C) and of synaptic boutons between (D) and (E). Neuronal cell bodies are represented by filled, or open triangles, growth cones by small triangles at the end of the axonal branches, synaptic boutons by dots. One of the neurones (open triangle) is eliminating its callosal axons, without dying, and presumably establishes permanent connections in the ipsilateral hemisphere (not shown in C–E). The arrow (in E) points to the border between visual areas 17 and 18. [Modified from Innocenti (1995).]

Innocenti, 1991). At this stage, individual callosal axons originating from cortical sites destined to remain callosally connected such as the region near the 17/18 border, and axons destined to be eliminated, those originating from area 17 show similarities in their behaviour with respect to their targets areas. Axons of both origins aim at the 17/18 border, which receives callosal axons in the adult, but also at more medial parts of area 17 or at more lateral parts of area 18 which receive no callosal axons in the adult.

The second stage involves branching in the white matter during the first and second postnatal weeks. It must be noticed that the branching is most abundant in the white matter underlying cortical target areas 17 and 18, although occasional branches can be found elsewhere along the trajectory of the axon. Both axons destined to be maintained, and those destined to be eliminated, branch in the white matter. A substantial proportion of the branches appears to terminate in the white matter without aiming clearly at a specific cortical area. The others point to either area 17, to area 18, or to the 17/18 border. The transient axons originating from area 17 branch less abundantly than those originating from the 17/18 border. Their branches terminate more often in the white matter without aiming clearly at one or the other cortical area. It must be noticed that, at this stage, the subcortical white matter contains a partially transient neuronal population, the cortical subplate, which is suspected to play a crucial role in guiding thalamic axons into the grey matter (Shatz et al., 1988), but whose role, if any, in the development of callosal connections is unknown.

The third stage consists in the invasion of the cortical grey matter and begins around the end of the first postnatal week. Interestingly, only axons originating near the 17/18 border, and presumably destined to be maintained, enter deeply into the grey matter and only near the 17/18 border. The vast majority of axons from area 17 remains confined to the white matter or to the intermediate region between grey matter and subplate, although a few engage into the lower third of the grey matter in area 17, 18 or near their common border. Some axons enter the cortex with a disjunctive distribution of branches recalling the columnar pattern seen in the adult.

The fourth stage involves the formation of branches in the cortical grey matter. This seems to begin almost as soon as the axons enter the grey matter, i.e. at the end of the first postnatal week in the most precocious examples found thus far. In the following weeks, and up to around the beginning of the third postnatal month, the number of branches increases above the numbers found in the adult. This growth blurs, somewhat, the previous disjunctive and quasi-columnar pattern of axonal ingrowth but remains confined to the region of the 17/18 border.

The fifth stage corresponds to synaptogenesis. This was assessed thus far by examining axonal swellings at the light microscopic level (for the morphological criteria used, see Aggoun-Zouaoui & Innocenti, 1994; Aggoun-Zouaoui et al., 1996). Although some boutons can be found at earlier ages in the region of the cortical subplate, boutons resembling those found in the adult appear in the grey matter at the end of the second postnatal week. Over the following weeks, the number of boutons increases reaching a peak, around the beginning of the third postnatal month, well above the number found in the adult. From the beginning, and over the whole period of synaptogenesis, the formation of boutons is specific in terms of their laminar distribution. Boutons appear initially in the infragranular layers but then they become more numerous in the supragranular layers. As it is mostly the case in the adult, they are sparse or absent in layer IV. Boutons acquire from the beginning a disjunctive 'columnar' distribution which they maintain during the whole phase of synaptogenesis.

The stages of axonal growth are identified, for the time being, on purely descriptive criteria.

Their temporal succession is schematized. For individual axons there may be overlap between the events ascribed to two successive stages (Fig. 2). Notably, growth into the grey matter and subcortical branching could overlap, at least in part. Also, branching in the grey matter from the end of the second week onwards, proceeds in parallel with the formation of synaptic boutons. Furthermore, different axons can, at the same point in time, be at different stages of their development.

Elimination of exuberant axonal structures

The growth stages listed above lead to overproduction of callosal axons, of branches in the white and in the grey matter, and of synapses. They are followed by selection of structures to be maintained and by elimination of the others. These eliminations are massive. Previous work has shown that at least 70 per cent of the callosal axons produced are eliminated in both cat and monkey (Berbel & Innocenti, 1988; LaMantia & Rakic, 1990b). Callosal axons from the 17/18 border (Aggoun-Zouaoui & Innocenti, 1994, Aggoun-Zouaoui et al., 1996) have established, on average, about ten branching points in the white matter during the second postnatal week, but these are reduced to about two in the adult. The number of branches in the grey matter was about 500 at the beginning of the third postnatal month and it was down to around 240 in the adult. The number of boutons reached about 2100 at the beginning of the third postnatal month and it was down to the average adult value of about 300 by the end of the fifth month. It should be noticed that these values are only indicative because the number of individual axons analysed by serial reconstruction is limited.

The stages of exuberant growth described above probably apply to other cortical axons although none, as yet, has been studied in comparable detail to the callosal ones. Evidence of exuberant branching in both the white and the grey matter, based on tracing of individual axons, exists for geniculo-cortical projections (Ghosh & Shatz, 1992; Antonini & Stryker, 1993), for intra-areal projections (Callaway & Katz, 1990; Assal & Innocenti, 1993), and for the hippocampus (Swann & Gomez-Di Cesare, 1994).

Exuberant development of cortical connections and epilepsy

The exuberant growth seems to be the expression of a search by trial-and-error that the axons perform of cues related to their targets and of the targets themselves. The selection of the axonal structures to be maintained and the elimination of the others sharpen the projection maps at increasing levels of topographical organization. In addition, the deletion of synaptic boutons might achieve the regulation of synaptic weights in different parts of the axonal arbor.

Within the frame of the present volume, it seems legitimate to wonder if some forms of juvenile cortical epilepsy might be due to an abnormal development of cortical connections. Abnormalities could involve the production as well as the selection of axons, axonal branches and synapses. Furthermore, periods of higher seizure susceptibility might be related to one or the other stage of axonal development, presumably those corresponding to an excess production of axonal branches and synapses. These periods might be naturally terminated by the regressive events which follow the exuberant growth. In agreement with the above interpretations, studies in the developing hippocampus demonstrated that the period of higher seizure sensitivity is correlated with the excess number of axonal branches and boutons in the recurrent collaterals of pyramidal neurones of the CA subfield (Swann & Gomez-Di Cesare, 1994). The interpretation of the data from the hippocampus, however, is complicated by the fact that axons were reconstructed from simple brain slices, which requires the axonal parameters to be scaled to neuronal density (Swann, 1995).

The overexcitability characteristic of the epileptic cortex does not necessarily imply production and maintenance of normally transient structures belonging to cortico-cortical axons. Over-elimination as well as impaired or delayed production of cortical or thalamic afferents to local inhibitory neurones could have the same effects of shifting the balance of connectivity towards excitation. Furthermore, the precise consequences of the exuberance of axonal branches and synaptic boutons remains speculative in the absence of information on the development of dendritic arbours of the target neurones, of quantal release properties of the juvenile versus adult boutons and of the electrophysiological properties of the post-synaptic neurones. Interestingly, the NMDA currents are prolonged in juvenile neurones (Carmignoto & Vicini, 1992) and there seems to be hypersensitivity to the NMDA (Tsumoto et al., 1987).

Along the lines discussed above, important progress in understanding the causes of juvenile epilepsy and its consequences for the developing brain might come from answering the following questions. First, what regulates the exuberant growth? Theories of development of connections have traditionally stressed the role of cues guiding axons to their targets. Exuberant growth, in addition, stresses the role of axonal growth itself as the expression of developmental programmes intrinsic to the neurone. In the course of development, axons might express one or several growth modes (Schneider et al., 1987; Bhide & Frost, 1991). Extrinsic signals might activate one or the other growth mode (Grumbacher-Reinert, 1989). In this context, the role of neurotrophic factors is potentially important as it appears to be the case for the geniculo-cortical axons (Carmignoto et al., 1993; Cabelli et al., 1995; Galuske et al., 1996). In addition to cues favouring axonal growth in specific directions, evidence of growth inhibiting signals has recently accumulated. These signals might play a role in preventing access of callosal axons to area 17 (Aggoun-Zouaoui & Innocenti, 1994).

The second crucial question is what regulates regressive events and selection? The fate of the juvenile axons, axonal branches and synapses is not rigidly pre-programmed but depends on local contingencies. Indeed, several examples exist that the fate of juvenile axons can be modified by epigenetic events including activity, early brain lesions, hormonal or dietary manipulations (reviewed in Innocenti, 1991). Thus, exuberant growth and regression appear to provide a remarkable degree of flexibility in the development of projection maps.

On the whole it appears that, in order to develop properly, juvenile cortico-cortical connections require an appropriate interplay with thalamic afferents. This interplay might require concurrent activation of the two sets of afferents as it has been suggested for intra-areal connections (Singer, 1995b). Whether activity conveyed through the thalamus controls only selection or also growth is presently not clear (discussed in Aggoun-Zouaoui et al., 1996).

The importance of activity in the development of cortical connections raises the important possibility that one or other of the growth and regression stages described above might be altered in the epileptic brain. On this issue, the available evidence is scanty. Nevertheless, an altered selection of juvenile callosal connections, with maintenance of connections which are normally eliminated, was reported as a result of the creation of epileptic foci in the cerebral cortex (Grigonis & Murphy, 1994). This might, in some cases, justify pharmacological treatment of the early epileptic seizures although the innocuity of these treatments on the developing cortical network remains to be assessed.

Acknowledgements

Supported by Swiss National Science Foundation grant (No. 3100–039707.93). I wish to thank Philippe Gaudard and Eric Bernardi for their help at various stages in the preparation of this manuscript.

References

Abeles, M. (1991): Corticonics. Neural circuits of the cerebral cortex, pp. 1–280. Cambridge: Cambridge University Press.

Aggoun-Zouaoui, D. & Innocenti, G.M. (1994): Juvenile visual callosal axons in kittens display origin- and fate-related morphology and distribution of arbors. *Eur. J. Neurosci.* **6**, 1846–1863.

Aggoun-Zouaoui, D., Kiper, D.C. & Innocenti, G.M. (1996): Growth of callosal terminal arbors in primary visual areas of the cat. *Eur. J. Neurosci.* **8**, 1132–1148.

Antonini, A. & Stryker, M.P. (1993): Development of individual geniculocortical arbors in cat striate cortex and effects of binocular impulse blockade. *J. Neurosci.* **13**, 3549–3573.

Assal, F. & Innocenti, G.M. (1993): Transient intra-areal axons in developing cat visual cortex. *Cereb. Cortex* **3**, 290–303.

Berbel, P. & Innocenti, G.M. (1988): The development of the corpus callosum in cats: a light- and electron-microscopic study. *J. Comp. Neurol.* **276**, 132–156.

Bhide, P.G. & Frost, D.O. (1991): Stages of growth of hamster retinofugal axons: implications for developing axonal pathways with multiple targets. *J. Neurosci.* **11**, 485–504.

Cabelli, R.J., Hohn, A. & Shatz, C.J. (1995): Inhibition of ocular dominance column formation by infusion of NT-4/5 or BDNF. *Science* **267**, 1662–1666.

Callaway, E.M. & Katz, L.C. (1990): Emergence and refinement of clustered horizontal connections in cat striate cortex. *J. Neurosci.* **10**, 1134–1153.

Carmignoto, G. & Vicini, S. (1992): Activity-dependent decrease in NMDA receptor responses during development of the visual cortex. *Science* **258**, 1007–1011.

Carmignoto, G., Canella, R., Candeo, P., Comelli, M.C. & Maffei, L. (1993): Effects of nerve growth factor on neuronal plasticity of the kitten striate cortex. *J. Physiol.* **464**, 343–360.

Conti, F. & Manzoni, T. (1994): The neurotransmitters and postsynaptic actions of callosally projecting neurons. *Behav. Brain Res.* **64**, 37–53.

Galuske, R.A.W., Kim, D.-S., Castrén, E., Thoenen, H. & Singer, W. (1996): Brain-derived neurotrophic factor reverses experience-dependent synaptic modifications in kitten visual cortex. *Eur. J. Neurosci.* **8**, 1554–1559.

Ghosh, A. & Shatz, C.J. (1992): Pathfinding and target selection by developing geniculocortical axons. *J. Neurosci.* **12**, 39–55.

Grigonis, A.M. & Murphy, E.H. (1994): The effects of epileptic cortical activity on the development of callosal projections. *Dev. Brain Res.* **77**, 251–255.

Grumbacher-Reinert, S. (1989): Local influence of substrate molecules in determining distinctive growth patterns of identified neurons in culture. *Proc. Natl. Acad. Sci. USA* **86**, 7270–7274.

Houzel, J.-C., Milleret, C. & Innocenti, G. (1994): Morphology of callosal axons interconnecting areas 17 and 18 of the cat. *Eur. J. Neurosci.* **6**, 898–917.

Hubel, D.H. & Wiesel, T.N. (1963): Shape and arrangement of columns in cat's striate cortex. *J. Physiol.* **165**, 559–568.

Hubel, D.H. & Wiesel, T.N. (1967): Cortical and callosal connections concerned with the vertical meridian of visual fields in the cat. *J. Neurophysiol.* **30**, 1561–1573.

Innocenti, G.M. (1981): Growth and reshaping of axons in the establishment of visual callosal connections. *Science* **212**, 824–827.

Innocenti, G.M. (1986): General organization of callosal connections in the cerebral cortex. In: *Cerebral Cortex*, vol. 5, eds. E.G. Jones & A. Peters, pp. 291–353. New York: Plenum Press.

Innocenti, G.M. (1991): The development of projections from cerebral cortex. In: *Progress in Sensory Physiology*, vol. 12, pp. 65–114. Berlin: Springer-Verlag.

Innocenti, G.M. (1994): Computational structure of central nervous system axons reflects developmental strategies. In: *Structural and functional organization of the neocortex*, eds. B. Albowitz, K. Albus, U. Kuhnt, H.-C. Nothdurft & P. Wahle, pp. 49–59. Berlin: Springer-Verlag.

Innocenti, G.M., Lehmann, P. & Houzel, J.-C. (1994): Computational structure of visual callosal axons. *Eur. J. Neurosci.* **6,** 918–935.

Innocenti, G.M. (1995): Exhuberant development of connections, and its possible permissive role in cortical evolution. *Trends Neurosci.* **4,** 397–402.

Kennedy, H., Meissirel, C. & Dehay, C. (1991): Callosal pathways and their compliancy to general rules governing the organization of corticocortical connectivity. In: *Vision and visual dysfunction*, vol. 3, *Neuroanatomy of the visual pathways and their development,* eds. B. Dreher & S. Robinson, pp. 324–359. London: Macmillan.

Koppel, H. & Innocenti, G.M. (1983): Is there a genuine exuberancy of callosal projections in development? A quantitative electron microscopic study in the cat. *Neurosci. Lett.* **41,** 33–40.

LaMantia, A.-S. & Rakic, P. (1990a): Cytological and quantitative characteristics of four cerebral commissures in the rhesus monkey. *J. Comp. Neurol.* **291,** 520–537.

LaMantia, A.-S. & Rakic, P. (1990b): Axon overproduction and elimination in the anterior commissure of the developing rhesus monkey. *J. Comp. Neurol.* **340,** 328–336.

O'Leary, D.D.M., Stanfield, B.B. & Cowan, W.M. (1981): Evidence that the early postnatal restriction of the cells of origin of the callosal projection is due to the elimination of axonal collaterals rather than to the death of neurons. *Dev. Brain Res.* **1,** 607–617.

Schneider, G.E., Jhaveri, S. & Davis, W.F. (1987): On the development of neuronal arbors. In: *Developmental neurobiology of mammals*, eds. C. Chagas & R. Linden, pp. 31–64. City of Vatican: Pontificia Academia Scientiarum.

Shatz, C.J., Chun, J.J.M. & Luskin, M.B. (1988): The role of the subplate in the development of the mammalian telencephalon. In: *Cerebral Cortex,* vol. 7, *Development and maturation of cerebral cortex*, eds. A. Peters & E.G. Jones, pp. 35–58. New York: Plenum Press.

Singer, W. (1995a): Time as coding space in neocortical processing: a hypothesis. In: *The cognitive neurosciences*, ed. M.S. Gazzaniga, pp. 91–104. Cambridge, Mass./London: MIT Press.

Singer, W. (1995b): Development and plasticity of cortical processing architectures. *Science* **270,** 758–764.

Softky, W.R. & Koch, C. (1993): The highly irregular firing of cortical cells is inconsistent with temporal integration of random EPSPs. *J. Neurosci.* **13,** 334–350.

Softky, W. (1994): Sub-millisecond coincidence detection in active dendritic trees. *Neuroscience* **58,** 13–41.

Swann, J.W. & Gomez-Di Cesare, C.M. (1994): Developmental plasticity and hippocampal epileptogenesis. *Hippocampus* **4,** 266–269.

Swann, J.W. (1995): Synaptogenesis and epileptogenesis in developing neural networks. In: *Brain development and epilepsy*, eds. P.A. Schwartzkroin, S.L. Moshé, J.L. Noebels & J.W. Swann, pp. 195–233. New York, Oxford: Oxford University Press.

Tettoni, L., Lehmann, P., Houzel, J.-C. & Innocenti, G.M. (1996): Maxsim, software for the analysis of multiple axonal arbors and their simulated activation. *J. Neurosci. Meth.* **67,** 1–9.

Tsumoto, T., Hagihara, K., Sato, H. & Hata, Y. (1987): NMDA receptors in the visual cortex of young kittens are more effective than those of adult cats. *Nature* **327,** 513–514.

Chapter 4

Cortical maturation and electroclinical expression of epileptic falls

Giuliano Avanzini, Flavio Villani, Laura Canafoglia and Tiziana Granata

Istituto Nazionale Neurologico C. Besta, via Celoria 11, 20133 Milan, Italy

Summary

Epileptic falls are here defined as those due to an epileptic discharge resulting in a sudden impairment of postural control. The definition includes astatic, myoclonic, tonic seizures and spasms that can occur in early epileptic encephalopathies, infantile spasms, myoclonic syndromes, myoclono-astatic epilepsy, Lennox–Gastaut syndromes and partial epilepsies of frontal origin. The clinical features of these types of seizures and epilepsies are analysed with reference to the maturational profile of cerebral structures involved in their generation and postural control mechanisms. Fragmentary or global postural lapses resulting from myoclonic seizures can be detected from the first month when a rudimentary control of head posture is already achieved. Further developmental stages are shown by the electroclinical phenomenology of myoclonus, tonic seizure, spasms and astatic (or akinetic or atonic) seizures, and by the types of epilepsies in which context they occur.

Introduction

That an epileptic seizure may throw a patient to the ground is so commonly perceived to justify the popular designation of 'falling sickness' for the epilepsies (Temkin, 1945). It is therefore meaningless to talk about epileptic falls unless the term is better defined. Here we refer to epileptic falls as those due to an epileptic discharge resulting in a sudden impairment of postural control. This definition typically applies to the astatic seizures which are thought to reflect a pure suppression of postural mechanisms. Myoclonic discharges can also abruptly impair the postural control leading the patient to slump to the ground. Myoclonic and astatic seizures are often associated in the same patient either independently or in combination as is the case for myoclono-astatic epilepsy, described by Doose (1985) and included in the ILAE classification of the epilepsies and epileptic syndromes (ICE, 1989). In addition, tonic seizures may impair the standing ability: the resulting fall can be difficult to differentiate from that induced by astatic seizures when the tonic seizure involves flexor muscles. Thus, even if we focus our attention seizures characterized by a sudden impairment of postural control, we have to take into account at least three different types of seizures – namely astatic, myoclonic and flexor tonic. It is reasonably assumed that the same pathophysiological mechanisms that can impair globally the postural control resulting in an epileptic fall, may also account for regional phenomena such as head drop and/or jaw slackening.

Such kind of fragmentary seizures will also be considered in this chapter in as much as they can be observed during development even before the baby is able to stand on its legs. The above mentioned types of seizures can be observed in the context of different epileptic syndromes such as West syndrome, different types of myoclonic epilepsies, Lennox–Gastaut syndrome, and focal cryptogenic/symptomatic epilepsies (namely of frontal origin). Most of them have a definite age-dependent expression in infancy suggesting a correlation between their typical electroclinical pattern and the developmental stages of the brain. In dealing with seizures that interfere with postural mechanisms it is mandatory to make reference to the time course of maturation of postural control.

Normal development of postural control

The developmental profile of postural control will be shortly reviewed with reference to the fundamental work of Touwen (1976). The ability to stand free in an upright position is normally attained by the baby between the 7th and the 12th month of postnatal life in 80 per cent of cases (Touwen, 1976). By the 18th postnatal month, 100 per cent of normally developed children can stand freely upright on their legs. Earlier maturational steps heralding the acquisition of the upright position are to be found in the development of head and trunk control (Fedrizzi & Bono, 1981). The newborn is able to keep its head in axis for more than 3 s; oscillatory movements reduce in the course of the first month in the majority of children and are observed in any child after the 4th month (Touwen, 1976). The ability to control the head is a prerequisite for the sequence of maturational steps of trunk and limb posture leading to the upright position. During the 4th month of postnatal life the control of trunk posture becomes sufficient to allow the child to sit with rounded back supporting itself with the arms. The arm support becomes unnecessary by the 7th month while the back changes progressively to a straight and then lordotic attitude between the 8th and 12th month. The control of leg extension becomes adequate to support the upright posture between the 8th and 9th month, when a predominantly flexor attitude is switched to a predominant extension. In this respect legs lag behind arms by about two months. Relevant to our topic is the preferential flexor attitude of the limbs that is found in the early months of postnatal life (3–4 months for arms and 6–8 months for legs). Its possible correlation with flexor tonic seizures or flexor spasms that occur in the early postnatal period will be discussed later.

The development of postural control is the result of maturational processes involving vestibular-proprioceptive systems, cerebellum, basal ganglia and cerebral cortex. A proper head posture in the setting position shows that immediately after birth the interaction between vestibular-proprioceptive afferences and muscle strength control is already effective. The reduction of head swaying from the second to the 4th month reflects the evolution of feed-back control systems of neck and trunk connected with the functional development of the cerebellum. The developmental stages of the upright position (kneeling being the first step) requires the integration of cerebellar, brainstem and basal ganglia activities whose maturational profiles largely overlap. The ability to stand up is time related to the transition from dorsi-flexor to plantar flexor foot sole response that is considered as evidence of an increase in suprasegmental

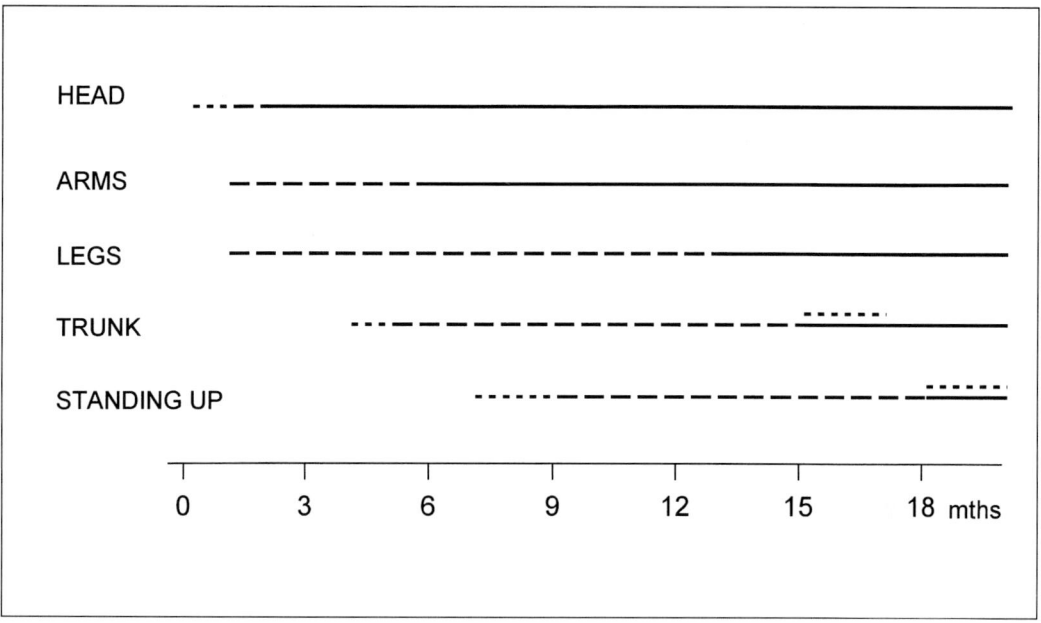

Fig. 1. Development of postural control for head trunk, arms, legs and global upright position in the first 18 postnatal months. For each item the degree of the achieved control is scored as rudimentary, shown by ·········, incomplete – – – –, complete with some variability ·········, and complete ———. [Based on Touwen (1976).]

influence on spinal mechanisms. This is due to the maturation of cerebrospinal integration as a result of which the dominance of the extensor activity in the motility of the toes is shifted to the flexor side (Touwen, 1976). The acquisition of the upright position is therefore considered to be correlated with the maturation of the cerebral cortex and cortico-spinal system.

The normal developmental profile of postural control is schematically outlined in Figure 1. It is clear that, in a restricted sense, epileptic falls cannot be observed before the 9th–12th month when the child is able to stand in an upright position. Fragmentary epileptic falls affecting trunk and head can however be detected from the 4th and 1st month respectively.

Maturation of physiological properties of cortical and thalamic neurons relevant to epileptogenesis

Since the cerebral cortex is particularly involved in epileptogenesis, we will focus our attention on the maturation of physiological properties of cortical neurons and of the interconnected thalamic structures. The maturational periods of some cellular properties relevant to epileptogenesis are schematically drawn in Figure 2. Most of the available information comes from experimental studies on animals, raising the problem of correlating the developmental stages in different animal species. Some indications can be drawn from the comparison of available maturational parameters of the neocortex in rat and man. Data on the time relationship between callosal reshaping, changes in synaptic density in visual area 17, and myelination of corpus callosum in rat and man, have been reviewed by Innocenti (1986). According to his scheme, the brain of the rat can be considered more immature than the human one at birth and to reach a common developmental stage around P5 corresponding to about 1 month of human postnatal

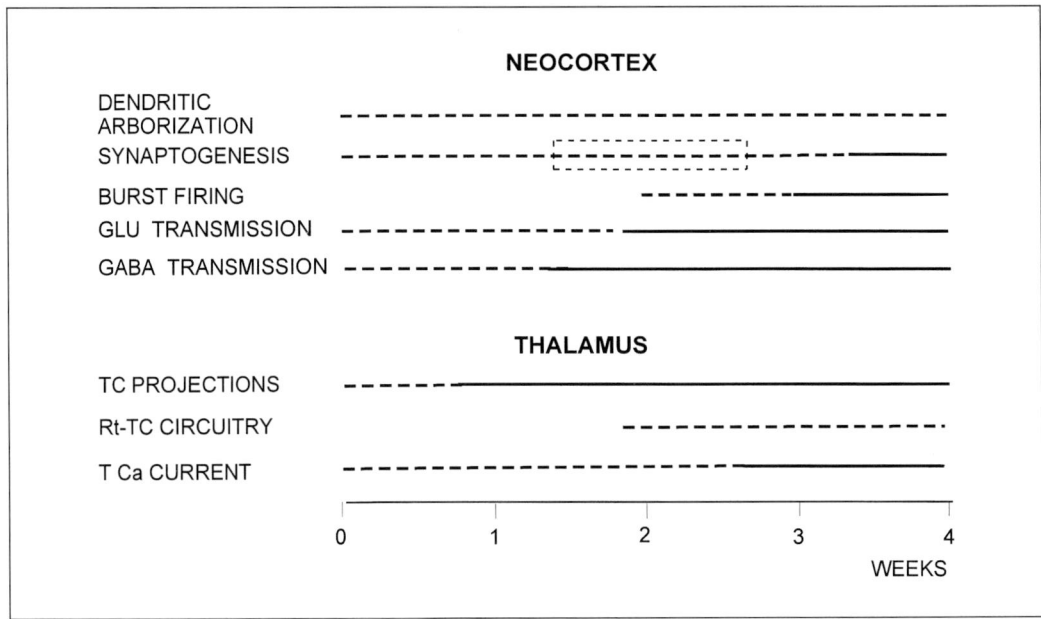

Fig. 2. Development of cortical and thalamic neuronal properties relevant to cell excitability. Maturational periods are marked by broken lines. On the course of synaptogenesis the period of reshaping of exhuberant synapses is marked by a box drawn by broken lines. [Based on Kriegstein et al., 1987; McCormick & Prince, 1987; Luhman & Prince, 1991; Avanzini et al., 1992; Franceschetti et al., 1993; Tsakiridou et al., 1995; De Biasi et al., 1996).]

life. From this point rat/man developmental rates diverge significantly so that the first year of postnatal life does not outlast the 25th day of rat postnatal life.

In this period membrane properties and synaptically evoked activities of rat neocortical neurons undergo significant changes (Kriegstein *et al.*, 1987; McCormick & Prince, 1987; Avanzini *et al.*, 1992).

During the first week, resting membrane potentials (V_M) are 10 per cent lower than in adults, while membrane resistance (R_N) and time constant are more than twofold higher than in mature neurons. All neurons show low frequency regular discharge with evidence of spike frequency adaptation of variable strength (Avanzini *et al.*, 1992). In spite of the presence of GABA immunoreactive neurons, hyperpolarizing inhibitory postsynaptic potentials (IPSPs) are not detectable. On the contrary, an immature excitatory aminoacid (EAA)-mediated neurotransmission is already effective the first days of life. Immature excitatory postsynaptic potentials (EPSPs) are highly fatiguable, long lasting and contain a N-methyl-D-aspartate (NMDA) component which is less sensitive to the voltage-dependent Mg^{2+} block than in adults (Avanzini *et al.*, 1992).

During the second week passive properties evolve towards mature values and GABA-mediated IPSPs become more and more pronounced. EAA-mediated monosynaptic EPSPs become shorter, although a late NMDA-mediated component is still evident at V_M until P10–15 V_M. In addition, the multisynaptic multiphasic EPSPs can be orthodromically elicited from P8 to P15, due to the relative immaturity of GABA-mediated inhibition, which fails to counteract them effectively (Luhman & Prince, 1991). Fast-firing (FS) putative GABAergic interneurons IB cells can occasionally be recorded.

During the third week NMDA-mediated neurotransmission evolves rapidly toward its mature characteristic (i.e. voltage-dependent Mg^{2+} sensitivity). A differentiation between regular spiking (RS) versus intrinsically bursting (IB) neurons according to the Connors & Gutnick (1990) definition becomes evident (Franceschetti et al., 1993). A significant proportion of IB neurons can be found in layer IV and V from P14. Rudimentary, two-spike bursts evolve rapidly toward more robust bursting behaviour which is seen at the end of the third week when firing properties and synaptic activities in the neocortex are comparable to those of mature animals (Franceschetti et al., 1995).

Several factors concur in making the cerebral cortex particularly susceptible to epileptogenic agents in this period. The NMDA-mediated neurotransmission is relatively facilitated due to its incomplete sensitivity to voltage-dependent Mg^{2+} block (Avanzini et al., 1992). Concurrently GABA transmission is poorly effective in the earliest stages and tends to induce depolarizing rather than hyperpolarizing IPSPs (Luhman & Prince, 1991).

In discussing the physiological properties of the neocortex, it should be borne in mind that cortical activities are by no means independent of subcortical, namely thalamic, influences that are particularly relevant to the generation of thalamo-cortical rhythms (e.g. sleep spindles). It has been shown that thalamic rhythmogenesis depends on the reciprocal interaction between thalamic reticular nucleus (Rt) and the other thalamic nuclei projecting to the neocortex (Thalamo-cortical nuclei: TC; Mulle et al., 1986; Avanzini et al., 1989). Thanks to a set of Ca^{2+}/K^+ membrane currents Rt neurons are in fact able to generate sequences of bursts-hyperpolarization complexes resulting in membrane rhythmic oscillations that are then transmitted to TC nuclei.

The interaction between Rt and TC depends on their reciprocal interconnections including the GABAergic (inhibitory) Rt–TC projection and the glutamatergic (excitatory) TC–Rt projection established by the axon collaterals of TC neurons. In rats it has been shown that low threshold T Ca^{2+} current is responsible for Rt rhythmogenic properties mature during the third postnatal week (Tsakiridou et al., 1995). During the same period the synaptic organization of both TC collaterals to Rt and Rt projection fibres to TC nuclei develops considerably, reaching the adult morphological features by P21 (De Biasi et al., 1996). However, the functional effectiveness of the system is still insufficient to generate highly synchronous activities such as the ones that are known to subserve spike-wave discharges (Avanzini et al., 1993), since in rats they appear only during the second month of postnatal life. According to our criteria of correspondence between rat and human development, the effectiveness of the thalamus as a pace-maker of bilateral synchronous rhythmic spikes and waves become marked only in the last part of the second year.

Intracortical mechanisms operated by IB and local circuit neurons may also contribute to some extent to generate regional EEG synchronous activities. IB neurons have been shown to generate a strong synchronized output which can recruit a large neuronal population through their widespread horizontal connectivity (Getting, 1983). Moreover recurrent synchronous IPSPs arising from GABAergic neurons are known to contribute in sculpting synchronous discharges such as generalized spikes and waves (Gloor & Fariello, 1988). The ineffectiveness of these two synchronizing mechanisms in the immature cortex accounts for the asynchronous erratic character of EEG epileptic discharges in early infancy. The possible implication of subcortical (namely brainstem) structures in the periodic expression of the EEG patterns will be further discussed.

Age-dependent expression of infantile epilepsies with epileptic falls

Early epileptic encephalopathies

Two main forms are known to develop in newborns or infants aged less than three months: the *early myoclonus encephalopathy* (EME, Aicardi & Gouthieres, 1978) and the *early infantile encephalopathy with suppression burst* (EIEE, Ohtahara, 1978; Ohtahara *et al.*, 1976). These two syndromes occur in infants with a severe neurological impairment. Both are associated with the suppression-burst (SB) EEG pattern but present with different types of seizures: mainly spasms in EIEE; partial motor seizures, tonic spasms (uncommon before 4 to 5 months of age) and myoclonus in EME, that is therefore particularly relevant to our topic. SB are commonly attributed to a disconnection of the cortex from subcortical (namely thalamic) afferents. This could release an 'idiocortical' rhythmic activity responsible for SB. In alternative SB have been suggested to be triggered by brainstem rhythmogenic structures that can influence the cortical activities through direct projections ending in the superficial cortical layers. The brainstem hypothesis for SB pathogenesis is therefore compatible with a cortical disconnection from thalamic structures. In any case the discontinuous character of SB resulting from high amplitude or rhythmic bursts of cortical activities interspersed by flat EEG correlates very well with the above reported physiological properties of immature cortical neurons. The facilitation of EAA mediated neurotransmission (due to the incomplete sensitivity to the voltage-dependent Mg^{2+} block of NMDA receptors) and the poor inhibitory effectiveness of GABA transmission (due to GABA depolarizing responses) together with the immaturity of intracortical IB dependent synchronizing mechanisms, would account for the characters of the bursts. The remarkable fatiguability of excitatory mechanisms would explain the suppression of the EEG activities following the bursts, that has been shown to reflect on inhibitory status of cortical neurons (Steriade *et al.*, 1994). The thalamo-cortical disconnection may result from different pathological mechanisms including the persistence of primitive spiny neurons in the white matter preventing the thalamic afferents from reaching their cortical target (Spreafico *et al.*, 1993).

West syndrome and related conditions

West syndrome is often considered as synonymous for *infantile spasms* (IS), a unique form of seizure disorder occurring in infants during the first year of life. Its usual age of onset is between 3 and 7 months. Spasms consist of sudden bilateral symmetrical or asymmetrical contractions of neck, trunk and arm muscles. They can predominantly involve either flexor or extensor muscle and can be unilateral in 6–8 per cent of the cases. IS are typically associated with the interictal pattern of hypsarrhythmia consisting of a very high-voltage slow EEG activity, irregularly interspersed with spikes and sharp waves occurring randomly in all cortical areas. Atypical patterns include preservation of portions of background rhythm, occurrence of spike-wave bursts, and periodic pattern in the awake-EEG. The most common ictal pattern is a high-voltage, frontal dominant generalized slow-wave transient, followed by profound voltage attenuation.

The age range of expression of hypsarrhythmia correlates well with differentiation of the intracortical synchronizing mechanism provided by IB neurons. The ability of such a subpopulation of layer V pyramidal neurons to recruit large populations of cortical neurons in synchronous activities may account for the generation of high-voltage slow and sharp waves or spikes. The erratic character of hypsarrhythmia is due to the persisting immaturity of projection systems capable of a more widespread synchronizing effect of different cortical regions.

Myoclonic epilepsies of infancy and early childhood

Myoclonic seizures with the characteristics described in the previous paragraph may occur in many different types of epilepsies and have therefore no specific nosographic value. Two main types of myoclonic epilepsy occurring in infancy or early childhood have been identified under the headings of benign and severe myoclonic epilepsies in infants (Dravet et al., 1985a, b).

Benign myoclonic epilepsy in infants presents exclusively or primarily with myoclonic attacks beginning in normal childhood between 5 months and 2 years according to Dravet et al. (1985a) and between 5 months and 5 years according to Aicardi (1994). The myoclonus involves the axis of the body and the limbs causing head drop and flexion of legs with falling. In the early stages the clinical phenomenology can be limited to head nodding. Myoclonic jerks are associated with bilateral, diffuse arrhythmic bursts of spike- and polyspike-waves of short duration on a normal background that may occur also interictally.

Severe myoclonic epilepsy in infants – in this form, myoclonic seizures are consistently associated with clonic seizures and multiple seizure types (Dravet et al., 1985b; Aicardi 1994). The onset is between 4 and 11 months of age in apparently normal children often with long-lasting emigeneralized (less frequently generalized) clonic seizures triggered by fever, which tend to recur within 2 months either during febrile episodes or without fever. During the second or third year of life myoclonic seizures, often photosensitive, appear and recur with variable frequency. Other types of seizures include atypical absences partial seizures with either autonomic or astatic phenomena, and episodes of non-convulsive status with erratic myoclonus.

Falling may result either from intense myoclonic or astatic seizures. The EEG is initially normal or shows 5–6 Hz central or vertex theta rhythms. From the second year of life, interictal and ictal discharges of fast spike-wave or polyspike waves appear sometimes predominant on one hemisphere and are associated with focal or multifocal spikes. Photoconvulsive response is typically found from the early stages. The prognosis is bad as both seizure control and psychomotor development (behavioural disturbances, mental retardation, ataxia and erratic myoclonus). Myoclonic seizures disappear in most cases after 4 to 7 years giving way to generalized tonic-clonic seizures, emiclonic alternating seizures or complex partial seizures.

These two types of infantile myoclonic epilepsies occur in apparently normal children at partially overlapping maturational stages but differ profoundly in their prognosis reflecting completely different pathogenic mechanisms. Their interaction with maturational processes in the brain can be considered in two ways: (1) how the maturational stage of the brain accounts for the clinical expression of the epileptic symptomatology; and (2) whether and how the epileptogenic process can interfere with further development of the brain in the severe but not in the benign myoclonic epilepsies.

A first point is that as early as the second semester of postnatal life the brain is able to generate bilateral synchronous discharges associated with massive myoclonus that in the benign form has electroclinical features quite similar to those of myoclonic epilepsies occurring later in life. As reported above, in this period the intracortical synchronizing mechanisms related to intrinsic neuronal properties (i.e. burst generation) and to cell to cell communication (i.e. excitatory and inhibitory synaptic transmission) are already developed. As far as the reciprocal connections between cerebral cortex and subcortical structures (i.e. thalamic nuclei), they are already functional at this stage thus providing the basis for bilateral synchronous discharges.

The fact that the intrathalamic Rt-TC circuitry is still incompletely developed (see above) does not prevent TC nuclei from participating in bilateral arrhythmic discharges such as the ones associated with myoclonic seizures. Only during the second year of life do the intrathalamic rhythmogenic systems attain a sufficient degree of maturation to support sustained rhythmic discharges of spike-waves. The presence of photosensitivity (especially frequent in the severe type) can also be correlated with the functional effectiveness of thalamo-cortical projection systems.

The second issue about the relationship between epileptogenesis and the impairment of brain development in severe myoclonic epilepsy can only be addressed speculatively. The high proportion of familial antecedents had led us to hypothesize the existence of unfavourable genetic factors that might cause secondary aggravation of a primary epilepsy (Dravet *et al.*, 1985b). On the other hand the polymorphic epileptic manifestations of severe myoclonic epilepsy including multifocal seizures and EEG discharges might be viewed as potentially harmful for brain development. Further progress in our understanding of the pathogenic factors will clarify the issue.

Lennox–Gastaut syndrome and myoclono-astatic epilepsy

The boundaries (if any) between these two syndromes are the subject of an unresolved debate that would not be appropriate to discuss here. Relevant to our topic are their general features that include onset in early childhood and polymorphic ictal phenomenology comprising atonic and tonic seizures, whereas myoclonic seizures are often considered to characterize *myoclono-astatic epilepsy* (MAE) but not *Lennox–Gastaut Syndrome* (LGS). A further defining element is the EEG pattern of diffuse interictal spike-wave complexes which should be less than 2.5 Hz in frequency in LGS (Gastaut *et al.*, 1966) while it can be faster (more than 2.5 Hz) in MAE. Doose *et al.* (1970) also emphasize the interictal pattern of monomorphic parietal theta rhythm as the hallmark of a genetic susceptibility to epilepsy in MAE.

Tonic seizures may provoke a sudden fall to the ground or a rhythmic step-by-step falling down, though it can be limited to a head drop or to a sagging of the body. The ictal discharge may feature polyspike waves or fast recruiting rhythms associated with a suppression of EMG postural activity. Tonic seizures may involve either extensor or flexor muscles throwing the patient to the ground in a rigid posture or by collapsing with triple flexion of lower extremities respectively. In this last case the flexor tonic seizure is indistinguishable from an atonic one. Very short flexor tonic seizures can mimic spasms. The ictal EEG may show simple flattening of all activity or fast activities (up to 20 Hz) of increasing amplitude.

Myoclonic seizures are brief muscle jerks associated with 20–150 ms bursts of bi- or polyphasic EMG potentials and ictal generalized spike-waves or polyspike-waves. The myoclonic jerks can be followed by tonic or atonic seizures (as typically described by Doose, 1992).

The consistent presence of highly synchronized discharges, featuring spikes and waves of different frequency usually bilateral and synchronous or Doose's theta rhythm, is to be correlated with the effectiveness of a subcortical, thalamic pace-maker capable of driving large cortical areas of both hemispheres in sustained rhythmic activities. Among the maturational factors discussed above, the abrupt increase in conductance velocity of Rt-TC-cortical loops which is associated with completion of myelinization should be taken into account.

Another interesting EEG aspect is the occurrence of high frequency discharges that reflect the increased effectiveness of regenerative mechanisms of membrane excitability (see above) allowing the rhythmogenic cortical cells of the layer V to attain much higher firing frequencies than in earlier maturational stages.

Myoclonic epilepsies of late childhood and adolescence

Spontaneous or provoked myoclonic jerks may occur in combination with other types of seizures in many types of generalized or multifocal epilepsies of late childhood and adolescence usually conferring them a less favourable prognosis.

This is typically the case of *epilepsy with myoclonic absences* (Tassinari *et al.*, 1969) presenting with rhythmic massive jerks time-locked to the spike component of typical 3 Hz spike-wave discharges. These myoclonic (or clonic) absence seizures are resistant to drug therapy and are often associated to mental deterioration. On the other hand, in other cases typically exemplified by *juvenile myoclonic epilepsy* (JME) the prominence of bilateral regional or massive myoclonic jerks, usually predominant at shoulders and arms, has by no means a bad prognostic significance, it being an idiopathic, putatively genetic type of epilepsy characterized by a very good outcome as both seizure control and neuropsychic status.

Partial epilepsies

Seizures affecting global, regional or segmental postural control may occur both in symptomatic/cryptogenic and idiopathic partial epilepsies. The postural loss may result from tonic, myoclonic or akinetic manifestations often combined in complex patterns. In general, epileptic falls in the context of epilepsies with partial seizures are particularly difficult to control with drug therapy. Their pathophysiology and relationship with brain development will be further discussed in the next paragraph.

Cerebral maturation and epileptic postural lapses

Myoclonic, tonic and astatic seizures may all occur from the earliest phases of life in the context of the different types of epilepsies reviewed above, but their clinical and EEG expression depend on the degree of maturation of the cerebral structures that are responsible for their generation.

Myoclonic seizures

Myoclonic jerks with erratic fragmentary expression can be observed as early as a few hours from birth in early myoclonic encephalopathy. Their brainstem versus cortical origin is discussed. Based on experimental data (Moshè *et al.*, 1994) a prominent involvement of brainstem structures has been suggested. A secondary involvement of the cerebral cortex is possible through the aminergic pathways: the immaturity of intracortical and thalamo cortical synchronizing mechanisms accounts for the continuous anarchic regional shifting of the jerks. Due to the limited ability of the infant to hold postural attitude, the effect of jerks on postural control is scarcely valuable.

Only after the fifth to sixth month of life, when thalamo-cortical projections become effective, bilateral myoclonic seizures affecting head and limb posture can be observed. The disturbing effect on postural control is due to both muscle jerk and suppression of muscular activity that often follows the jerk. Pure 'negative myoclonus' inducing sequential or massive drops is reported only later in life. Recent observations suggest that the discharges responsible for negative myoclonus arise in the pre-motor cortex that exert a suppressive effect on motor cortex (see below).

Tonic seizures

A primary involvement of brainstem structures has also been demonstrated for tonic seizures. Experimental observations in rats with seizures induced by acoustic stimulation (Jobe et al., 1995) or by pentylenetetrazol injection (Browning & Nelson, 1989) have shown that brainstem structures are both necessary and sufficient to generate tonic seizures. The occurrence of tonic seizures in early stages of life is therefore to be expected. Detailed studies of seizures induced in developing rats by N-methyl-D-aspartate and homocysteine (Mares & Velisek, 1992; Kubova et al., 1995) have characterized a special type of flexor or tonic seizures occurring between the 7th and 18th postnatal day. Although a strict correlation with the typical age of expression of *infantile flexor spasms* is difficult to establish, these experimental results suggest that the cerebral structures responsible for spasms can generate flexor spasms only during a critical maturational phase. In a general sense, spasms could be considered a special type of tonic seizures: however there are several reasons to keep distinct the two types of seizure. As discussed elsewhere in this volume (Franceschetti et al., Chapter 8) the interictal and ictal EEG pattern, the association with other types of cortically generated seizures and the neuropathological finding, suggest spasms with a cortical rather than subcortical generator. According to the above reviewed data, during the critical age of expression for spasms (3–7 months) the maturational processes going on in the cortex are far less advanced than in brainstem and cerebellar structures responsible for head, trunk and limb posture. Whether and how the maturational stage of the cortex can account for the peculiar character of the discharge, cannot be resolved at present. Suffice to say that the fatiguability of excitatory cortical mechanisms is consistent with the much shorter duration of spasms with respect to brainstem generated tonic seizures observed at the same age.

Wherever generated, the discharge will eventually affect the subcortical structures responsible for postural control resulting in the typical stereotyped response of neck, trunk and limb muscles. The functional result of the integratory activity taking place in subcortical motor structures between 3 and 8 months determines a prevalence of flexor attitude and may explain the typical flexor pattern of spasms. Reasons for extensor or mixed patterns that are not infrequently observed are unknown.

It has to borne in mind that infantile spasms occur frequently in the context of severe encephalopathies that can impair the normal developmental profile of postural control mechanisms. The consequences can be so severe as to result in a developmental arrest that makes possible a persistence of spasm generating mechanisms long after their usual age of expression.

Astatic, akinetic, atonic seizures

These terms (neither one completely satisfactory) are the most frequently employed to designate seizures characterized by a transient suppression of muscle activity. This definition includes also short interruptions of muscular activity causing a sudden postural pause, referred to as *negative myoclonus* (see above).

Evidence for a cortical origin of the discharge responsible for a suppressory effect on muscle activity, either in isolation or combined with positive motor phenomena, has been repeatedly provided (Tassinari et al., 1968; Guerrini et al., 1993; Shibasaki et al., 1994). In principle, a cortical suppressor effect on muscular activity may be due to: (1) inhibition of corticospinal neurons depriving spinal motoneurons from cortical excitatory input; or (2) activation of corticofugal pathways that selectively excite inhibitory spinal interneurons. With reference to observations on the silent period induced by magnetic cortical stimulations (Uncini et al., 1993;

Wilson et al., 1993), Shibasaki et al. (1994) conclude that cortical inhibitory mechanisms play a major role in stimulus-sensitive negative myoclonus. Recently Rubboli et al. (1995) have demonstrated the negative myoclonus-related cortical potential to map the contralateral frontal region that may exert an inhibitory effect on the motor system resulting in negative myoclonus (Tassinari et al., 1995). The involvement of frontal areas in seizures affecting postural control is further demonstrated by the frequent occurrence of epileptic falls in frontal lobe partial epilepsies. Postural lapses due to frontal localized discharges are thought to depend on rapid spread of the discharges to the contralateral side (Bancaud & Telairach, 1992).

Conclusions

The cerebral maturation processes going on during infancy and childhood determine both the special susceptibility to epileptogenic agents and the age-dependent expression of epileptic manifestations. Fragmentary or massive postural lapses due to astatic, myoclonic, tonic seizures and spasms occur in several epilepsies of infancy and childhood including early epileptic encephalopathies, infantile spasms, myoclonic syndromes, myoclono-astatic epilepsy, Lennox–Gastaut syndrome and partial epilepsies of frontal origin.

The clinical expression of these different types of epilepsy depends on the interaction between the epileptogenic factor(s) and the maturational stage of the brain according to modalities that are only incompletely understood. The different electroclinical patterns of seizures that impair postural control can be correlated with the maturational profile of cerebral structures responsible for their generation and for the subsequent axial and global postural control.

References

Aicardi, J. & Gouthieres, F. (1978): Encéphalopathie myoclonique néonatale. *Rev. EEG Neurophysiol.* **8,** 99–101.

Aicardi, J. (1994): *Epilepsy in children.* New York: Raven Press.

Avanzini, G., de Curtis, M., Panzica, F. & Spreafico, R. (1989): Intrinsic properties of nucleus reticularis thalami of the rat studied *in vitro. J. Physiol.* **416,** 111–122.

Avanzini, G., Franceschetti, S., Panzica, F. & Buzio, S. (1992): Age-dependent changes in excitability of rat neocortical neurons studied *in vitro.* In: *Molecular neurobiology of epilepsy,* eds. J. Engel, Jr, C. Wasterlain, E.A. Cavalheiro, U. Heinemann & G. Avanzini, *Epilepsy Res.* Suppl. 9, pp. 95–105. Amsterdam: Elsevier.

Avanzini, G., Vergnes, M., Spreafico, R. & Marescaux, C. (1993): Calcium-dependent regulation of genetically determined spikes and waves by the reticular thalamic nucleus of rats. *Epilepsia* **34,** 1–7.

Browning, R.A. & Nelson, D.K. (1989): Modification of electroshock and pentylenetetrazol seizure patterns in rats after precollicular transections. *Eur. Neurol.* **93,** 546–556.

Connors, B.W. & Gutnick, M.J. (1990): Intrinsic firing patterns of diverse neocortical neurons. *Trends Neurosci.* **13,** 99–104.

Bancaud, J. & Teleirach, J. (1992): Clinical semiology of frontal lobe seizures. In: *Frontal lobe seizures and epilepsies,* eds. P. Chauvel, A.V. Delgado-Escueta, E. Halgren & J. Bancaud, *Advances in Neurology,* vol. 57, pp. 3–58. New York: Raven Press.

De Biasi, S., Amadeo, A., Arcelli, P., Frassoni, C., Meroni, A. & Spreafico, R. (1996): Ultrastructural characterization of the postnatal development of the thalamic ventrobasal and reticular nuclei in the rat. *Anat. Embryol.* **193,** 341–353.

Doose, H., Gerken, H., Leohardt, R., Volzke, E. & Volz, C. (1970): Centrencephalic myoclonic-astatic petit mal. *Neuropaediatrie* **4,** 162–171.

Doose, H. (1985): Myoclonic astatic epilepsy of early childhood. In: *Epileptic syndromes in infancy, childhood and adolescence,* eds. J. Roger, C. Dravet, M. Bureau, F.E. Dreifuss & P. Wolf, pp. 78–88. London: John Libbey.

Doose, H. (1992): Myoclonic astatic epilepsy of early childhood. In: *Epileptic syndromes in infancy, childhood and adolescence,* eds. J. Roger, M. Bureau, C. Dravet, F.E. Dreifuss, A. Perret & P. Wolf, 2nd edn., pp. 103–114. London: John Libbey.

Dravet, C., Bureau, M. & Roger, J. (1985a): Benign myoclonic epilepsy in infants. In: *Epileptic syndromes in infancy, childhood and adolescence,* eds. J. Roger, C. Dravet, M. Bureau, F.E. Dreifuss & P. Wolf, pp. 51–57. London: John Libbey.

Dravet, C., Bureau, M. & Roger, J. (1985b): Severe myoclonic epilepsy in infants. In: *Epileptic syndromes in infancy, childhood and adolescence,* eds. J. Roger, C. Dravet, M. Bureau, F.E. Dreifuss & P. Wolf, pp. 58–67. London: John Libbey.

Fedrizzi, E. & Bono, R. (1981): Evolution of head control. *Rehabilitation and learning* **2,** 129–142.

Franceschetti, S., Buzio, S., Sancini, G., Panzica, F. & Avanzini, G. (1993): Expression of intrinsic bursting properties in neurons of maturing sensorimotor cortex. *Neurosci. Lett.* **162,** 25–28.

Franceschetti, S., Guatteo, E., Panzica, F., Sancini, G., Wanke, E. & Avanzini, G. (1995): Ionic mechanisms underlying burst firing in pyramidal neurons: intracellular study in rat sensorymotor cortex. *Brain Res.* **696,** 127–139.

Franceschetti, S., Granata, T., Binelli, S., Canafoglia, L. & Avanzini, G. (1997): Infantile spasms and tonic seizures. In: *Falls in epileptic and non-epileptic seizures during childhood,* eds. F. Andermann, G. Avanzini, A. Beaumanoir, L. Mira & L. Martini, pp. 75–82. Sydney: John Libbey.

Gastaut, H., Roger, J., Soulayrol, R., Tassinari, C., Régis, H., Dravet, C., Bernard, R., Pinsard, N. & Saint-Jean, M. (1966): Childhood epileptic encephalopathy with diffuse slow spike-waves (otherwise known as 'petit mal variant') or Lennox syndrome. *Epilepsia* **7,** 139–179.

Getting, P. (1983): Emerging principles governating the operation of neural networks. *Ann. Rev. Neurosci.* **12,** 185–204.

Gloor, P. & Fariello, R.G. (1988): Generalized epilepsy: some of its cellular mechanisms differ from those of focal epilepsy. *Trends Neurosci.* **11,** 63–68.

Guerrini, R., Dravet, C., Genton, P., Bureau, M., Roger, J., Rubboli, G. & Tassinari, C.A. (1993): Epileptic negative myoclonus. *Neurology* **43,** 1078–1083.

Innocenti, G.M. (1986): General organization of callosal connections in the cerebral cortex. In: *Sensory-motor areas and aspects of cortical connectivity,* eds. E.G. Jones & A. Peters, *Cerebral Cortex.*, vol. 5, pp. 291–353. New York: Plenum Press.

ICE (1989): Proposal for revised classification of epilepsies and epileptic syndromes. Commission on classification and terminology of the International League against Epilepsy. *Epilepsia* **30,** 389–399.

Jobe, P.C., Mishra, P.K., Adam-Curtis, L.E., Deoskar, V.U., Ko, K.H., Browning, R.A. & Dailey, J.W. (1995): The genetically epilepsy-prone rat (GEPR). *Ital. J. Neurol. Sci.* **16,** 91–99.

Kriegstein, A.R., Suppes, T. & Prince, D.A. (1987): Cellular and synaptic physiology and epileptogenesis of developing rat neocortical neurons *in vitro. Dev. Brain Res.* **34,** 161–171.

Kubova, H., Folbergrova, J. & Mares, P. (1995): Seizures induced by homocysteine in rats during ontogenesis. *Epilepsia* **36,** 750–756.

Luhman, H.J. & Prince, D.A. (1991): Postnatal maturation of the GABAergic system in rat neocortex. *J. Neurophysiol.* **65,** 247–263.

Mares, P. & Velisek, L. (1992): N-methyl-D-aspartate (NMDA)-induced seizures in developing rats. *Dev. Brain Res.* **65,** 185–189.

McCormick, D.A. & Prince, D.A. (1987): Post-natal development of electrophysiological properties of rat cerebral cortical pyramidal neurones. *J. Physiol.* **393,** 743–762.

Moshè, S.L., Velisek, L. & Holmes, G.L. (1994): Developmental aspects of experimental generalized seizures induced by pentylenetetrazol, bicuculline and flurothyl. In: *Idiopathic generalized epilepsies,* eds. A. Malafosse, P. Genton, E. Hirsch, C. Marescaux, D. Broglin & R. Bernasconi, pp. 51–64. London: John Libbey.

Mulle, C., Madariaga, A. & Deschenes, M. (1986): Morphology and electrophysiological properties of reticularis thalami neurons in cat: *in vivo* study of a thalamic pacemaker. *J. Neurosci.* **6**, 2134–2145.

Ohtahara, S., Ishida, T., Oka, E., Yamatogi, Y., Inique, H., Ohtsuka, Y. & Kanda, S. (1976): On the age-dependent epileptic syndromes: the early infantile encephalopathies with suppression-burst. *Brain Dev.* **8**, 270–288.

Ohtahara, S. (1978): Clinico-electrical delineation of epileptic encephalopathies in childhood. *Asian Med. J.* **21**, 7–17.

Rubboli, G., Parmeggiani, L. & Tassinari, C.A. (1995): Frontal inhibitory spike component associated with epileptic negative myoclonus. *Electroencephalogr. Clin. Neurophysiol.* **95**, 201–205.

Shibazaki, H., Ikeda, A., Nagamine, T., Mima, T., Terada, K., Nishitani, N., Kanda, M., Takano, S., Hanazono, T., Kohara, N., Kaji, R. & Kimura, J. (1994): Cortical reflex negative myoclonus. *Brain* **117**, 477–486.

Spreafico, R., Angelini, L., Binelli, S., Granata, T., Rumi, V., Rosti, D., Runza, L. & Bugiani, O. (1993): Burst suppression and impairment of neocortical ontogenesis: Electroclinical and neuropathologic findings in two infants with early myoclonic encephalopathy. *Epilepsia* **34**, 800–808.

Steriade, M., Amzica, F. & Contreras, D. (1994): Cortical and thalamic cellular correlates of electroencephalographic burst suppression. *Electroencephalogr. Clin. Neurophysiol.* **90**, 1–16.

Tassinari, C.A., Régis, H. & Gastaut, H. (1968): A particular form of muscular inhibition in epilepsy: the related epileptic silent period (RESP). *Proc. Aust. Ass. Neurol.* **5**, 595–602.

Tassinari, C.A., Lyagoubi, S., Santos, V., Gambarelli, F., Roger, J., Dravet, C. & Gastaut, H. (1969): Etude des décharges de pointes ondes chez l'homme. II: Les aspects cliniques et électroencéphalographiques des absences myocloniques. *Rev. Neurol.* **121**, 379–383.

Tassinari, C.A., Rubboli, G., Parmeggiani, L., Valzania, F., Plasmati, R., Riguzzi, P., Michelucci, R., Volpi, L., Passarelli, D., Meletti, S., Fontana, E. & Dalla Bernardina, B. (1995): Epileptic negative myoclonus. In: *Negative motor phenomena*, eds. S. Fahn, M. Hallett, H.O. Luders & C.D. Marsden, *Advances in neurology* vol. 67, pp. 181–197. Philadelphia: Lippincott-Raven.

Temkin, O. (1945): *The falling sickness.* Baltimore: Johns Hopkins Press.

Touwen, B. (1976): Neurological development in infancy. *Clinics in Developmental Medicine.* **58**, Spastic International Medical Publications, London: Heinemann.

Tsakiridou, E., Bertollini, L., de Curtis, M., Avanzini, G. & Pape, H.C. (1995): T-type calcium conductance in the reticular thalamic nucleus: a contribution to absence epilepsy. *J. Neurosci.* **15**, 3110–3117.

Uncini, A., Treviso, M., Di Muzio, A., Simone, P. & Pullman, S. (1993): Physiological basis of voluntary activity inhibition induced by transcranial cortical stimulation. *Electroencephalogr. Clin. Neurophysiol.* **89**, 211–220.

Wilson, S.A., Lockwood, R.J., Thickbroom, G.W. & Mastaglia, F.L. (1993): The muscle silent period following transcranial magnetic cortical stimulation. *J. Neurol. Sci.* **114**, 216–222.

PART II

Chapter 5

Muscular silent period following transcranial magnetic stimulation: contribution of peripheral and central mechanisms

Paolo M. Rossini*†° and Simone Rossi*

*I Divisione Neurologia, Ospedale Fatebenefratelli, Isola Tiberina, Rome;
†I.R.C.C.S. 'S. Lucia', via Ardeatina, Rome;
°IRCCS Centro San Giovanni di Dio Istituto Sacro Cuore, Brescia

Summary

Brain transcranial stimulation (TCS) is followed by periods of increasing (= excitatory = motor-evoked potentials = MEPs) and decreasing (= inhibitory = silent periods = SPs) firing probability of motoneurons, often followed by a rebound acceleration. Thus, the SP represents an epoch in which the electromyographic (EMG) activity voluntarily exerted in the muscle is suppressed. Even though excitatory and inhibitory effects are usually combined in a sequential order, descending pathways mediating MEPs and SPs might not coincide and/or might be excited at a different threshold. Several mechanisms can be responsible for the suppression of EMG activity following TCS, operating at different levels of corticospinal pathways, including cortical, supra-segmental and spinal-segmental sites. In the present paper, these neurophysiological mechanisms are revised, together with other inhibitory effects of brain TCS.

Introduction

Non-invasive electrical transcranial stimulation (TCS) of the human brain was introduced in the early 1980s (Merton & Morton 1980; Merton et al., 1982) and immediately became the most important tool for researchers studying motor pathways and brain responsiveness (Rossini et al., 1985; 1987), despite the fact that high-voltage electric shocks delivered by the first-generation stimulators rendered the procedure uncomfortable. After that, Barker et al., (1985) introduced electromagnetic stimulation of nerves, brain and spinal cord; in this way, discharging a high current through a coil it was possible to produce short-lasting magnetic fields, inducing – on their own – a current flow circulating within the brain with an orientation opposite to that of the current circulating within the coil, so that cortical neurones could be excited. Since the induction of current within the brain bypasses extracerebral tissues

– including scalp muscles and pain receptors – the stimulating procedure is nearly painless for the subject. This great advantage with respect to previous electric TCS, together with the proven safety of the method even in epileptic patients (Tassinari et al., 1990), gave to this technique the chance to become one of the most commonly applied neurophysiological tests in routinely clinical applications (see for review Rossini & Caramia 1992; International Standard Guidelines, Rossini et al., 1994).

It has been shown that by recording from the target muscle – defined as the prime mover for a given motor programme (Tomberg & Caramia, 1991) – or by other synergistic muscles, brain TCS is followed by periods of increasing (= excitatory = motor evoked potentials = MEPs) and decreasing (= inhibitory = silent periods = SPs) firing probability, often followed by a rebound acceleration (Rossini et al., 1995). Even though clinical applications mainly focused on excitatory events together with the evaluation of motor central transit times, suppressory/inhibitory effects of TCS have now been thoroughly investigated by researchers, both in healthy subjects and in those with neurological disorders. In the present paper we will concentrate on SPs, the epoch generally following a MEP, in which the voluntary activation (EMG) of a given muscle is totally suppressed.

For a long time it has been known that following electrical stimulation of the peripheral nerve trunk during sustained voluntary EMG activity, SPs can take place in the muscle(s) more distally supplied by that nerve. Electric TCS is able *per se* to induce nonspecified SPs. This short-lasting inhibitory phenomenon can be observed even after the stimulation of a scalp site outside the motor area triggering contralateral MEPs; since it is not present if a magnetic stimulus is delivered on the same points, this effect is thought to be mediated by reflex pathways related to a nonspecific activation of trigeminal receptors after the painful electric shock.

On the other hand, following magnetic TCS of motor cortex, it is possible to observe SPs in contralateral tonically activated muscles (Fig. 1), which start directly after the initial early

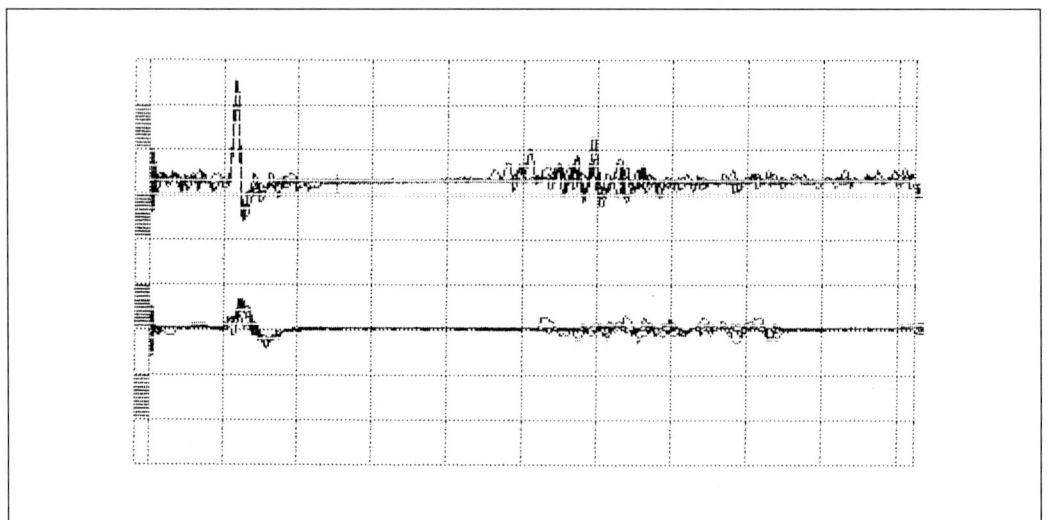

Fig. 1. MEPs and silent periods simultaneously recorded from the first dorsal Interosseous (upper trace) and abductor digiti minimi (lower trace) muscles, during near-threshold magnetic TCS stimulation and slight voluntary contraction of the two muscles. Each trace contains three trials to show reproducibility. The analysis time is 20 ms/div; the calibration is 2 mV/div.

response and last up to 300 ms; but, at variance with peripheral SPs, their recurrence and duration are both largely dependent upon the stimulus intensity (Rossini *et al.*, 1987; Claus *et al.*, 1988; Cohen *et al.*, 1990; Fuhr *et al.*, 1991; Mariorenzi *et al.*, 1991; Uncini *et al.*, 1993; Rossini *et al.*, 1995; 1996) rather than by the amplitude of the muscular response or by the amount of the voluntary exerted contraction.

Periods of suppression of EMG activity can be triggered following TCS both in distal and proximal muscles, lasting longer in the former than in the latter. However, it should be remembered that this longer duration of the SP is partly biased by differences in the excitability threshold, that is known to be lower for distal than for proximal muscles. Therefore, due to the straight correlation between intensity of TCS and duration of the SP, the same suprathreshold stimulus would lead to longer SPs in distal than in proximal muscle groups.

Some year ago, Caramia *et al.* (1991) demonstrated that in different neurological diseases, SPs can appear without being preceded by a MEP, provided that specific cerebral areas were stimulated. This aspect was more recently confirmed also in healthy subject by recording the firing properties of individual motor units (Rossini *et al.*, 1995). In other words, since subthreshold stimuli for MEP elicitation are able to introduce SPs, descending pathways and cerebral areas involved in the generation of excitatory and inhibitory events could be different.

Neurophysiological mechanisms

Several mechanisms can be responsible for the suppression of EMG activity following TCS, acting at different levels – and with different timing – of corticospinal pathways, including cortical, supra-segmental and spinal-segmental sites. An important factor is now thought to be the inaccessibility of the corticospinal projection to voluntary motor output (Fuhr *et al.*, 1991; Cantello *et al.*, 1992). These authors demonstrated that the inhibitory epoch recorded from the first dorsal Interosseus muscle is longer than the SP evoked by a single or a repetitive electrical stimulation delivered on the ulnar nerve. Moreover, both the F and H waves – markers of spinal excitability – had recovered by the last quarter of the SP despite the fact that no voluntary EMG activity was present. EMG responses produced by weak electrical stimuli to the cortex were also only slightly inhibited during the late SP. Therefore, authors suggested that the latter part of the SP is not due to inexcitability of spinal mechanisms, but is mainly due to inhibitory or suppressive phenomena at the cerebral cortex. Interestingly, this phenomenon can be disrupted in Parkinsonian patients (Cantello *et al.*, 1991), in whom SPs are shorter than normal, and frontal components of somatosensory evoked potentials – arising from a complex loop involving the supplementary motor area – are generally depressed or absent (Rossini *et al.*, 1989).

Fuhr *et al.* (1991) have studied the excitability of spinal motoneuronal pool during the SP by measuring the H-reflex amplitude at different intervals after TCS; the H-reflex was depressed at the beginning of the SP, while it regained its normal amplitude in the later part, thus indicating that both a reduction of spinal motoneurons excitability (in the early SP) and a lack of cortical drive (in the late SP) concur to explain the EMG silence, the latter hypothesis being supported also by experiments of paired magnetic shocks applied to the cortex (Inghilleri *et al.*, 1993).

In a recent paper Classen & Benecke (1995) demonstrated that the suppression of the firing of a single motoneuron after TCS can last up to 1000 ms; authors hypothesized that at least the later part of this SP is likely to result from GABAergic intracortical inhibitions rather than by other spinal inhibitory actions. According to a series of experimental studies cited in the article, in fact, inhibitory post-synaptic potentials generated by inhibitory spinal interneurons can last no more than 100 ms.

At 'muscular' level, during the contraction induced by the descending TCS volley, the muscle is shortened and spindle activity, as reflected by a reduction of their inputs mediated by group I and II fibres, can transiently modulate spinal excitability by lowering the frequency discharge, and consequently the threshold, of spinal alpha-motoneurons. However, other spinal inhibitory mechanisms can act together in lowering spinal motoneurons excitability, either through excitatory pathways activating the Renshaw inhibitory circuit or by the direct activation of specific cortical inhibitory centres.

The cortical 'drive' of SPs was further supported by a recent investigation of Von Giesen *et al.* (1994), in which authors demonstrated that in focal lesions of the primary motor cortex induced by ischaemia there is a decrease in SP duration or even a complete lack of SP, even though spinal inhibitory mechanisms tested by peripheral nerve stimulation were unaffected.

Although TCS-linked excitatory and inhibitory effects are usually combined in sequential order, descending pathways mediating MEPs and SPs might not coincide and/or might be excited at a different threshold. In fact, using near-threshold intensity of TCS and needle recordings of individual motor unit action potentials (MUAPs), SP can be present during which the MUAP is silenced without any preceding MEP (Rossini *et al.*, 1995, 1996; Classen & Benecke, 1995). Therefore, this again suggests that the SP after TCS is not merely generated by peripheral and spinal mechanisms linked with the unloading effects of muscle contraction (= less excitatory input from muscle spindle afferents) and with the action of Renshaw cells (Calancie *et al.*, 1987; Cantello *et al.*, 1992). It should be reminded that inhibition of hand motor unit firing was solely triggered by intracortical microstimulation in monkeys (Liddel & Phillips, 1952; Ranck, 1975); similarly, both in healthy and neurologically diseased humans, SPs without preceding MEPs have been described after contra- and ipsilateral magnetic TCS, including the focal type with a 'butterfly' coil (Caramia *et al.*, 1991; Wassermann *et al.*, 1991). After discharge, motoneuronal hyperpolarization, recurrent inhibition by Renshaw cells, block of fusimotor reafferent flow on alpha-motoneurons due to 'spindle unloading' after MEP, inhibitory volleys from the motor cortex, reciprocal inhibition due to coactivation of antagonists are all not mutually exclusive mechanisms which might contribute to spinal depression following the arrival of the corticospinal volley triggered by brain stimulation (Rothwell *et al.*, 1984; Caramia *et al.*, 1991; Cantello *et al.*, 1992; Fuhr *et al.*, 1991; Triggs *et al.*, 1991; Uncini *et al.*, 1993; Rossini *et al.*, 1995, 1996; Classen & Benecke, 1995).

Recently, mapping studies concerning the topography of excitatory and inhibitory corticospinal outputs following 'focal' TCS of several scalp positions have been carried out. Wilson *et al.* (1993) showed by surface EMG recordings that the 'centre of gravity' of the map constructed for the duration of the SP and that of the MEP amplitude evoked by contralateral hemiscalp magnetic stimulation had very similar co-ordinates. By TCS mapping procedures, Wasserman *et al.* (1994) showed that SPs can be represented also in the motor cortex ipsilateral to the hand and arm.

Other inhibitory effects of TCS

The cortical origin of inhibitory phenomena following TCS is also strongly suggested by a number of evidences of suppressory effects on strictly cortical functions such as the perception of a visual stimulus (Amassian *et al.*, 1989) or by the possibility of delaying voluntary reaction times to acoustic, visual or somatosensory stimuli when a suprathreshold magnetic stimulus is given in the reaction period (Pascual-Leone et al., 1992). Moreover, magnetic TCS is able to interfere with the execution of complex motor programmes; in fact, Day et al. (1989) showed that TCS of the motor cortex could delay the onset of a voluntary wrist repetitive movement, but the subject was able to carry out in an appropriate way the whole motor programme. Further evidences of the storage of the motor programme and of the possibility of externally delaying it by TCS have been provided by Priori et al. (1993): visually guided saccadic eye movements could be delayed up to 100 ms by a single transcranial magnetic stimulus delivered trough a circular coil centred on the vertex, whilst more focal stimuli did not lead to the same effects.

Using repetitive magnetic stimuli, reproducible speech arrest can be induced only by stimulation of infero-lateral posterior frontal areas of the left hemisphere (Broca's area) (Pascual-Leone et al., 1991). In addition, magnetic TCS of the sensorimotor cortex – appropriately timed in relation to an electric stimulus applied to a finger of the contralateral hand – can attenuate the detection of the sensory stimulus (Cohen et al., 1991). Finally, Amassian et al. (1991) showed that a single magnetic stimulus delivered on the scalp overlying the supplementary motor area could cause errors in a sequential finger tapping task.

Some interesting observations in epileptic patients have recently been performed by studying cortico-cortical inhibitory phenomena through pairs of magnetic stimuli applied to the skull. The MEP recovery cycle as revealed by the analysis to paired shocks of different intensity, showed in normal a period of total refractoriness lasting 1 to 4 ms, followed by a progressive

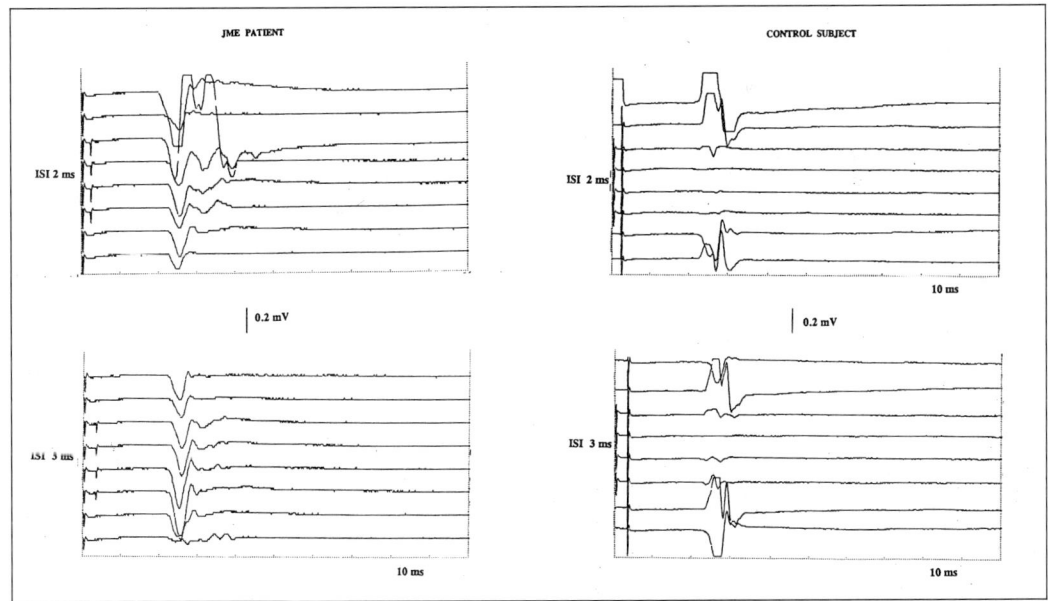

Fig. 2. Right side: MEP recordings from a single control subject. MEPs to magnetic TCS in relaxed thenar muscles are inhibited by a prior subthreshold conditioning stimulus (ISIs = 2 ms top panel, 3 ms bottom panel). The first two traces as well as the lower two traces, in each panel, show the response to the test stimulus alone. In the remaining middle traces, conditioned MEPs are dramatically suppressed. Left side: same organization as in the control subject. MEP recordings in a patient with JME. Here, at 2 ms and 3 ms ISIs, the inhibition is absent, with conditioned MEPs matching the amplitude of the test MEP. [Caramia et al. (1996) with permission.]

recovery of baseline excitability threshold. Caramia *et al.* (1996) have combined threshold measurement using individual TCS with a protocol employing paired stimuli (= conditioning-subthreshold + test-suprathreshold (Fig. 2); in order to measure excitatory and inhibitory aspects of altered brain excitability in patients with juvenile myoclonic epilepsy (JME) and grand mal seizures.

In one case with JME, recordings were also obtained before and after the initiation of a specific therapy with valproate. In JME patients undergoing anti-epileptic treatment, threshold values were higher, while in the untreated case it was the opposite. Unlike normal control, MEP inhibition was greatly diminished during paired shocks stimulation (Fig. 2); this was ascribed to loss of intracortical inhibitory mechanisms. Another interesting aspect was represented by the progressively larger MEPs elicited by a cascade of consecutive stimuli of the same intensity. This goes in the opposite way than for normal cases, in whom a 'physiological' decremental trend of MEPs amplitude has been found (Rossini *et al.*, 1991) and ascribed to a progressive increase of inhibition, possibly due to self-protection against overstimulation; this protective mechanism is evidently altered in JME patients, in which other 'markers' of cortical hyperexcitability are generally found, as giant components of somatosensory evoked potentials or larger than normal MEPs following conditioning electrical pre-stimulation of the peripheral nerves (Mariorenzi *et al.*, 1991; Reutens *et al.*, 1993). In the two cases with grand mal seizures the recovery cycle matched that of controls in the range of 1 to 4 ms. The authors (Caramia *et al.*, 1996) suggest that the pattern of cortical inhibition, as investigated with the paired stimuli protocol, could be related to GABA influences on neuronal firing level (Kujirai *et al.*, 1993), probably – as known from experimental studies – by hyperpolarization mechanisms at postsynaptic cell membrane level (on cortical inhibitory interneurons?), by increasing the conductance of the Cl– ions and/or modulating the neuronal firing level.

References

Amassian, V.E., Cracco, J.B., Cracco, R.Q. & Maccabee, P.J. (1990): Magnetic coil stimulation of human pre-motor cortex affects sequential digital movements. *J. Physiol.* **424**, 65.

Amassian, V.E., Cracco, R.Q., Maccabee, P.J., Bigland-Ritchie, B. & Cracco, J.B. (1991): Matching focal and non-focal magnetic coil stimulation to properties of human nervous system: mapping motor unit fields in motor cortex contrasted with altering sequential digit movements by pre-motor SMA stimulation. In: W.J. Levy *et al.* (eds.) *Magnetic motor stimulation: Basic principles and clinical experience.* vol. 3, 28. Amsterdam: Elsevier B.V.

Barker, A.T., Jalinous, R. & Freenston, I.I. (1985): Non-invasive magnetic stimulation of the human motor cortex. *Lancet*, **i**, 1106–1107.

Calanicie, B., Nordin, M., Wallin, U. & Hagbarth, K.E. (1987): Motor unit responses in human wrist flexor and extensor muscles to transcranial cortical stimuli. *J. Neurophysiol.* **58**, 1168–1185.

Cantello, R., Gianelli, M., Bettucci, D., Civardi, C. & Mutani, R. (1991): Parkinson's disease rigidity: magnetic motor evoked potentials in a small hand muscle. *Neurology*, **41**, 1449–1456.

Cantello, R., Gianelli, M., Civardi, C. & Mutani, R. (1992): Magnetic brain stimulation: the silent period after the motor evoked potential. *Neurology* **42**, 1951–1959.

Caramia, M.D., Cicinelli, P., Paradiso, C., Mariorenzi, R., Zarola, F., Bernardi, G. & Rossini, P.M. (1991): 'Excitability' changes of muscular responses to magnetic brain stimulation in patients with central motor disorders. *Electroenceph. Clin. Neurophysiol.* **81**, 243–250.

Caramia, M.D., Gigli, G.L., Iani, C., Desiato, M.T., Diomedi, M., Palmieri, M.P. & Bernardi, G. (1996): Distinguishing forms of generalized epilepsy using magnetic brain stimulation. *Electroenceph. Clin. Neurophysiol.* (in press).

Classen, J. & Benecke, R. (1995): Inhibitory phenomena in individual motor units induced by transcranial magnetic stimulation. *Electroenceph. Clin. Neurophysiol.* **97**, 264–274.

Claus, D., Mills, K.R. & Murray, N.M.F. (1988): Facilitation of muscles responses to magnetic brain stimulation by mechanical stimuli in man. *Exp. Brain Res.* **71**, 243–278.

Cohen, L.G., Roth, B.J., Nillson, J., Dang, N., Panizza, M., Bandinelli, S., Frianf, W. & Hallett, M. (1990): Effects of coil design on delivery of focal magnetic stimulation. *Electroenceph. Clin. Neurophysiol.* **75**, 350–357.

Cohen, L.G., Bandinelli, S., Sato, S., Kufta, C. & Hallett, M. (1991): Attenuation in detection of somatosensory stimuli by transcranial magnetic stimulation. *Electroenceph. Clin. Neurophysiol.* **81**, 366–376.

Day, B.L., Rothwell, J.C., Thompson, P.D., Maertens de Noordhout, A., Nakashima, K., Shannon, K. & Marsden, C.D. (1989): Delay in the execution of voluntary movement by electrical or magnetic brain stimulation in intact man. Evidence for the storage of motor programmes in the brain. *Brain* **112**, 649–663.

Fuhr, P., Agostino, R. & Hallett, M. (1991): Spinal motor neuron excitability during the silent period after cortical stimulation. *Electroenceph. Clin. Neurophysiol.* **81**, 257–262.

Kujirai, T., Caramia, M.D., Rothwell, J.C., Day, B.L., Thompson, P.D., Ferbert, A., Wroe, S., Asselmann, P. & Marsden, C.D. (1993): Corticocortical inhibition in human motor cortex. *J. Physiol.* **471**, 501–519.

Inghilleri, M., Berardelli, A., Cruccu, G. & Manfredi, M. (1993): Silent period evoked by transcranial stimulation of the human motor cortex and cervicomedullary junction. *J. Physiol.* **34**, 521–534.

Liddel, E.G.T. & Phillips, C.G. (1952): The cortical representation of motor units. *Brain* **75**, 510–525.

Mariorenzi, R., Zarola, F., Caramia, M.D., Paradiso, C. & Rossini, P.M. (1991): Non-invasive evaluation of central motor tract excitability changes following peripheral nerve stimulation. *Electroenceph. Clin. Neurophysiol.* **81**, 90–101.

Merton, P.A. & Morton, H.B. (1980): Stimulation of the cerebral cortex in the intact human subject. *Nature* **285**, 277.

Merton, P.A., Hill, D.K., Morton, H.B. & Marsden, C.D. (1982): Scope of a technique or electrical stimulation of the human brain. *Lancet* **ii**, 597–600.

Pascual-Leone, A., Gates, J.R. & Dhuna, A. (1991): Induction of speech arrest and counting errors with rapid-rate transcranial stimulation. *Neurology* **41**, 697–702.

Pascual-Leone, A., Brasil-Neto, J.P., Valls-Solé, J., Cohen, L.G. & Hallett, M. (1992): Simple reaction time to focal transcranial magnetic stimulation. *Brain* **115**, 109–122.

Priori, A., Bertolasi, L., Rothwell, J.C., Day, B.L. & Marsden, C.D. (1993): Some saccadic eye movements can be delayed by transcranial magnetic stimulation of the cerebral cortex in man. *Brain* **116**, 355–367.

Ranck Jr., J.B. (1975): Which elements are excited in electrical stimulation of mammalian central nervous system: a review. *Brain Res.* **98**, 417–440.

Reutens, D.C., Puce, A. & Berkovic, S.F. (1993): Cortical hyperexcitability in progressive myoclonic epilepsy: a study with transcranial magnetic stimulation. *Neurology* **43**, 186–192.

Rossini, P.M., Marciani, M.G., Caramia, M.D., Roma, V. & Zarola, F. (1985): Nervous propagation along 'central' motor pathways in intact man: characteristics of motor responses to 'bifocal' and 'unifocal' spin and scalp non-invasive stimulation. *Electroenceph. Clin. Neurophysiol.* 272–286.

Rossini, P.M., Caramia, M.D. & Zarola, F. (1987): Central motor tract propagation in man: studies with non-invasive, unifocal, scalp stimulation. *Brain Res.* **415**, 211–225.

Rossini, P.M., Babiloni, F., Bernardi, G., Cecchi, L., Johnson, P.B., Malentacca, A., Stanzione, P. & Urbano, A. (1989): Abnormalities of short-latency somatosensory evoked potentials in Parkinsonian patients. *Electroenceph. Clin. Neurophysiol.* **74**, 277–289.

Rossini, P.M., Desiato, M.T., Lavaroni, F. & Caramia, M.D. (1991): Brain excitability and electroencephalographic activation: non-invasive evaluation in healthy humans via transcranial magnetic stimulation. *Brain Res.* **567**, 111–119.

Rossini, P.M. & Caramia, M.D. (1992): Central conduction studies and magnetic stimulation. *Curr. Opin. Neurol. Neurosurg.* **5,** 697–703.

Rossini, P.M., Barker, A.T., Berardelli, A., Caramia, M.D., Caruso, G., Cracco, R.Q., Dimitrijevic, M.R., Hallett, M., Katayama, Y., Lucking, C.H., Maertens de Noordhout, A.L., Marsden, C.D., Murray, N.M.F., Rothwell, J.C., Swash, M. & Tomberg, C. (1994): Non-invasive electrical and magnetic stimulation of the brain, spinal cord and roots: basic principles and procedures for routine clinical application. Report of a IFCN committee. *Electroenceph. Clin. Neurophysiol.* **91,** 79–92.

Rossini, P.M., Caramia, M.D., Iani, C., Desiato, M.T., Sciarretta, G. & Bernardi, G. (1995): Magnetic transcranial stimulation in healthy humans: influence on the behavior of upper limbs motor units. *Brain Res.* **676,** 314–324.

Rossini, P.M., Rossi, S., Tecchio, F., Sciarretta, G., Caramia, M.D., Iani, C. & Finazzi-Agrò, A. (1996): A method to evaluate the effects of transcranial stimulation on upper limbs motor units. *Neurosci. Prot.* **70,** 1–15.

Rothwell, J.C., Day, B.L., Berardelli, A. & Marsden, C.D. (1984): Effects of motor cortex stimulation on spinal motoneurons in intact man. *Exp. Brain Res.* **54,** 382–384.

Tassinari, C.A., Michelucci, R., Forti, A. & Rubboli, G. (1990): Transcranial magnetic stimulation in epileptic patients: usefulness and safety. *Neurology* **40,** 1132–1133.

Tomberg, C. & Caramia, M.D. (1991): Prime mover muscle in finger lift or finger flexion reaction times: identification with a transcranial magnetic stimulation. *Electroenceph. Clin. Neurophysiol.* **81,** 319–322.

Triggs, W.J., Macdonnel, R.A.L. & Cross, D.P. (1991): Inhibitory effect of magnetic cortical stimulation in the upper motor neuron syndrome. *Ann. Neurol.* **30,** 317–321.

Uncini, A., Treviso, M., Di Mascio, A., Simone, P. & Pullman, S. (1993): Physiological basis of voluntary activity inhibition induced by transcranial cortical stimulation. *Electroenceph. Clin. Neurophysiol.* **89,** 211–226.

Von Giesen, H.J., Roick, H. & Benecke, R. (1994): Inhibitory actions of motor cortex in hemispheric brain lesions studied by magnetic brain stimulation. *Exp. Brain Res.* **99,** 84–96.

Wassermann, E.M., Fuhr, P., Cohen, L.G. & Hallett, M. (1991): Effects of transcranial magnetic stimulation on ipsilateral muscles. *Neurology* **41,** 1795–1799.

Wassermann, E.M., Pascual-Leone, A. & Hallett, M. (1994): Cortical motor representation of the ipsilateral hand and arm. *Exp. Brain Res.* **100,** 121–132.

Wilson, S.A., Thickbroom, G.W. & Mastaglia, F.L. (1993): Topography of excitatory and inhibitory muscle responses evoked by transcranial magnetic stimulation in the human motor cortex. *Neurosci. Lett.* **154,** 52–56.

Chapter 6

Clinical and neurophysiological features of different forms of epileptic falls

Guido Rubboli, Roberto Michelucci, Franco Valzania,
Lucio Parmeggiani, Stefano Meletti, Elena Gardella,
Romana Rizzi, Anna Zaniboni and Carlo Alberto Tassinari

Department of Neurology, University of Bologna, Bellaria Hospital, via Altura 3, 40139 Bologna, Italy

Summary

Falling seizures are a heterogeneous group of epileptic seizures in which the fall represents the main or only clinical manifestation. In this chapter, we discuss the clinical and neurophysiological characteristics of focal atonic epileptic events, such as epileptic negative myoclonus, and of different types of epileptic falling seizures, occurring in generalized and partial epilepsies. Pathophysiological hypotheses on epileptic negative myoclonus indicate the involvement of frontal areas with inhibitory effect on the motor system. Current knowledge on basic mechanisms of epileptic falling seizures is still limited; subcortical as well as cortical mechanisms have been suggested to play a role in the origin of these types of seizures. Appropriate neurophysiological investigations, particularly video-polygraphic recordings, have been, so far, extremely useful to describe the electroclinical characteristics of these phenomena, and it is conceivable that a more diffuse application of these techniques will provide further insights on the different types of falling seizures and their pathophysiological mechanisms.

Introduction

Falling seizures are a heterogeneous and poorly understood group of epileptic seizures. They can occur in a variety of epileptic conditions and different pathophysiological mechanisms have been postulated responsible for falling seizures in epileptics. Video-polygraphic recordings were found crucial in the investigation and analysis of the clinical and electrophysiological phenomenology of these events. However, in the literature only a few polygraphic studies of falling seizures have been published (Dravet *et al.*, 1988; Egli *et al.*, 1985; Gastaut & Broughton, 1972; Gastaut & Régis, 1961; Gastaut *et al.*, 1966a; Ikeno *et al.*, 1985; Oguni *et al.*, 1992; Yaqub, 1993). In this chapter we outline the clinical aspects and neurophysiological features of different types of falling seizures in epileptic patients. The neurophysiological data have been obtained by means of different neurophysiological techniques, such as video-polygraphic monitoring and computerized EEG-polygraphic analysis techniques allowing assessment of cortical and spinal excitability. Two main groups of phenomena are discussed: focal 'atonic' epileptic events, i.e. epileptic negative myoclonus, and epileptic falling seizures, considered to be those seizures in which the fall is the main or only clinical manifestation.

Epileptic negative myoclonus

Epileptic negative myoclonus (ENM) is defined as an interruption of tonic muscular activity, time-locked to a spike or a sharp wave on the EEG, without evidence of an antecedent myoclonia (Fig. 1) (Tassinari *et al.*, 1995a). The first description of a phenomenon characterized by brief interruptions of muscular activity, temporally related to a paroxysmal EEG event, was reported by Tassinari *et al.* 1968 under the label of related epileptic silent period (RESP). A similar phenomenon, clearly focal, involving either one or both limbs on the same side of the body, and associated with a contralateral spike, was described later (Tassinari, 1981). The term epileptic negative myoclonus was recently introduced by Tassinari *et al.* (1990) and Guerrini *et al.* (1993).

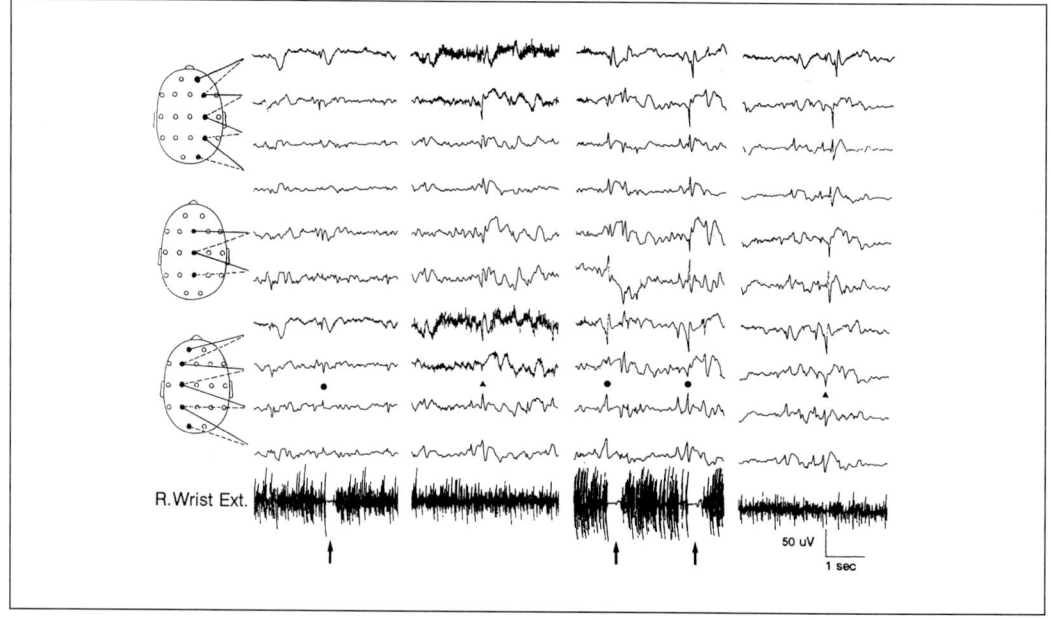

Fig. 1. Epileptic negative myoclonus (ENM) in the right upper limb in a patient with epileptic encephalopathy due to birth anoxia. ENM appears as an abrupt flattening of EMG activity (arrows) in the right wrist extensor, associated with a spike in the left fronto-central regions (black dots). The same tracing also shows spikes unrelated to ENM (black triangles). (R.Wrist Ext. = right wrist extensor.)

Clinical aspects

Clinically, ENM is characterized by brief postural lapses of a body segment. This disorder can be discrete, and should be carefully looked for and investigated by means of simultaneous

EEG–EMG polygraphic recording, particularly to ascertain the absence of any previous myoclonia, on agonist and antagonist muscles. It can be, sometimes, almost undetected, the patient complaining of just an 'instability'. More often, it can cause dropping of objects from the hands, head nodding, or even falls to the ground. In children, particularly when it is frequent, it can be so disturbing as to cause change of handedness or a motor neglect.

Tassinari et al. (1995a) reviewed the relationship between ENM and epilepsy. They found ENM in a group of epileptic subjects suffering from different epileptic conditions, classified, according to an aetiological criterion, as idiopathic, cryptogenic and symptomatic. In the idiopathic group, all patients were children presenting with a condition identifiable or resembling benign epilepsy with centro-temporal spikes. The mean ages of onset, for both epilepsy and ENM, were similar, at 4.8 years. In these cases, ENM usually lasted 1 – 2 years; prognosis of epilepsy was good as well. The cryptogenic group was composed of a group of children showing neuropsychological disorders, absence seizures and, most of them presenting with 'ESES or electrical status epilepticus during sleep' (Tassinari et al., 1992). In the symptomatic group, ENM was present in children with some degree of neuropsychological impairment, absence seizures and ESES, and in patients with disorders such as Lafora disease, or epileptic encephalopathy due to birth anoxia. Other examples of patients with ENM, associated with a symptomatic aetiology, included cases of progressive myoclonus epilepsies (Yokota & Tsukagoshi, 1992; Shibasaki et al., 1994; Thomas et al., 1994), mitochondrial diseases (Guerrini et al., 1993), neuronal migration disorders (Guerrini et al., 1993; Colamaria et al., 1989; Dalla Bernardina et al., 1996). In the symptomatic group, the evolution of epilepsy and ENM was related to aetiology.

Neurophysiological features

Several techniques have been used to investigate ENM (Tassinari et al., 1995a). Polygraphic recordings were essential to correlate the muscular phenomena to the EEG event. In children with ENM and benign epilepsy with centro-temporal spikes, ENM in one upper limb was associated with a triphasic spike in contralateral central regions. The EMG silent periods lasted from 200 to 400 ms; the associated spikes could spread to the homologous regions of the opposite hemisphere, causing the appearance of ENM in the contralateral upper limb. In patients with progressive myoclonus epilepsies, polygraphic investigation demonstrated the association of both positive and negative myoclonus; sometimes, the EMG silent period could precede the positive myoclonic burst. The brief muscular suppressions could be associated with a small spike in contralateral central regions or, in some cases, they could be devoid of any EEG correlate.

Computerized analysis of EEG-polygraphic signals allowed a more precise correlation between the EEG and the EMG events. Rubboli et al. (1995) used a spike-averaging technique to distinguish spikes associated with ENM from spikes unrelated to ENM, in a patient with epileptic encephalopathy due to birth anoxia and ENM in the right upper limb. ENMs were associated with left fronto-central spikes. A relationship between spike amplitude and EMG silent period duration was observed. Spikes associated with ENM were characterized, as compared to spikes unrelated to ENM, by a 'double peak' morphology, with the second peak following the first one by about 40 ms and preceding the onset of the EMG silent period by about 30 ms (Fig. 2). Topographical analysis showed that the first peak of the spike associated with ENM had the same voltage field distribution of the spikes unrelated to ENM; the second peak, presumably related to ENM, had a more frontal and midline topography, suggesting the involvement of the frontal areas in the generation of ENM. Recently, Suisse et al. (1995), by

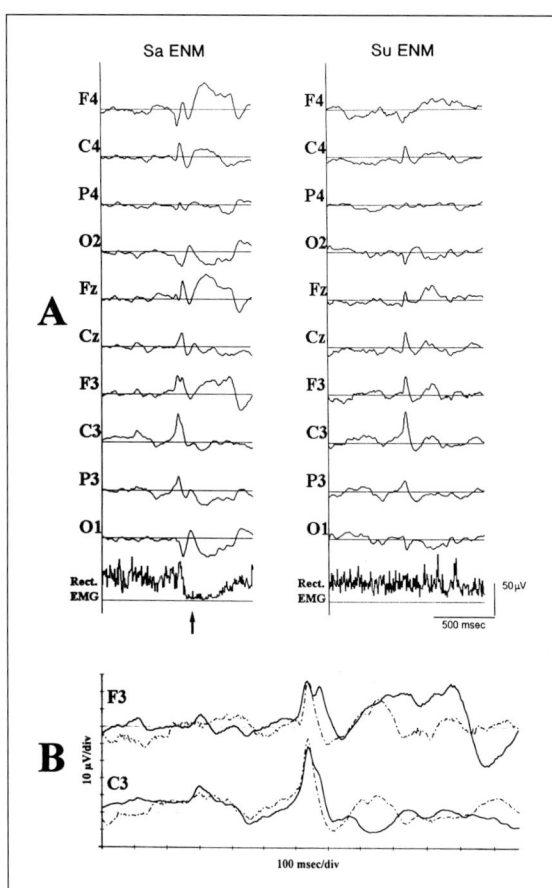

Fig. 2. Same tracing as in Figure 1. (a) On the left, averaged spikes associated with ENM (SaENM); on the right, averaged spikes unrelated to ENM (SuENM). Distinctive feature between SaENM and SuENM is the presence in SaENM, at F3 and C3, of a 'double peak', preceding the onset (arrow) of the EMG silent period of ENM of about 30 ms. (b) Superposition of SaENM (solid line) and SuENM (dotted line), demonstrating the presence of the second peak only in SaENM, particularly prominent at F3. Rect.EMG = rectified EMG of the right wrist extensor. Average potential reference; negative is up. [From Rubboli et al. (1995) with permission.]

using a back-averaging technique triggered at the onset of the muscular silent period, and Baumgartner et al. (1996), by means of EEG-SPECT co-registration and superposition to MRI images, have confirmed the role of frontal areas in the origin of this motor phenomenon. These data are in keeping with the results obtained by Luders et al. (1988), with electrical cortical stimulations of epileptic subjects, that demonstrated the existence of negative motor areas involving frontal and supplementary motor areas.

Cortical excitability during ENM was explored by means of transcranial magnetic stimulation (TMS) (Tassinari et al., 1995a). TMS was performed during ENM, at rest and during tonic activation. The motor evoked potentials were recorded from the right extensor carpi radiali. During ENM, TMS failed to evoke a motor evoked response in the right extensor carpi radiali muscle; on the contrary, in control conditions, at rest or during tonic activation, a motor evoked potential was easily obtainable from the same muscle (Fig. 3(a)). These results suggest a pronounced cortical inhibition during ENM silent period. Assessment of spinal excitability was performed evaluating F-wave of the ulnar nerve at the 1st and 2nd interosseus, elicited 30–120 ms from the onset of ENM, in a series of about 20–30 trials (Tassinari et al., 1995a). F-wave during ENM showed the same mean latency, amplitude and frequency, either in agonist and antagonist muscles, as compared to tonic activation (Fig. 3(b)). These findings are consistent

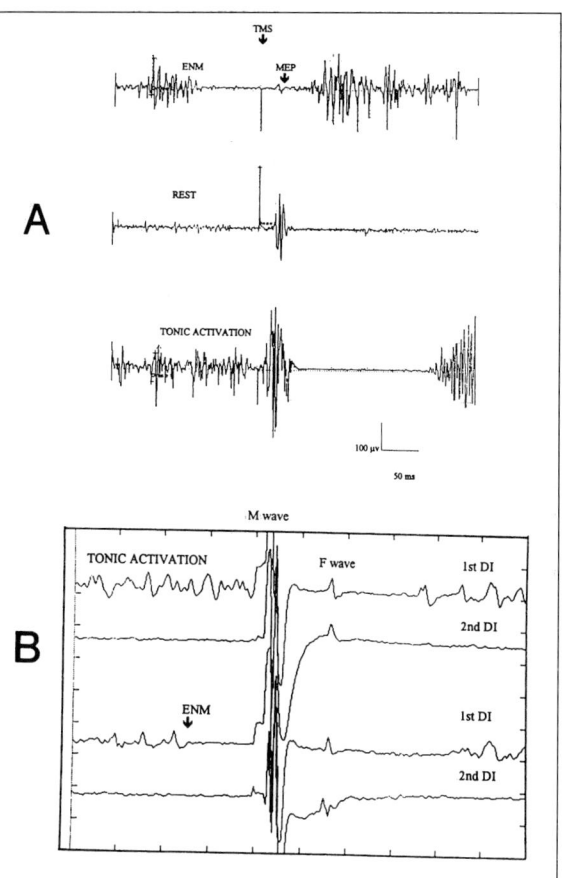

Fig. 3. (a) Motor evoked potentials elicited by transcranial magnetic stimulation (TMS) from the right extensor carpi radiali muscle during ENM silent period (upper trace), muscular rest (middle trace), and tonic activation (bottom trace). A significant inhibition of the motor evoked potentials is evident during ENM, compared with muscular rest and tonic contraction. (b) F-wave assessment during tonic activation (top pair of traces) and ENM (bottom pair of traces) in the first and second dorsal interossues. In both conditions, F-wave latency and amplitude in agonist and antagonist muscles were similar. Stimulation of the right ulnar nerve at the wrist. [From Tassinari et al. (1995a) with permission.]

with a preserved spinal excitability during 30–120 ms after the onset of muscular suppression, and suggest that ENM cannot be attributed to spinal mechanisms, but it is presumably related to the activation of supraspinal cortical areas with inhibitory effects on the motor system. Summarizing these data, ENM appears to be an aetiologically heterogeneous phenomenon that can occur in different epileptic disorders, ranging from benign syndromic conditions, such as benign epilepsy with centro-temporal spikes, to focal static lesional epilepsy or to severe progressive myoclonic encephalopathies. Neurophysiological findings are consistent with a cortical origin, and suggest the participation of an inhibitory active mechanism related, primarily or secondarily, to the involvement of frontal, particularly supplementary motor, areas.

Epileptic falling seizures (EFS)

In the International Classification of Epileptic Seizures proposed by the Commission on Classification and Terminology of the International League Against Epilepsy (1981), EFS are classified using only three terms, i.e. atonic, astatic and drop seizures, each of them implying a sudden loss of tone as the cause of the EFS. However, these terms and their pathophysiological implications cannot account for the vast majority of falling seizures. EFS have been recently reviewed by Tassinari et al. (1997). Under the label of EFS, a heterogeneous group of epileptic seizures in which the fall is the main or only clinical feature, without any other major motor event, can be included. EFS can occur in patients suffering from generalized as well as partial epilepsies.

Electroclinical features of EFS in generalized epilepsies

Generalized epilepsies with EFS recognize mostly a cryptogenic or symptomatic aetiology, such as Lennox–Gastaut syndrome and myoclonic-astatic epilepsy. The first description of the electroclinical aspects of EFS, by means of video-polygraphic recordings, was reported by Gastaut *et al.* (1966b) in three patients with Lennox–Gastaut syndrome. Since then, other authors have reported descriptions of EFS in generalized epilepsies (Egli *et al.*, 1985; Ikeno *et al.*, 1985; Dravet *et al.*, 1988; Oguni *et al.*, 1992; Yaqub, 1993). Based on the results reported in these studies, four different types of EFS can be identified in generalized epilepsies: (a) pure atonic seizures; (b) myoclonic-atonic seizures; (c) myoclonic seizures; (d) tonic seizures.

Atonic seizures

The International Classification of Epileptic Seizures (1981) defines as atonic seizures those seizures in which 'a sudden diminution in muscle tone occurs which may be fragmentary, leading to head drop with slackening of the jaw, the dropping of a limb or loss of all muscle tone leading to a slumping to the ground'. In reality, as has been proven by video-polygraphic findings (Dravet *et al.*, 1988; Gastaut & Broughton, 1972; Gastaut *et al.*, 1966a; Gastaut *et al.*, 1974; Ikeno *et al.*, 1985), EFS caused by pure loss of muscular tone are remarkably rare.

Clinically, they can be of short duration (also called 'effondrements épileptiques' or 'drop seizures'), with the loss of tone limited to the head, or involving all postural muscles and causing fall to the ground, and sometimes associated with a brief loss of consciousness. They can be also of longer duration ('akinetic' seizures), lasting from 1 min up to several minutes, with prolonged loss of consciousness and generalized atonia.

Gastaut *et al.* (1966a) observed that brief atonic seizures could occur in less than 1 s, characterized by a drop of the head, followed by loss of tone of the trunk and the legs (Fig. 4). The standing position was recovered after about 2 s. The ictal polygraphic recording showed a generalized discharge of polyspikes and waves, with the interruption of the postural tone associated with the slow wave component; bradycardia or modification of respiration could be observed. Other ictal patterns were represented by high-voltage fast activity, EEG flattening, or polyspikes preceding a discharge of spikes and waves.

Myoclonic-atonic

This type of EFS is characterized by a sudden fall, preceded by some symmetrical myoclonic jerks of the face, the trunk or the arms. Myoclonic-atonic falls are the distinctive seizure type of myoclonic epilepsy of early childhood described by Doose (1985). The ictal polygraphic findings showed discharges of generalized slow spike and wave complexes (at 2–3 Hz), with the myoclonic phenomena associated with the spike, and the following atonia with the slow wave.

Myoclonic seizures

Only few cases have been documented, showing a massive axial myoclonic jerk, not followed by loss of tone, causing violent fall to the ground (Dravet *et al.*, 1988; Yaqub, 1993). On the EEG, the myoclonic jerks were associated with generalized 3–3.5 c/s spike and wave activity.

Chapter 6 Clinical and neurophysiological features of different falls

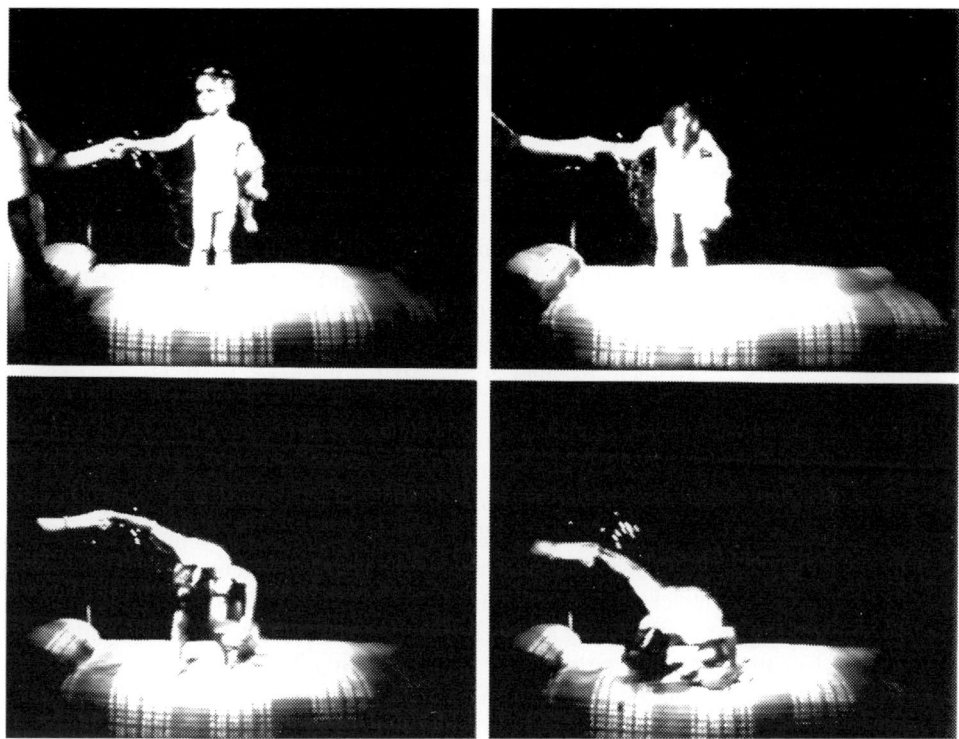

Fig. 4. Photographic sequence of an atonic epileptic falling seizure. The child is standing (top row, left picture); the first event is represented by an abrupt drop of the head onto the chest (top row, right picture); then a flexion of the trunk (bottom row, left picture) and of the legs (bottom row, right picture), due to loss of muscular tone, occurs. Interval between each photogram is about 200–240 ms. [Photographs taken from the original film by Prof. Gastaut and Tassinari; also reported in Gastaut et al. (1966a).]

Tonic seizures

The typical clinical characteristics of the tonic seizures are the abduction and extension of the extremities associated with a rigid stretching of the body. Other phenomena that can be observed are a sudden flexion of the neck and the body, rising of the semiflexed arms, extension of the lower limbs, rolling of the eyes, apnoea, tachi- or bradicardia, change of the facial expression with facial flushing, dilatation of the pupils and, sometimes, enuresis. They can be symmetrical or asymmetrical, occurring either during wakefulness or during sleep (Tassinari & Ambrosetto, 1988), and represent the most common cause of fall in Lennox–Gastaut syndrome. Under the label of 'axial spasms', Egli *et al.* (1985) described short tonic seizures, that can also be induced by unexpected stimuli. Clinically, they are characterized by a sudden muscular contraction of the whole body, with abduction of the upper limbs, mild extension of the legs and forward flexion of the head and the trunk at the hips, that cause the violent fall. Polygraphic recordings have shown a slight EEG attenuation or no change at all, whereas the EMG channel demonstrated a sudden, massive increase of muscular tone, particularly in the neck and shoulders. Ikeno *et al.* (1985) reported similar manifestations, in some cases associated with generalized slow waves. Tonic seizures can be also of longer duration, with a progressively increasing stiffness of the whole body, until the patient falls to the ground. In these cases, the most frequent ictal EEG patterns are represented by a low-voltage fast activity, or a discharge of rhythmic polyspikes, ending in spike and wave complexes.

Electroclinical features of EFS in partial epilepsies

EFS in patients with partial seizures can cause an extremely abrupt and violent fall, such as to cause severe damage to the patient. Essentially, two types can be recognized: a first one, characterized by a preceding stiffening or tonic posturing, and a second type, characterized by a sudden onset, without any evident associated motor phenomenon. The first type of EFS is usually considered to depend on the involvement of the frontal or the supplementary motor areas (Broglin *et al.*, 1992; Delgado-Escueta *et al.*, 1987; Ethelberg, 1950; Geier *et al.*, 1977; Waterman & Wada, 1990; Williamson *et al.*, 1985). In some respects, this type of seizure resembles tonic seizures and may be accompanied by automatisms, vocalizations, and head or eyes turning. Ictal EEG shows a diffuse flattening, followed by a fast activity discharge, more prominent in the bilateral fronto-temporal regions. In the interictal EEG, unilateral or bilateral paroxysmal abnormalities can be detected, mainly in frontal and vertex regions, sometimes with diffuse spikes and waves associated. The second type of EFS in patients with partial epilepsy (also called epileptic drop attacks) consists of an abrupt fall to the ground and rapid recovery, without any preceding or accompanying signs. This form of EFS is generally considered to be of atonic nature, although adequate polygraphic documentation is lacking. An extratemporal or bitemporal origin has been suggested by Delgado-Escueta *et al.* (1982, 1987). Interictal EEG can show focal or multifocal abnormalities, in frontal or temporal leads. Gambardella *et al.* (1994) provided stereo-EEG documentation of a drop attack in a patient with temporal lobe epilepsy. The paroxysmal discharge originated in the left amygdala and hippocampus, and spread rapidly to the contralateral hippocampus and both orbito-frontal regions.

Diagnostic issues

Due to the evidence that EFS can occur in different epileptic conditions and seizure types, an adequate neurophysiological investigation by means of video-polygraphic recording is mandatory. Analysis of video-polygraphic data renders possible the recognition of the different motor manifestations of a given EFS, revealing phenomena hardly observable by clinical observation of the event, such as mild and brisk myoclonic contractions preceding the fall. By using video-polygraphic techniques, it is possible to correctly classify the different types of EFS, and these methods can be expected to provide further insights on the mechanisms of EFS. Furthermore, video-polygraphic monitoring is essential to differentiate EFS from non-epileptic falling seizures, such as cataplectic attacks, syncopes, breath-holding spells, psychogenic seizures.

Pathophysiological considerations on EFS

The complexity of the clinical manifestations of EFS suggests that different pathophysiological mechanisms are involved in the generation of these types of seizures. Subcortical mechanisms, with participation of brainstem structures, have been postulated by Egli *et al.* (1985) in patients with Lennox–Gastaut. This hypothesis was based on the predominant axial and flexor muscular involvement, consistent with an archaic motor pattern, and it was supported by experimental findings demonstrating the existence of self-sustained brainstem seizures in animals (Kreindler *et al.*, 1958; Cesa-Bianchi *et al.*, 1967). Velasco *et al.* (1991) provided data in favour of the subcortical theory, showing the absence of thalamic or surface EEG events during the brief atonic seizures, suggesting the participation, in these EFS, of cerebral structures outside the thalamo-cortical system. A role for brainstem structures in the generation of atonic seizures has been proposed, also following the identification of the pontine brainstem reticular formation mediating REM sleep atonia and cataplexy (Siegel et al., 1991).

Cortical mechanisms were suggested by Gastaut & Broughton (1972) who proposed that intense, short-lasting cortical inhibitory phenomena could be implicated in epileptic drop attacks. The existence of cortical inhibitory or negative motor areas has been convincingly demonstrated (Penfield & Jasper, 1954; Luders et al., 1988), even though their involvement in atonic EFS is still a matter of discussion. Other clues in favour of a cortical origin of EFS are the positive results of callosotomy in patients with EFS, that suggest a possible role, in provoking the fall, of bilateral synchronization of epileptic discharge via corpus callosum, and the evidence of phenomena of recurrent cortical inhibition, mediated by thalamo-cortical circuits, that can interfere with and disrupt cortical activity (Gloor, 1979).

Investigations on the modulatory effects on the motor system of fast polyspike discharges during tonic seizures have been performed by Tassinari et al. (1995b) by means of H-reflex assessment and evaluation of motor evoked potentials, elicited by transcranial magnetic stimulation. They observed a facilitation of both H-reflex and motor evoked potentials at the beginning of the tonic seizures, when no changes were observable yet in the EMG polygraphic channels. During the tonic contraction of the tonic seizure, H-reflex and motor evoked potentials were further increased; a significant decrement was seen only in the postictal phase. These data demonstrated that in tonic seizures the initial, apparently 'subclinical', EEG paroxysmal activity could modify spinal excitability, raising new issues on the distinction between 'ictal' and 'interictal' EEG abnormalities.

Concluding remarks

Falling seizures still represent a puzzling phenomenon, and clearly our knowledge on these complex paroxysmal motor events is limited. These seizures can occur in a variety of epileptic conditions, and it is conceivable that video-polygraphic recordings of EFS will contribute to improve the comprehension of the different mechanisms underlying these motor phenomena, also providing data useful for classification purposes. Whatever the origin and the mechanisms underlying EFS, these seizures have a poor prognosis, mainly because of resistance to pharmacological treatment and risk of injuries due to the frequent falls. Because of these diagnostic and prognostic reasons, Tassinari et al. (1997) suggest that EFS might deserve a recognition as an individual seizure type.

References

Baumgartner, C., Podreka, I., Olbrich, A., Novak, K., Serles, W., Aull, S., Almer, G., Lurger, S., Pietrzyk, U., Prayer, D. & Lindinger, G. (1996): Epileptic negative myoclonus: an EEG-single-photon emission CT study indicating involvement of pre-motor cortex. *Neurology* **46**, 753–758.

Broglin, D., Delgado-Escueta, A.V., Walsh, G.O., Bancaud, J. & Chauvel, P. (1992): Clinical approach to the patient with seizures and epilepsies of frontal origin. In: *Frontal lobe seizures and epilepsies, Advances in Neurology,* vol. 17, eds. P. Chauvel, A.V. Delgado-Escueta, E. Halgren & J. Bancaud, pp. 59–88. New York: Raven Press.

Cesa-Bianchi, M.G., Mancia, M. & Mutani, R. (1967): Experimental epilepsy induced by cobalt powder in lower brainstem and thalamic structures. *Electroencephalogr. Clin. Neurophysiol.* **22**, 525–536.

Colamaria, V., Grimau-Merino, R., Sgro' V., Caraballo, R., Simeone, M., Residori, E., Terzano, M.G., Calzetti, S., Faienza, C., Prati, L. & Sani, E. (1989): Epilessia focale con stato di punta-onda continua in sonno lento: asterixis critico in soggetto con emipachigiria. *Boll. Lega. Ital. Epil.* **66/67,** 267–268.

Commission on Classification and Terminology of the International League Against Epilepsy (1981): Proposal for revised clinical and electroencephalographic classification of epileptic seizures. *Epilepsia* **22,** 489–501.

Dalla Bernardina, B., Perez-Jimenez, A., Fontana, E. *et al.* (1996): Electroencephalographic findings associated with cortical dysplasias. In: *Dysplasias of the cerebral cortex and epilepsy,* eds. R. Guerrini, F. Andermann, R. Canapicchi, J. Roger & P. Pfanner. Philadelphia: Lippincott-Raven.

Delgado-Escueta, A.V., Enrile Bacsal, F. & Treiman, D.M. (1982): Complex partial seizures on closed-circuit television and EEG: a study of 691 attacks in 79 patients. *Ann. Neurol.* **11,** 292–300.

Delgado-Escueta, A.V., Swartz, B.E., Maldonado, H.M., Walsh, G.O., Rand, R.W. & Halgren, E. (1987): Complex partial seizures of frontal lobe origin. In: *Presurgical evaluation of epilepsies,* eds. H.G. Wieser & C.E. Elger, pp. 267–299. Berlin Heidelberg: Springer-Verlag.

Doose, H. (1985): Myoclonic astatic epilepsy of early childhood. In: *Epileptic syndromes in infancy, childhood and adolescence,* eds. J. Roger, C. Dravet, M. Bureau, F. E. Dreifuss & P. Wolf, pp. 78–88. London: John Libbey.

Dravet, C., Bureau, M., Tassinari, C.A. & Roger, J. (1988): Different types of epileptic drop seizures in children. *Neurologia et Psychiatria* **11 (suppl. 1),** 7–16.

Egli, M., Mothersill, I., O'Kane, M. & O'Kane, F. (1985): The axial spasm – the predominant type of drop seizure in patients with secondary generalized epilepsy. *Epilepsia* **26,** 401–415.

Ethelberg, S. (1950): Symptomatic 'cataplexy' or chalastic fits in cortical lesion of the frontal lobe. *Brain* **53,** 499–511.

Gambardella, A., Reutens, D.C., Andermann, F., Cendes, F., Gloor, P., Dubeau, F. & Olivier, A. (1994): Late-onset drop attacks in temporal lobe epilepsy: a reevaluation of the concept of temporal lobe syncope. *Neurology* **44,** 1074–1078.

Gastaut, H. & Régis, H. (1961): On the subject of Lennox's 'akinetic' petit mal. *Epilepsia* **2,** 298–305.

Gastaut, H., Tassinari, C.A. & Bureau-Paillas, M. (1966a): Étude polygraphique et cliniques des 'effondrements atoniques épileptiques'. *Riv. Neurol.* **36,** 5–21.

Gastaut, H., Roger, J. Soulayrol, R., Tassinari, C.A., Régis H. & Dravet C. (1966b): Childhood epileptic encephalopathy with diffuse slow spike-waves (otherwise known as 'Petit mal variant') or Lennox syndrome. *Epilepsia* **7,** 139–179.

Gastaut, H. & Broughton, R. (1972): *Epileptic seizures.* Springfield IL: Charles C. Thomas.

Gastaut, H., Broughton, R., Roger, J. & Tassinari, C.A. (1974): Generalized non-convulsive seizures without local onset. In: *The epilepsies – Handbook of clinical neurology.* vol. 15, eds. P.J. Vinken & G.W. Bruyn, pp. 130–144. Amsterdam: North-Holland.

Geier, S., Bancaud, J., Talairach, J., Bonis, A., Szikla, G. & Enjelvin, M. The seizures of frontal lobe epilepsy: a study of clinical manifestations. *Neurology* **27,** 951–958.

Gloor, P. (1979): Generalized epilepsy with spike-and-wave discharge: a reinterpretation of its electrographic and clinical manifestations. *Epilepsia* **20,** 571–588.

Guerrini, R., Dravet, C., Genton, P., Bureau, M., Roger, J., Rubboli, G. & Tassinari, C.A. (1993): Epileptic negative myoclonus. *Neurology* **43,** 1078–1083.

Ikeno, T., Shigematsu, H., Miyakashi, M., Ohba, A., Yagi, K. & Seino, M. (1985): An analytic study of epileptic falls. *Epilepsia* **26,** 612–621.

Kreindler, A., Zuckermann, E., Steriade, M. & Chimion, D. (1958): Electroclinical features of the convulsive fit induced experimentally through stimulation of the brainstem. *J. Neurophysiol.* **21,** 430–436.

Luders, H. O., Lesser, P., Dinner, D. S., Morris, H. H. Wyllie, E. & Godoy, J. (1988): Localization of cortical function: new information from extraoperative monitoring of patients with epilepsy. *Epilepsia* **29 (suppl. 2),** S56–S65.

Oguni, H., Fukuyama, Y., Imaizumi, Y. & Uehara, T. (1992): Video-EEG analysis of drop seizures in myoclonic-astatic epilepsy of early childhood (Doose syndrome). *Epilepsia* **33**, 805–813.

Penfield, W. & Jasper, H.H. (1954): *Epilepsy and the functional anatomy of the human brain.* Boston: Little, Brown.

Rubboli, G., Parmeggiani, L. & Tassinari, C.A. (1995): Frontal inhibitory spike component associated with epileptic negative myoclonus. *Electroencephalogr. Clin. Neurophysiol.* **95**, 201–205.

Shibasaki, H., Ikeda, A., Nagamine, T., Mima, T., Terada, K., Nishitani, N., Kanda, M., Takano, S., Hanazono, T., Kohara, N., Kaji, R. & Kimura, J. (1994): Cortical reflex negative myoclonus. *Brain* **117**, 477–486.

Siegel, J.M., Nienhuis, R., Fahringer, H.M., Paul, R., Shiromani, P., Dement, W.C., Mignot, E. & Chiu, C. (1991): Neuronal activity in narcolepsy: identification of cataplexy-related cells in the medial medulla. *Science* **252**, 1315–1318.

Suisse, G., Thomas, P., Borg, M. & Dolisi, C. (1995): Myoclonies négatives épileptiques. Application de la technique du moyennage rétrograde. *Epilepsies* **7**, 409–417.

Tassinari, C.A., Régis, H. & Gastaut, H. (1968): A particular form of muscular inhibition in epilepsy: the related epileptic silent period (RESP). *Proc. Aust. Ass. Neurol.* **5**, 595–602.

Tassinari, C.A. (1981): New perspectives in epileptology. In: *Trends in modern epileptology,* ed. Japanese Epilepsy Association, pp. 42–59. Tokyo: International Public Seminar on Epileptology.

Tassinari, C.A. & Ambrosetto, G. (1988): Tonic seizures in the Lennox Gastaut syndrome: semiology and differential diagnosis. In: *The Lennox–Gastaut syndrome,* eds. E. Niedermeyer & R. Degen, pp. 109–124. New York: Alan R. Liss.

Tassinari, C.A., Michelucci, R. & Rubboli G. (1990): Negative epileptic myoclonus. *Mov. Disord.* **5 (suppl. 1)**, 44.

Tassinari, C.A., Bureau, M., Dravet, C., Dalla Bernardina, B. & Roger, J. (1992): Epilepsy with continuous spikes and waves during slow sleep – otherwise described as ESES. In: *Epileptic syndromes in infancy, childhood and adolescence,* 2nd ed., eds. J. Roger, M. Bureau, C. Dravet, F.E. Dreifuss, A. Perret & P. Wolf, pp. 245–256. London: John Libbey.

Tassinari, C.A., Rubboli, G., Parmeggiani, L., Valzania, F., Plasmati, R., Riguzzi, P., Michelucci, R., Volpi, L., Passarelli, D., Meletti, S., Fontana, E. & Dalla Bernardina, B. (1995a): Epileptic negative myoclonus. In: *Negative motor phenomena,* eds. S. Fahn, M. Hallett, H. O. Luders & C. D. Marsden, pp. 181–197. Philadelphia: Lippincott-Raven.

Tassinari, C.A., Rubboli, G., Valzania, F., Parmeggiani, L., Michelucci, R., Meletti, S., Borghi, A.M., Vetrugno, R., & Volpi L. (1995b): Effets modulateurs décharges paroxystiques intercritiques sur le système moteur. *Neurophysiol. Clin.* **25**, 238.

Tassinari, C.A., Michelucci, R., Shigematsu, H. & Seino, M. (1997): Atonic and falling seizures. In: *Epilepsy. A comprehensive textbook,* eds. J. Engel & T. Pedley, in press. Philadelphia: Lippincott-Raven.

Thomas, P., Meneguz, C., Alchaar, H., Suisse, G. & Desnuelle, C. (1994): Pure cortical negative action myoclonus showing Lafora disease. *Epilepsia* **35 (suppl. 7)**, 37–38.

Velasco, M., Velasco, F., Alcala', H., Davila, G., Diaz-de-Leon, A.E. (1991): Epileptiform EEG activity of the centromedian thalamic nuclei in children with intractable generalized seizures of the Lennox–Gastaut syndrome. *Epilepsia* **32**, 310–321.

Waterman, K. & Wada, J.A. (1990): Frontal lobe epilepsy. In: *Comprehensive epileptology,* eds. M. Dam & L. Gram, pp. 197–213. New York: Raven Press.

Williamson, P.D., Spencer, D.D., Spencer, S.S., Novelly, R.A. & Mattson, R.H. (1985): Complex partial seizures of frontal lobe origin. *Ann. Neurol.* **18**, 497–504.

Yaqub, B.A. (1993): Electroclinical seizures in Lennox–Gastaut syndrome. *Epilepsia* **34**, 120–127.

Yokota, T & Tsukagoshi, H. (1992): Cortical activity-associated negative myoclonus. *J. Neurol Sci.* **111**, 77–81.

Chapter 7

Study of epileptic falls: methodologies and polygraphies

Michelle Bureau and Henri Régis

Centre Saint Paul, 300 boulevard Sainte Marguerite, 13009 Marseille, France

The polygraphic recording of a fall must not be done blindly. It requires first a careful clinical examination of the phenomenon. All details and documents must be taken into account in order to inform the clinician. One can use both the collapsing patient's picture and the polygraphic signs. The instrumental approach must be modified to suit each different case and take the clinical context into account.

We will consider successively visual means, (i.e. picture study) and then technical means, to obtain an EEG and EMG representation of the movement.

The picture

Visualizing the fall in optimal conditions requires knowledge of probable occurrence time, motor facilitating circumstances, behavioural situation, patient's position ... In a medical environment, a previous observation of the phenomenon is necessary.

Different ways may then be used to fix and transmit the picture. Rhythmic photography shows a good frame succession of the fall (24 frames/s), motion pictures (Fig. 1) (film or camcorder) with an overlaying clock showing a time reference (Gastaut *et al.*, 1966).

In the laboratory, one must use the EEG video, which is the patient's camcorder filmed picture and the EEG recording with a possibility of mixing. In such conditions, it is necessary to have a time cursor on the EEG picture in order to indicate the time corresponding to the video picture. The time correlation between EEG and visual representation must be as precise as possible. The presence of a physician or a technician is indispensable during the EEG video recording. On line juxtaposition of computer memorized comments is very useful for an *a posteriori* data analysis.

Technical means

An abnormal epileptic motor phenomenon that may produce a fall depends on three different mechanisms, which are sometimes associated with one another: a sudden tonic contraction

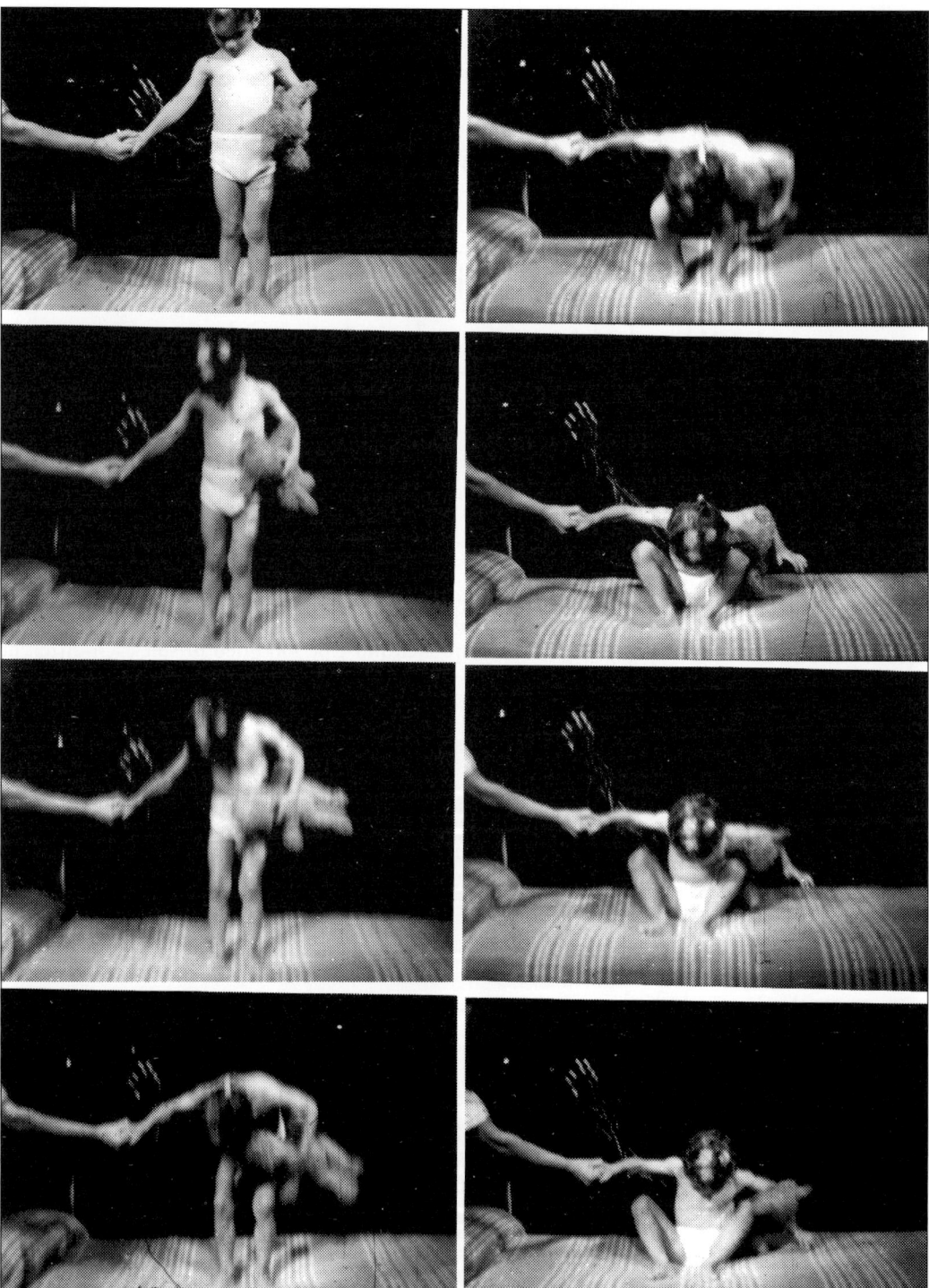

Fig. 1. Different cinematographic sequences of a global atonic drop. Each sequence is separated from the previous one by an interval of 40 ms, giving a good analysis during the different fall components.

(relatively uncommon), a myoclonia (much more frequent), and, shown by perturbing walking or by it's abruptness, an atonia. These manifestations are probably more often associated with one another than first apparent. Therefore, the movement must be displayed graphically and its corresponding EMG–EEG translation simultaneously recorded.

Movement – graphic representations

These may be obtained by physical instruments: quartz, piezoelectric cell, accelerometer (which shows a good representation of the movement, if it isn't directional), goniometer, which shows a good translation of articular movements. Finally, with a simple photo-cell and a beam of light, it is easy to see a massive displacement.

The collapse of the body was recorded by placing a photo-cell on the patient's forehead; when the head drops, less light falls on the photo-cell and the excursion reading from it with each flash (for example) became smaller (Fig. 2) (Gastaut & Régis, 1961).

These graphic representations of movement are easy to obtain, inexpensive, and may represent a good polygraphy synchronizer, especially in the use of back-averaging.

However, this is overall information about pathological movement, which must be linked to an electrographic study for a better analysis of the chronology and topography of muscle implication.

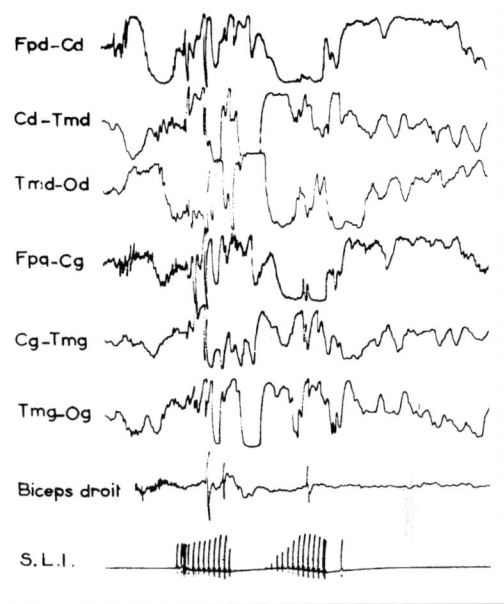

Fig. 2. The ILS provokes on the EEG a burst of spike-waves accompanied by myoclonias easily seen on the biceps; the previous tonism disappearance is announced by a myoclonia. The spikes are followed by slow waves (masked by an artefact) concomitant to the fall. The head drop is indicated by means of the non-inscription of the ILS. The progressive reappearance of the light inscription indicates the straightening of the subject. Fpd-cd = Fp2-C4; Cd-Tmd = C4T4; Tmd-Od = T4-O2; Fpg-Cg = Fp1-C3; Cg-Tmg = C3-T5; Tmg-Og = T5-O1; Biceps droit = Right biceps; SLI = ILS.

Electromyography

Electrode positioning (Fig. 3)

Surface electrodes (capsules) are nearly always used. There must be a minimum distance of twice their diameter between each of them and they must be placed along the axis of muscle fibres, within the fleshy mass of the muscle. If the muscle is too short, one electrode will be placed on the median area and the other on its tendinous insertion.

The choice of explored muscles depends on clinical data, but usually topographical distribution of electrodes follows a certain systematization, meant to ease the understanding of pathological movement organization.

For massive axial falls, electrodes must be placed on the back of the neck and on paravertebral muscles. In the case of head dropping, it is necessary to add electrodes on sternocleidomastoidus muscles (rotation movements are often associated).

In connection with the trunk, it may be useful to record lumbar and rectus abdominis muscles in the same time (infants, while sitting, may have a trunk flexion either by lumbar muscle hypotonus or, more often, by hypertonic contraction of the rectus abdominis muscles).

In connection with the limbs, it is interesting to compare proximal (axorhizomelic) and distal musculatures. Moreover, it is useful to oppose antagonistic muscles at different levels (for an upper limb, put, from top to bottom on the graphic: trapezius, deltoideus, brachial biceps, brachial triceps, flexor digitorum, extensor digitorum). It is often necessary to record both limbs, symmetrically and simultaneously.

Running the examination

The position and functioning of the electrodes should always be checked first, by a successive contraction of every selected muscle, in order to verify the quality of the electrophysiological recording and produce a reference picture of voluntary activity, that will later be compared with pathological activity.

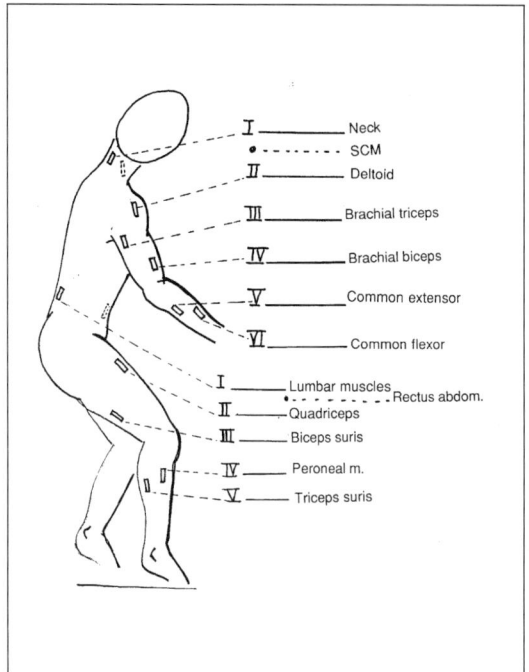

Fig. 3. Different muscles are required for the EMG-polygraphy recording.

The patient's position during the recording is chosen according to clinical symptoms; with an attempt to find an antigravidic position for the part of the body affected by the fall (e.g. standing, Mingazzini, upper limb abduction, lower limb raising . . .).

Depending on the patient's co-operation, several motor situations are successively explored: rest, passive mobilization, stance keeping, progressively increasing voluntary contraction, ballistic movement and pursuit movement.

Finally, the examination must be ended with an unexpected application of stimulations, mostly tactile and auditory. The pathological response will either be a hypotonia or a reflex hypertonia. If the patient is standing when the stimulation occurs, it will be proven that the clinical consequence of this stimulation really is a fall, whatever the mechanism.

Types of EMG manifestations (Fig. 4)

At rest, there is no EMG activity; electric 'silence' is the electrophysiological condition of normal rest.

During a myoclonia, it is common to notice, clearly coming out of the baseline activity, a short lasting group of ample phasic potentials followed by a postmyoclonic silence which can last 200 ms. Thus, this picture contains the two opposite elements most commonly associated in a myoclonia: the positive element (hypersynchrone activation) and the negative element (postmyoclonic inhibition).

Chapter 8

Infantile spasms and tonic seizures

Silvana Franceschetti, Tiziana Granata, Simona Binelli, Laura Canafoglia and Giuliano Avanzini

Istituto Nazionale Neurologico C. Besta, via Celoria 11, 20133 Milan, Italy

Summary

Infantile spasms and tonic seizures are both characterized by sustained contraction of neck, trunk and limb muscles but differ as to duration, EEG ictal pattern, mode of presentation and electroclinical background. Spasms tend to cluster with a quasi-periodic time course, as is typically seen in West syndrome and related disorders. The typical EEG pattern associated with each spasm consists of slow waves followed by an abrupt attenuation of the activity, whereas tonic seizures are typically associated with high frequency (up to 20 Hz) repetitive spikes. A brainstem generator has been suggested for spasms on the basis of neurophysiological and neuropathological evidence. On the other hand a possible cortical origin is supported by the not-infrequent association of partial seizures and/or focal EEG discharges with spasms. Moreover, spasms are frequently observed in infants with neocortical lesions such as neuronal migration disorders, phakomatoses, etc., and are reported to benefit from lesionectomy.

Tonic seizures are considered to be a typical model of generalized seizures; however a focal cortical generator (namely located in the supplementary motor area) can be detected also in several patients showing symmetric or asymmetric tonic seizures, suggesting that different physiopathological mechanism can sustain this seizure type.

Further improvement in our understanding of neurological bases for spasms and tonic seizures are expected to lead to a rational pharmacological treatment and to a better definition of criteria for a surgical approach.

Introduction

Infantile spasms and tonic seizures are both characterized by a sudden 'tonic' contraction involving the muscles of the neck, trunk and extremities. The motor pattern of the seizure depends on the extent of muscle involvement and whether the flexor or extensor muscles are principally involved. On the basis of the prevailing distribution of the muscle contraction, they can be classified as flexor, extensor or mixed.

Differences in the intensity and location of the muscle contraction lead to varying degrees of ictal phenomena: if only the neck muscle is involved (as is often the case), the result may be just a sudden head bob, but if a number of different segments are recruited, this may give rise to a massive contraction and to complex postural changes depending on the prevalence of flexion or extension. Both spasms and tonic seizures can lead to a sudden fall as a result of an abrupt change in postural tone, due to involuntary muscle contraction. However, although these characteristics are common to both spasms and tonic seizures, there are a number of elements which suggest that the two types of seizure should be considered as being semeiologically distinct. From a merely observational point of view the main difference lies in their duration: spasms are very brief, with the muscle contraction lasting from some hundred milliseconds to a few (usually 1–2) seconds; whereas the duration of tonic seizures, although variable, is generally longer. In fact, it was precisely the brevity of spasm seizures that led to their early definition as infantile 'myoclonic' spasms, even though the duration of muscle activation during spasms is usually greater than that of myoclonic jerks, and its onset is generally more gradual. Even more substantial distinctions between spasms and tonic seizures concern the EEG ictal pattern, the time course of the seizures, and the electroclinical backgrounds in which the two different seizure patterns typically occur. Nevertheless, in some cases very brief tonic seizures cannot be easily differentiated from spasms; tonic seizures may well occur in children who had experienced spasms in their early infancy, and, as recently observed by Romeo et al. (1995), spasms and tonic seizures may concurrently occur in children affected by Lennox–Gastaut syndrome.

Spasms

Spasms typically occur in early infancy (usually between the third and twelfth month), and have a remarkable tendency to cluster with a quasi-periodic time course. These features are so typical that the term of 'infantile spasm' (properly referred to a seizure type) is frequently used as a synonym for the West syndrome (West, 1841) and related disorders, which typically present with seizures in series. Spasms rarely persist (Talwar et al., 1995) or even start in older children affected by severe epilepsies (Gobbi et al., 1987), and when they do are usually associated with other seizure types.

Polygraphic studies (Kellaway et al., 1979) and extensive video-EEG recording (Donat & Wright, 1991), have shown that more than one type of spasm may occur in the same infant, and that the motor phenomena may be asymmetric (Kellaway et al., 1979). A considerable body of literature concerning unusual presentations of infantile spasm has been accumulated over the past few years, suggesting that fragmentary motor phenomena, often presenting with unilateral or focal features (Donat & Wright, 1991; Watanabe et al., 1994; Gaily et al., 1995) may replace (or occur with) typical spasms. Furthermore, episodes of behavioural 'arrest' accompanying or replacing the spasms have been reported as ictal phenomena (Kellaway et al., 1979). There are various reasons for classifying these disparate ictal symptoms and massive 'spasms', as homogeneous expressions of early infantile epilepsies: both massive ictal phenomena more properly called 'spasms', on which the original definition of West was based, and fragmentary, sometimes focal motor fits or even ictal 'arrests' can occur in the same series; moreover, series of both subtle and massive motor phenomena can occur, and individual fits can increase in strength over time, and often terminate with a 'decreasing' trend, a sequence that suggests a common physiopathological substrate for each individual ictal event making up the series. In addition, long-lasting electrographic changes (i.e. a marked decrease in interictal activity or focal slowing) often precede the onset and then persist between the individual ictal events, until the end of a series, thus suggesting that the spasms (and/or their subtle substitute) take place during the course of a long lasting change in the physiological (or physiopathological) state of the brain, that is interrupted by periodic phenomena.

Within a series, the interval between spasms may be regular or irregular, often over a period of many minutes. The maximum frequency of spasms within a series evaluated by Kellaway et al. (1979) was 13/min, and the maximum number of spasms making up a series was 125. The duration of a series may vary in the same infant, and an isolated spasm can occasionally occur in an infant who usually has seizures in series. Spasms predominantly occur soon after arousal, although they can also appear during wakefulness and sleep.

The typical ictal EEG change associated with each spasm consists of a complex wave which includes a generalized slow-wave transient, followed by an abrupt attenuation of background activity lasting from one to a few seconds. In many cases the slow wave complex may be replaced by a more complex wave form that consists of more than one slow and/or sharp transient, followed by attenuation and short discharges of fast activity. Several studies have shown that the ictal EEG event can consist of a fragment of the above-mentioned patterns, and that fast activity, alone or superimposed over background attenuation, may be the only seizure pattern. In the study of Kellaway et al. (1979), characteristics of the ictal EEG events did not strictly correlate with the type of spasm (flexor, extensor or mixed), but 'arrest' and asymmetrical seizures were typically associated with attenuation and fast activity discharges.

The interictal EEG pattern typically associated with infantile spasms (or associated subtle seizures) is traditionally defined as 'hypsarrhythmia'. The classical expression of hypsarrhythmia consists of high-amplitude polymorphic slow activity associated with multifocal spikes, sharp waves, and spike and wave discharges in every brain region. West syndrome is typically characterized by the concomitant occurrence of spasms and hypsarrhythmic EEG activity, generally associated with impaired psychomotor development, in infants aged from three months to one year. However, a number of variants of hypsarrhythmia have been described and these have been classified by Hrachovy et al. (1984) as 'modified' hypsarrhythmic patterns: hemi-hypsarrhythmia or hypsarrhythmia with consistent focus when there is evidence of a lateralized or focal prevalence of interictal epileptic activity or, 'hypsarrhythmia with increased synchronization' when there is a tendency to generate almost synchronous discharges. Two additional 'variants' have been defined on the basis of episodes of generalized or local attenuation, or dominant slow, asynchronous activity with very little sharp-wave or spike activity. A possible change from one modified pattern to another in the same infant, often in relation to the sleep–wake cycle, was underlined by the authors.

The physiopathological substrate of infantile spasms is still unclear; despite repeated electrophysiological and neuropathological studies of infants with West syndrome or related epileptic disorders, the main controversy concerns the location of the primary generator of the spasms. Some authors (Kellaway et al., 1983; Hrachovy & Frost, 1989), have proposed a brainstem generator as the only source of spasms, on the basis that a dysfunction of brainstem nuclei (i.e. pontine reticular formation) can generate spasms interfering with the cortico-spinal afferences controlling spinal reflex. According to this model, both ictal and interictal phenomena (i.e. hypsarrhythmia) may be due to an abnormal input to cortical (or thalamic) structures. Some evidence supporting this model comes from the occasional observation of pathological changes affecting the pontine nuclei in infants affected by West syndrome (Satho et al., 1986), and from electrophysiological evidence of altered brainstem auditory potentials, suggesting a local dysfunction (Kaga et al., 1982). In addition the specific involvement of axial structures has been suggested by biochemical evidence indicating a specific serotonergic neurotransmission impairment (Colemann, 1971; Langlais et al., 1991).

On the contrary, a considerable body of clinical and neuropathological evidence supports the primary involvement of cortical structures in the generation of both the ictal and interictal patterns, that characterize the epileptic encephalopathies presenting with spasms. The following points should be stressed:

(1) prominent focal or diffuse cerebral damage involving the cerebral cortex is evident in many cases of infant symptomatic epilepsies presenting with spasms, and many cases of West syndrome have been attributed to neuropathological lesions specifically involving the neocortex (i.e. neuronal migration disorders, acquired disruptive lesions, phakomathoses, etc.);

(2) several reports describe the therapeutic effect of surgical resection of localized cortical lesions (Uthman et al., 1991; Shields et al., 1992). Moreover the observation that callosotomy may interrupt a bilateral hypsarrhythmia suggests that a cortico-cortical pathway through the corpus callosum is involved in the diffuse expression of interictal activity in West syndrome (Pinard et al., 1993);

(3) early in life, other seizure types (often focal seizures) can precede the onset of spasms;

(4) subtle lateralized motor fits presenting in series (and subsequently evolving into massive spasms), as well as asymmetric spasms, can be time locked with a contralateral ictal EEG discharge thus suggesting a focal cortical origin (Watanabe et al., 1994; Gaily et al., 1994). We recorded subtle seizures, focal signs or asymmetric spasms in 20 out of 26 infants with symptomatic West syndrome cases, 14 of whom had detectable focal ictal EEG changes (Fig. 1). In all of the infants with asymmetric or unilateral ictal signs, the localized ictal discharge (mainly fast activity) was located in the contralateral hemisphere, thus suggesting the existence of a cortical generator.

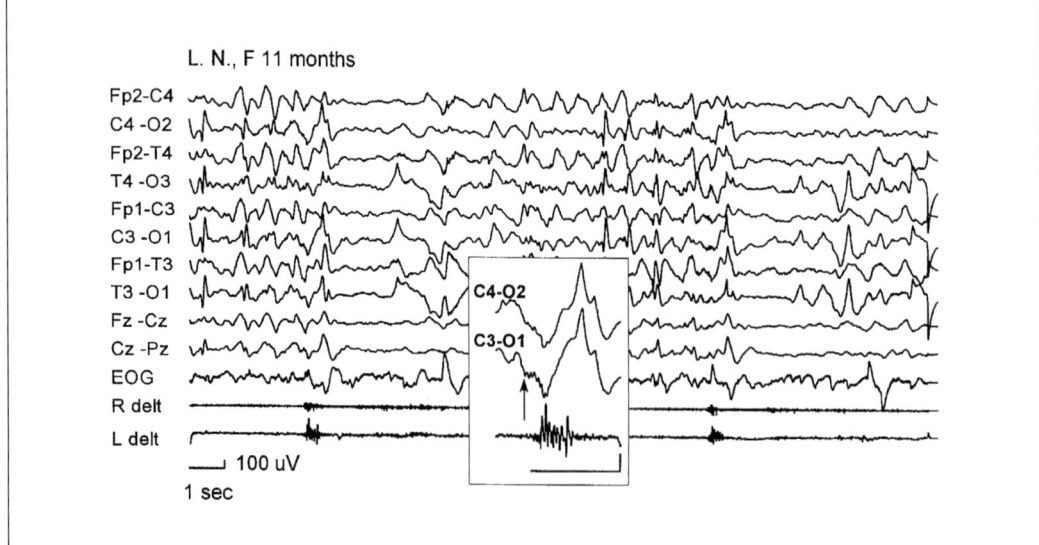

Fig. 1. Polygraphic recording performed on an infant with West syndrome. The slow wave complex associated with spasms is preceded by a short run of very low-amplitude fast activity with a presumed left onset (see inset) that is well recognizable on the centro-occipital leads.

In conclusion, on the basis of the available data, and in the absence of any suitable animal models that would provide a better understanding of spasm physiopathology, the opposing hypotheses of a brainstem or a cortical generator cannot be resolved. Axial structures apparently play a crucial role in the behavioural ictal phenomena characterizing massive spasms and their diffuse EEG ictal correlates. The involvement of brainstem (or thalamic) structures would also make it easier to explain the periodic occurrence of the seizures within a series, because subcortical structures are known to be especially capable of generating more or less periodic physiological (i.e. spindle) and pathological (i.e. burst suppression pattern) activities. On the contrary, the frequent observation of 'subtle' and presumably focal seizure patterns (e.g. eye deviation) or unilateral segmental activation, associated with a contralateral EEG discharge, suggest that the neocortex is the probable *primum movens* of seizure generation. While awaiting the results of further electrophysiological studies capable of definitively resolving the controversy, the hypothesis of Dulac & Plouin (1993) – who suggest that cortical discharges can trigger the disinhibition of brain structures, that thus become able to generate massive spasms in series – appears to be the most appropriate.

Tonic seizures

In principle, tonic seizures are a typical expression of generalized epilepsies, and an initial tonic stage marks the onset of the typical expression of generalized tonic-clonic seizures. However, the expression of tonic seizures can vary both in duration and in the extent of the involved segments, ranging from tonic eye opening and/or the almost 'subclinical' activation of axial and proximal muscles, sometimes only detected by means of contemporary EEG and polygraphic recordings (Fig. 2), to the massive contraction characterizing the onset of a convulsive seizure.

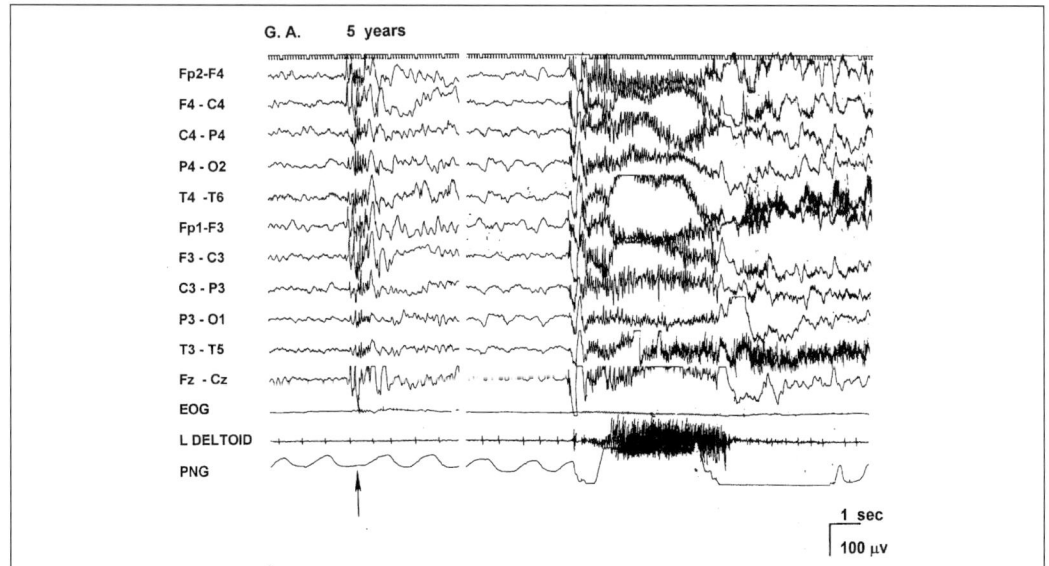

Fig. 2. Polygraphic recording performed on a child with Lennox–Gastaut syndrome. Left: a brief discharge of diffuse spikes is not associated with any detectable tonic contraction but leads to a just detectable delay in rhythmical breathing (arrow). Right: a few minutes later, a prolonged discharge of repetitive spikes concurs with a tonic seizure, leading to a concomitant apnoea.

Moreover, the term 'tonic' seizure often refers to a unilateral (hemi-tonic) or focal 'tonic contraction', that characterizes various types of essentially focal seizures in both adults and children; finally, the neonatal seizures consisting of the sustained asymmetric posturing of the limbs or trunk that are usually associated with focal EEG discharges, are usually classified as 'focal tonic'.

Even if the definition of a 'tonic seizure' is restricted to bilateral and symmetric muscle contractions, the physiopathological generating mechanism cannot be certainly referred to a 'generalized' discharge, since symmetric tonic seizures have been attributed to ictal discharges arising from supplementary motor area (Fusco et al., 1990; Connolly et al., 1994). Given the possibility that ictal tonic posturing can be due to either primary generalized or focal discharges, tonic seizures may be the main symptom of a heterogeneous clinical condition and different epileptic syndromes. Given the difficulty of differentiating the focal or generalized origin of tonic seizures, careful accurate evaluation of the electroclinical background appears to be particularly necessary in order to reach a precise diagnosis.

A high frequency discharge (typically close to 20 Hz) of repetitive spikes is the most characteristic ictal EEG pattern associated with tonic seizures: on a number of occasions, the spikes may be replaced by a run of rhythmic beta activity or an 'attenuation', often associated with superimposed low-amplitude fast activity. This low-amplitude variant of the tonic ictal pattern of very short tonic seizures is similar to that associated with spasms or seizures in series (see above).

Particular presentation of tonic seizures characterizes the expression of severe symptomatic or cryptogenic generalized epilepsies in childhood. Tonic seizures of variable duration and strength typically occur in cases of Lennox–Gastaut syndrome, for which the appearance of tonic seizures during sleep (sometimes replaced by 'subclinical' ictal phenomena detected by means of EEG recordings) is one of the diagnostic hallmarks. The appearance of tonic seizures during the course of other severe epileptic syndromes in childhood is quite common, and often considered to be associated with a worse prognosis. In severe forms of childhood epilepsy, very brief tonic seizures during wakefulness may provoke the repeated falls that are frequently observed in these clinical conditions, and these must be differentiated from other associated seizure types causing falls (e.g. massive 'myoclonic' jerks) by means of polygraphic studies. In children with Lennox–Gastaut syndrome (or other severe epileptic syndromes), recurrent tonic seizures can often sustain a 'tonic' epileptic status, during which individual seizures become progressively less evident, and the tonic phenomena tend to reduce their extent and duration. However, an increase in the autonomic disturbances that often accompany tonic status (mainly tracheobronchial hypersecretion) frequently represents the main medical problem in the management of tonic status. Repeated subtle tonic seizures can persist for many days, and can sometimes only be detected by polygraphic recordings.

Conclusions

Spasms and tonic seizures may be expressions of both focal and diffuse brain damage, and often constitute the predominant seizure type in severe encephalopathies and/or difficult to control epilepsies; pure tonic seizures are very rare in idiopathic epilepsies and spasms are the expression of a presumably idiopathic age-related epilepsy in very few cases (Vigevano et al., 1993). More than one 'variant' of both spasms and tonic seizures are known to occur, and occasionally the two seizure types can co-exist. Despite the great contribution made by many recent studies, there are still many open questions regarding the classification and physiopathological definition of spasms and tonic seizures. The semeiologic and nosographic categories used to classify these seizure types are largely insufficient: the Clinical and Electroencephalographic Classification of Epileptic Seizures proposed by the ILAE Commission (1981) did not classify spasms as a separate seizure type and, since then, they have usually been classified together with tonic seizures in a single category, although the ILAE Commission of Paediatric Epilepsy (1992) has suggested they should be separated. In addition, the consistent inclusion of spasms and tonic seizures in the class of generalized seizures often appears to be inadequate, since a focal onset is frequently detected (or suspected) for both seizure types, on the basis of evidence of focal EEG discharges or neuropathological and clinical signs unequivocally suggesting a focal brain lesion. Consequently, a possible focal origin cannot be ruled out even in some cases of age-related, generalized encephalopathies (Giroud et al., 1993).

The correct categorization of spasms and tonic seizures is often difficult, and more pertinent categories would be useful in helping to differentiate electroclinical pictures with a different pathophysiology and prognosis. This is especially true for spasms, for which separate classification categories are needed to distinguish patients with a typical picture of cryptogenic or idiopathic West syndrome from those with other or mixed types of seizures in series, in whom spasms are probably an age related presentation of localized (or multifocal) brain damage. Finally, further physiopathological studies are needed to define the generators of spasms and improve our understanding of the neurobiological basis of their peculiar time-course and presentation in infancy. An improvement in our knowledge of this field is essential in order to make it possible to outline a rational pharmacological treatment and, especially, define the extent of the applicability of surgical procedures in early infancy.

References

Colemann, M. (1971): Infantile spasms associated with 5-hydroxytryptophan administration in patients with Down's syndrome. *Neurology* **21**, 911–919.

Commission on classification and terminology of the International League Against Epilepsy (1981): Proposal for revised clinical and electroencephalographic classification of epileptic seizures. *Epilepsia* **22**, 489–501.

Commission on paediatric epilepsy of the International League Against Epilepsy (1992): Workshop on infantile spasms. *Epilepsia* **33**, 195.

Connolly, M.B, Langill, L., Wonget, K.H. & Farrell, K. (1994): Seizures involving the supplementary sensorimotor area in children: a video-EEG analysis. *Epilepsia* **36**, 1025–1032.

Donat, J. F. & Wright, F.S. (1991): Unusual variants of infantile spasms. *J. Child. Neurol.* **6**, 313–318.

Dulac, O. & Plouin, P. (1993): Infantile spasms and West syndrome. In: *The treatment of epilepsy: Principles and practices*, ed. E. Wyllie, pp. 464–491. Philadelphia: Lea & Febiger.

Fusco, L., Iani, C., Faedda, T. & Manfredi, M. (1990): Mesial frontal lobe epilepsy: a clinical entity not sufficiently described. *J. Epilepsy* **3**, 123–135.

Gaily, E.K., Shewmon, D.A., Chugani, H.T. & Curran, J.G. (1995): Asymmetric and asynchronous infantile spasms. *Epilepsia* **36**, 873–882.

Giroud, M., Fayolle, H., Gras, P., Vion, Ph., Baudoin, N., Brunotte, F. & Dumas, R. (1993): So-called generalized epilepsy in children leading to frontal epilepsy with frontal syndrome in adulthood: a clinical, EEG and radiological study in 10 cases. *Neurol. Res.* **15**, 299–303.

Gobbi, G., Bruno, L., Pini, A., Giovanardi Rossi, P. & Tassinari, C.A. (1987): Periodic spasms: an unclassified type of epileptic seizures in childhood. *Develop. Med. Child Neurol.* **29**, 766–775.

Hrachovy, R.A., Frost, J.D. & Kellaway, P. (1984): Hypsarrhythmia: variations on the theme. *Epilepsia* **25**, 317–325.

Hrachovy, R.A. & Frost, J.D. (1989): Infantile spasms: a disorder of the developing nervous system. In: *Problems and concepts in developmental neurophysiology,* eds. P. Kellaway & J.L. Noebels, pp. 131–147. Baltimore: J. Hopkins University Press.

Langlais, P.J., Mark, L.W. & Hitoshi, Y. (1991): Changes in CSF neurotransmitters in infantile spasms. *Pediatr. Neurol.* **7,** 440–445.

Kaga, K., Marsh, R.R. & Fukuyama, Y. (1982): Auditory brainstem responses in infantile spasms. *J. Pediatr. Otorhinolaryngol.* **4,** 57–67.

Kellaway, P., Hrachovy, R.A., Frost, J.D. Jr., & Zion, T. (1979): Precise characterization and quantification of infantile spasms. *Ann. Neurol.* **6,** 214–218.

Kellaway, P., Frost, J.D. & Hrachovy, R.A. (1983): Infantile spasms. In: *Antiepileptic drug therapy in pediatrics,* eds. P.D. Morselli, C.E. Pippenger & J.K. Penry, pp. 115–136. New York: Raven Press.

Pinard, J.M., Delande, O., Plouin, P. & Dulac, O. (1993): Callosotomy in West syndrome suggests a cortical origin of hypsarrhythmia. *Epilepsia* **34,** 780–787.

Romeo, A., Viri, M., Gonano, E.F. & Viani, F. (1995): Spasmi epilettici intercalati a crisi toniche nella sindrome di Lennox–Gastaut. *Boll. Lega It. Epil.* **91/92,** 67–69.

Satho, J., Mizutani, T. & Morimatsu, Y. (1986): Neuropathology of the brainstem in age-dependent epileptic encephalopathy especially in cases of infantile spasms. *Brain Dev.* **8,** 443–449.

Shields, W.D., Shewmon, D.A., Chugani, H.T. & Peacock, W.J. (1992): Treatment of infantile spasms: medical or surgical? *Epilepsia* **33 (suppl. 4),** s26–s21.

Talwar, D., Baldwin, M. A., Hutzler, R. & Griesemer, D. A. (1995): Epileptic spasms in older children: persistence beyond infancy. *Epilepsia* **36,** 151–155.

Vigevano, F., Fusco, L., Cusmai, R., Claps, D., Ricci, S. & Milani, L. (1993): The idiopathic form of West syndrome. *Epilepsia* **34,** 743–746.

Watanabe, K., Toshiko, H., Tamiko, N., Kousaburo, A. & Norihide, M. (1994): Focal spasms in clusters, focal delayed myeliantion, and hypsarrhythmia: unusual variant of West Syndrome. *Pediatr. Neurol.* **11,** 47–49.

West, W.J. (1841) On a peculiar form of infantile convulsions. *Lancet* **I,** 724–725.

Chapter 9

Semeiological features of non-epileptic falls

Giuseppe Gobbi and Antonella Pini

*Servizio di Neuropsichiatria Infantile, Arcispedale Santa Maria Nuova, viale Risorgimento 80,
42100 Reggio Emilia, Italy*

Summary

Sudden fall is usually considered as an epileptic event, but non-epileptic falls (NEFs) are also frequent in infancy and childhood. NEFs may be divided in NEFs with loss of consciousness and NEFs without loss of consciousness. The syncope is the most frequent cause of NEFs with loss of consciousness. Syncopes may be due to cardiac disease (cardiac syncopes) or to reflex mechanism (neuromediated – reflex – vasovagal syncopes). Usually, the syncope is preceded by subjective sensations, and the loss of tone is progressive. In some cases the premonitory phase is extremely brief or absent, and the patient may fall abruptly. In more severe cases the syncope is convulsive. Breath-holding spells (of pallid or cyanotic type) and the self-induced syncope by the Valsalva manoeuvre in children with behaviour disturbances with or without mental impairment are also included in this group. NEFs without loss of consciousness are less frequent and occur in some rare neurological conditions. Hyperekplexia, paroxysmal kinesigenic choreoathetosis and narcolepsy-cataplexy are heterogeneous conditions characterized by sudden impairment of the standing position. The pathogenesis of these attacks, whether epileptic or not, is not completely clear.

In order to reach a correct diagnostic approach to these paroxysmal disorders, detailed information has to be obtained about familial and personal clinical history and the situations in which the fall attacks have occurred, stimulus which has preceded the falls, prodromic symptoms, onset, ictal outcome, postictal state and after-effects. Clinical differentiation between epileptic and non-epileptic falls is very important for a correct therapeutical approach. NEFs may occur in children affected by epileptic seizures as well.

Finally, pure psychological mechanisms have to be considered as a possible cause of NEFs in the context of convulsive pseudo-seizures, with or without loss of consciousness.

Introduction

Sudden falls are usually considered as an epileptic event, but non-epileptic falls (NEFs) also frequently occur in infancy and childhood. As the main topic here is to discuss those abrupt falls whose semeiology is suggestive of epileptic seizures, this study will report only NEFs caused by an abrupt impairment of the postural tone due to a sudden disfunction of any structure (in the central nervous system or in the neuromuscular system) functionally related to the maintenance of the standing and sitting position. Other NEFs causing stumbles and falls such as gait disturbances (such as in spastic paraparesis, movement disorders or myotonia), benign paroxysmal vertigo and attention deficit disorders with hyperactivity have been excluded.

In an attempt to give practical suggestions for the diagnostic therapeutical approaches as well as differential diagnosis with epileptic seizures, NEFs are divided into NEFs with consciousness loss and NEFs without consciousness loss (Table 1).

Table 1. Classification of non-epileptic falls (NEFs)

NEFs with consciousness loss:	syncope
	breath-holding spell
	other conditions
NEFs without consciousness loss:	hyperekplexia
	paroxysmal kinesigenic choreoathetosis
	narcolepsy – cataplexy
Psychogenic seizures with or without loss of consciousness	

NEFs with consciousness loss

Syncope

The typical cause of NEFs is syncope or anoxic seizure. Syncope is defined as a sudden temporary loss of consciousness, associated with loss of postural tone followed by spontaneous recovery, which is due to an abrupt lack of energy substrates to the cerebral cortex and upper brainstem (Gastaut, 1974; Stephenson, 1990; Kapoor, 1991). This usually results from a sudden reduction in the cerebral blood flow or from reduced oxygen content. If the decrease in cerebral blood flow is not sufficient to cause a complete consciousness loss, one can feel like fainting, have equilibrium disorders, asthenia, blurred vision, perspiration and paleness. When loss of consciousness and postural tone occur in short-lasting hypoxia or ischaemia, the event is commonly described as fainting of simple syncope. Longer anoxia leads to motor seizure or convulsion – the so-called 'convulsive syncope'. In this latter condition seizures are mainly tonic fits and a few jerks might follow the tonic phase.

Apart from the drug-induced syncopes (such as vasodilators, barbiturates, diuretics, adrenergic antagonists, phenotiazines, antidepressants etc.), low blood pressure might result from cardiac events, so-called cardiogenic syncopes, or from peripheral vascular reflex mechanisms, so-called neuromediated or reflex or vaso-vagal syncopes. Cardiogenic syncopes occur in 8–35 per cent of the cases. They are due to cardiac diseases such as sick sinus syndrome, prolonged Q-T syndrome, arrhythmia, valvular stenosis and so on (Kapoor, 1991). Frequently they are of the convulsive type, and the prognosis may be severe as sudden death could occur at any time. Neuromediated (reflex-vasovagal) syncopes are more frequent in teenagers and females. Neuromediated syncopes may be emotional (such as those due to the sight of blood, minor pain or an injection), situational (such as those due to micturition, defecation, cough or swallow), or due to orthostatic hypotension, carotid sinus stimulation and glossopharyngeal and trigeminal neuralgia. At times, reflex syncopes are provoked by the same stimuli. Usually, the reflex syncope occurs when the patient is in a standing or sitting position. It is preceded by subjective sensations, and the loss of tone is progressive. In some cases, however, the premonitory phase is extremely brief or absent, and the patients might fall abruptly. In more severe cases the syncope is convulsive. In these cases urinary incontinence is frequent and the patients may be injured. Rarely, a true epileptic seizure may follow a syncopal attack (Stephenson, 1990).

The EEG picture of syncope has been studied by Gastaut during vaso-vagal reflex syncope induced by ocular compression (Gastaut & Gastaut, 1958). This manoeuvre results in prolonged asystole. Six to seven seconds after the asystole, diffuse slow waves occur for about 3 s and pallor occurs. Then there is a flattening of EEG activity which corresponds to the spasm and to the cyanosis for about 8 s. Then monomorphous slow waves (lasting from 2 to 5 s), which can be concomitant to clonic contractions, reappear before the EEG becomes normal again.

The diagnosis of syncope is often difficult and many different causes should be considered. Apart from collecting the family history, determining the setting in which the episode (or episodes) has occurred and carrying out a physical examination, often neurological, cardiological and metabolic examinations are required. An EKG should be performed in each case. Long-term EKG monitoring and other more sophisticated tests (such as the head-up Tilt-test, carotid sinus massage, ocular compression, Valsalva's manoeuvre and the electrophysiologic studies of the autonomic nervous system) can be required to differentiate cardiovascular reflex neuromediated syncope (Brignole *et al.*, 1995). In such circumstances well-equipped laboratories are required, but these tests cannot be performed on very young children. For the evaluation of syncope in older children and adults, see Kapoor (1991). An EEG examination is not necessary on the case of simple and single syncope; on the contrary, if convulsive syncope occurs, an EEG examination should be indicated.

When syncopes recur and consist of tonic contraction, they must be differentiated from generalized epileptic seizures, and especially from those tonic-clonic seizures in which the tonic phase predominates. It has to be noted that one-third of syncopes are misdiagnosed as epileptic seizures (Gastaut, 1974) and differential diagnosis is not always easy (Blume, 1990), especially when urination occurs during syncopes and the biting of the tip of the tongue may result from the fall of the patient. The characteristics of the person's position (usually upright or after standing up), the presence of precipitating factors (micturition, defecation, pain, emotion, anger), the gradual onset of a fainting feeling, the presence of pallor and sweating, the occurrence of only a few jerks, if any, and the quick recovery, typically suggest a syncopal origin of the consciousness loss. Moreover, opisthotonus is much more common in syncopal attacks than in tonic-clonic epileptic seizures, and downward deviation of gaze is an important feature (Stephenson, 1990).

Syncope must be obviously differentiated from those consciousness losses due to cerebrovascular disorders causing stroke or transitory ischaemic attacks (Butler, 1993), including migraine (Sacquegna, *et al.*, 1989). Personal history and the presence of sudden onset focal neurological deficit eventually associated with neuro-imaging confirmation of cerebral infarction define the diagnosis.

Breath-holding spell

Syncope due to the so-called breath-holding spell is most frequent in infancy. This condition has been distinguished into two different types: cyanotic and pallid type (Lombroso & Lerman, 1967). In the majority of the cases the attacks do not recur after the age of five years and there are not relationships with later epilepsy. In some patients the attacks may be stereotyped and repetitive.

In the cyanotic breath-holding spells, provocative emotional event-induced crying can determine, after two or three loud cries, a permanence of the spell in expiration with a period of apnoea. If the apnoea lasts from 5 to 10 s, only a colour change occurs and thereafter the respiration is resumed. If the apnoeic spell is prolonged, cerebral anoxia develops and it is the ultimate factor responsible for the loss of consciousness observed in the severe forms of the breath-holding spell (Di Mario, 1992; Stephenson, 1990). In these severe forms, a brief stiffening of the body and/or a true brief convulsive phase (two or three jerks) and incontinence of urine may follow giving rise to differential diagnostic problems with epileptic seizures. Polygraphic recordings have shown that apnoea is associated with tachycardia followed by bradycardia, while anoxic EEG-slowing appears only at the time of clinical manifestations (Gastaut, 1974). Oxygen desaturation and reduction of cerebral blood flow due to an increased intrathoracic pressure with decreased venous return have been suggested as pathogenetic mechanisms. Impaired autonomic nervous system regulation has been suggested (Di Mario, 1992).

The pallid breath-holding attacks are less common than cyanotic ones. Minor injuries instead of emotional events are the provoking factors. A loss of consciousness may or may not be preceded by crying and, more frequently than in cyanotic attacks, is associated with opisthotonus or stiffening, downward deviation of gaze, and jerking of the limbs. Clinical seizure is concomitant with a period of asystole (Lombroso & Lerman, 1967; Gastaut, 1974; Stephenson, 1990) so that the syncope is the result of acute cerebral anoxia secondary to a vagal cardiac arrest due to an excessive vagal reflex ('vagotonia'). This type of breath-holding attack is more frequently misdiagnosed as an epileptic event.

The differential diagnosis from epileptic seizures poses the same problems as in syncopes. An EEG examination is not necessary, since the situation and the typical sequence of the different breath-holding spell phases (always well described by the parents) allow for correct diagnosis.

Other conditions

A condition which has some pathogenetic aspects in common with the breath-holding spell is the syncope which is self-induced by the Valsalva manoeuvre. In children with mental retardation or prepsychotic behavioural disorders, Gastaut (1980) reported a peculiar symptomatological picture characterized by sudden abdominal swelling (due to forced expiration against a closed-glottis Valsalva manoeuvre), blue facial pallor, contact impairment and, sometimes, loss of muscular tone and consciousness loss. He hypothesized a self-induced mechanism.

Girls with Rett syndrome present with an impaired spell rhythm regulation can also undergo a consciousness loss due to cerebral hypoxia (Kerr, 1992). In this disorder hyperventilation bursts alternate with apnoeic spells. On the EEG a theta monomorphic activity appears, at first on central regions, then diffuses. Recurrent apnoeic-polypnoeic spells can also occur in patients affected by severe lesional encephalopathy.

The pathogenesis of this respiratory apraxia is not well understood. A dysfunction of the forebrain followed by gradual involvement of the thalamic nucleus and of the frontal cerebral cortex has been hypothesized (Cirignotta *et al.*, 1990).

The differential diagnosis from epileptic seizures might be especially difficult in these cases. In fact, one should consider that children with mental retardation and girls with Rett syndrome might have true epileptic manifestations and that epileptic seizures can be induced by paroxysmal spell rhythm. In these cases, therefore, polymyographic ictal EEG recording is necessary for a correct diagnosis of the nature of these phenomena.

NEFs without consciousness loss

Being startled is a common emotional reaction to a sudden unexpected stimulus, producing a stereotyped motor response which can cause falling. When this response is exaggerated (i.e. is elicited by stimuli that do not induce similar startle-reactions in a normal subject because the motor response is more violent or because there is no habituation), and such that it interferes with normal activities, it is termed as pathological startle.

Pathological startle is considered as synonymous with hereditary startle-disease hyperekplexia. However, other pathological conditions can include pathological startle; for example, cerebral palsy (syncinesie-sursaut), the Gilles de la Tourette Jumping Frenchmen of Maine syndrome (Hillion & Beaumanoir, 1989) and degenerative diseases.

Hyperekplexia

Hereditary startle disease or hyperekplexia (Suhren et al., 1966) is a rare disease, often confused with epilepsy in the first year of life. It is characterized by transient congenital hypertonia and hypokinesia in the waking state, exaggerated startle response (sometimes associated with falls), markedly hyperactive brainstem reflexes, marked nocturnal myoclonic jerks, hip dislocation and umbilical-epigastric-inguinal hernia. It is an autosomal dominant- or recessive-hereditary disorder which has been localized on chromosome 5 (Ryan et al., 1992). Sporadic cases have been reported in the past (Gastaut & Villeneuve, 1967).

The first description of the condition is that of Suhren et al. in 1966. An increase in muscle tone is the first sign after birth. In the first months of life, flexing spasms appear to stimuli such as being lifted out of the cradle. After learning to walk these children stumble readily, occasionally becoming stiff all over and falling on to their face without extending the arms. The falls are already related to an abnormal startle-reaction, most frequently following an unexpected auditory stimuli.

Electrophysiological studies show '... a stereotyped response on the EEG, consisting of a sequence of one or more fast spikes, a prominent electropositive sharp wave and one or more medium-amplitude slow waves, each complex lasting 0.5 to 1 s; with prominent startle, the complex was followed by flattening of the background rhythms for 1 to 2 s' (Markand et al., 1984). On polygraphic studies other phenomena can be observed: variable tachycardia, rise in arterial pressure (mainly systolic), very brief apnoea and a fall in arterial peripheral blood flow.

The true nature of the EEG response accompanying being startled is still controversial. Gastaut & Villeneuve (1967) considered the EEG complex discharge as an electrical event of cortical origin, i.e. an evoked response to a sensory stimulus. Markand et al. (1984) thought that the spike potentials and the electropositive sharp waves were essentially of myogenic and ocular origin respectively, i.e. that the EEG activity was artefact. These authors, studying the long-loop reflexes, found a prominent C-response after the F-wave (and before the end of the silent period). This is a late, probably transcortically mediated, response which occurs after stimulation of a mixed nerve. Normally a C-response does not appear in relaxed conditions. A small and inconsistent C-response may only occur during isotonic and (less) isometric contraction. In patients with startle disease, these authors recorded consistent C-responses after median nerve stimulation in the isometric condition and, in some, even in the relaxed position. Similar responses occurred in cortical, reflex and postanoxic myoclonus. These findings suggested an increased cortical neuronal excitability. More recently, Matsumoto *et al.* (1992), studying the muscular activation pattern after auditory and sensory stimulation, concluded that diffuse hyperexcitability at the brainstem and spinal cord levels could be present in startle disease, while cortical hyperexcitability could be an inconstant phenomenon. On the contrary, Ferri *et al.* (1994), according to Markand *et al.* (1984), when analysing the somatosensory evoked potentials in startle disease, demonstrated a clear change in cortical excitability mediated by the classical somatosensory pathway with contralateral projection. In fact, after an N20 wave with normal latency and amplitude, great amplitude P25 and N45 waves appear. In conclusion, electrophysiological studies suggest that in startle disease there exists a combination of cortical and brainstem hyperexcitability, which, on one hand, could explain the increased amplitude of evoked potential response and the decreased latency of muscular response to sensory stimuli, and, on the other hand, could also determine the generalized tonic contractions triggered by unexpected environmental stimuli (Ferri *et al.*, 1994).

The clinical and electrophysiological findings in startle disease and the effectiveness of benzodiazepines, suggest possible involvement of neurotransmitters, especially GABA or its receptors. According with this hypothesis it is extremely interesting that in the q33–q35 region of chromosome 5 there is the gene for the alfa sub-unit of the GABA-A receptor, the gene for the receptor dopamine-1 and the genes which encode adrenergic receptors; a genetic defect in this region was therefore suggested (for a review of these data, see Ferri *et al.*, 1994). Unfortunately, a therapeutic approach with GABA agonists was unsuccessful (Berthier *et al.*, 1994; Ferri *et al.*, 1994).

Startle disease must be differentiated from reflex myoclonic epilepsy, myoclonic epilepsies, *épilepsie-sursaut* and from startle-induced epilepsy. The polygraphic EEG ictal recording of the seizure is determining for a differential diagnosis.

Paroxysmal kinesigenic choreoathetosis (PKC)

This syndrome is a clinical condition in which sudden voluntary movements after rest characteristically precipitate tonic, dystonic or choreoathetotic attacks which can provoke falling (Kersetz, 1967; Lance, 1977). This is an entity which, probably, has to be considered as a functional age-dependent disorder with autosomal dominant or recessive inheritance. However, similar attacks have been reported in patients affected by basal ganglia or pre-motor cortex disease, cerebral palsy and multiple sclerosis.

In hereditary PKC the attacks start in childhood between the ages of 8 to 15 years, and last less than 1–2 min with unimpaired consciousness. The choreoathetoid movements are usually unilateral; when bilateral, the axial and antigravitary musculature is also involved and falling occurs. The attacks may be preceded by a prodrome of limb heaviness or tightness and they can occur many times in the day. The course of the disease is benign. Neuro-imaging investigations and electrophysiological studies failed to demonstrate the presence of cerebral lesions (Busard *et al.*, 1984).

The pathogenesis of the attacks, whether epileptic or not, is not completely clarified. Benefits with both anticonvulsants or L-Dopa (Loong & Ong, 1973) or dopamine blocking agent (Busard *et al.*, 1984) have been obtained. The choreoathetotic nature of the attacks, the absence of troubles of the contact during the attacks and the electrophysiological studies provided arguments in support of an extrapyramidal origin. Busard *et al.* (1984) suggested that the right-posterior P-T region 4–5 Hz rhythm observed in one of their patients which disappeared at the beginning of every PKC attack and which is replaced in postictal phase by a 9–10 Hz rhythm '... is generated by a non-inhibited subcortical nuclear structure'. The authors hypothesized that these '... findings are in support of the opinion that PKC is caused by dysmaturitas or dysbalance of the extrapyramidal system'. However, the hypothesis that PKC is a form of reflex epilepsy involving the basal ganglia (so-called 'basal ganglia epilepsy' or 'striatal epilepsy' or 'extrapyramidal epilepsy') is still being debated. Arguments in favour of an epileptic origin are the presence of sensory prodroma, the reflex and paroxysmal nature of the attacks and the high incidence of epilepsy in the relatives. Moreover, recently Lombroso (1995), recording a PKC attack with deep electrodes in a patient, found that the attack of PKC was an epileptic event originating from the supplementary motor region then involving the nucleus caudatus. The author suggested that '... this may be one way to explain how cortically originated ictal discharges would cause symptomatology characteristic for basal ganglia disorders'.

Narcolepsy – cataplexy

Cataplexy consists of an abrupt loss of muscle tone resulting in a complete fall, without consciousness impairment, precipitated by a sudden emotion such as laughter or surprise. It usually begins in adolescence or early adulthood and is a cardinal manifestation of the narcolepsy syndrome. Narcolepsy, that is, irresistible attacks of sleepiness due to a generalized disorganization of sleep–waking functions, is instead usually the presenting symptom. However, isolated cataplexy without narcolepsy can, very rarely, occur.

Family studies showing excessive sleep disturbances among the parents, siblings and children of probands with narcolepsy indicate genetic factors. However, to our knowledge, a precise pattern of inheritance has not been identified. Cases with symptomatic cataplexy (and narcolepsy) have also been reported (D'Cruz et al., 1994).

Atonic epileptic falls might be confused with cataplexy. The presence of precipitating factors and the associated sleep disorders are the most typical findings in cataplexy, which also suggest the correct diagnosis. Neuro-imaging investigations are therefore indicated, focusing on the brainstem and the hypothalamus. Multiple sclerosis must also be investigated.

Psychogenic seizures with or without loss of consciousness

This is a wide field which goes beyond the limits of this presentation. We only mean to mention that patients with emotional disturbances, neurosis or psychosis can have syncopal consciousness loss caused by ventilatory impairment during anxiety attacks (Blume, 1990). Moreover, hysterical seizures mimicking convulsive seizures or cataplexy do occur. Differential diagnosis can sometimes be difficult. Usually the characteristics of the time of onset, the longitudinal history of recurrent multiple complaints, the manner and attitude of the patient and the absence of symptoms and signs of other medical and surgical disease will allow for an accurate diagnosis in the majority of cases. However, prolonged EEG recording during the seizure (which may be provoked) is definitely clarifying, especially in epileptic patients with associated psychiatric disorders.

Conclusions

The chapter of the so-called paroxysmal non-epileptic manifestations is extremely important for its prognostic and therapeutical consequences. Since epileptic falls commonly have a very severe prognosis, differential diagnosis between epileptic and non-epileptic falls is especially important. Moreover the epileptic or non-epileptic nature of some of NEFs without loss of consciousness is not yet clarified, and NEFs may occur also in epileptic patients. As the NEF-triggering circumstances are very suggestive for a correct diagnosis, neurologists and child neurologists must obtain detailed information about the familial and personal clinical history, the settings in which the fall attacks have occurred, the stimuli which have preceded the falls, prodromic symptoms, the onset, the ictal outcome, postictal state and the after-effects. Psychic mechanisms have to be considered as a possible cause of NEFs as well. In general, EKG and/or long-term EKG monitoring are sufficient for a correct diagnosis, but in the misleading cases, more sophisticated tests such as the head-up tilt-test, carotid sinus massage, ocular compression, Valsalva's manoeuvre, the electrophysiologic studies of the autonomic nervous system and prolonged EEG recording have to be recommended.

References

Blume, W.T. (1990): Differential diagnosis of epileptic seizures. In: *Clinical neurophysiology of epilepsy. EEG Handbook* (revised series, vol. 4), eds. J.A. Wada and R.J. Ellingson, pp. 407–431. Amsterdam: Elsevier Science.

Berthier, M., Bonneau, D., Desbordes, J-M., Chevrel, J., Oriot, D., Jaeken, J. & Laborit, H. (1994): Possible involvement of gamma-hydroxybutyric acid receptor in startle disease. *Acta. Paediatr.* **83**, 678–680.

Brignole, M., Menozzi, C., Bottoni, N., Gianfranchi, L., Lolli, G., Oddone, D. & Gaggioli, G. (1995): Mechanisms of syncope caused by transient bradycardia and the diagnostic value of electrophysiologic testing and cardiovascular reflexivity maneuvers. *Am. J. Cardiol.* **76**, 273–278.

Busard, H.L.S.M., Renier, W.O., Gabreels, F.J.M., Vos, A.J.M., Declerck, A.C. & Verhey, F.H.M. (1984): Autosomal dominant paroxysmal kinesigenic choreoathetosis. *Clin. Neurol. Neurosurg.* **86–4**, 281–289.

Butler, I.J. (1993): Cerebrovascular disorders in children. *J. Child. Neurol.* **8**, 197–200.

Cirignotta, F., Sforza, E., Burroni M., Zappella, M. & Lugaresi, E. (1990): Breathing disorders in males with acquired encephalopathy. *Brain Dev.* **12**, 69–72.

D'Cruz, O'Neill F., Vaughan, B.V., Gold, S.H. & Greenwood, R.S. (1994): Symptomatic cataplexy in ponto-medullary lesions. *Neurology* **44**, 2189–2191.

Di Mario, F. (1992): Breath-holding spells in childhood. *A. J. D. C.* **146**, 125–131.

Ferri, R., Elia, M., Masumeci, S.A., Colamaria, V., Dalla Bernardina, B., Del Gracco, S. & Bergonzi, P. (1994): Giant somatosensory evoked potentials and pathophysiology of hyperekplexia. Neurophysiological study of one patient. *Neurophysiol. Clin.* **24**, 318–324.

Gastaut, H. & Gastaut, Y. (1958): Electroencephalographic and clinical study of anoxic convulsions in children. *Electroencephalography Clin. Neurophysiol.* **10**, 607–620.

Gastaut, H. & Villeneuve A. (1967): The startle disease or hyperekplexia. Pathological surprise reaction. *Journal Neurol. Sci.* **5**, 523–542.

Gastaut, H. (1974): Syncopes: generalized anoxic seizures. In: *Handbook of Clinical Neurology*, vol. 15, eds. P.J. Vinken and G.V.B.W. Bruyn, pp. 815–835. Amsterdam: Elsevier Science.

Gastaut, H. (1980): Un syndrome névrotique méconnu de l'enfant oligophréne. Les syncopes autoprovoquées de façon compulsive par manoeuvre de Valsalva. *Bull. Acad. Nat. Med.* **164**, 713–717.

Hillion, C. & Beaumanoir A. (1989): Startle disease. Report of a case. In: *Reflex seizures and reflex epilepsies*, eds. A. Beaumanoir, H. Gastaut, R. Naquet, pp. 415–419. Editions Médecine et Hygiène: Genève.

Kapoor, W. (1991): Diagnostic evaluation of syncope. *Am. J. Cardiol.* **90**, 91–106.

Kerr, A. M. (1992): A review of the respiratory disorder in the Rett syndrome. *Brain Dev.* **14 (suppl.)**, S43–S45.

Kertesz, A. (1967): Paroxysmal kinesigenic choreoathetosis. An entity within the paroxysmal choreoathetosis syndrome. Description of 10 cases, including 1 autopsied. *Neurology* **17**, 680–690.

Lance, J.W. (1977): Familial paroxysmal dystonic choreoathetosis and its differentiation from related syndromes. *Ann. Neurol.* **2**, 285–293.

Lombroso, C.T. & Lerman, P. (1967): Breath-holding spells (cyanotic and pallid infantile syncopes). *Pediatrics* **39**, 563–581.

Lombroso, C.T. (1995): Paroxysmal choreoathetosis: an epileptic or non-epileptic disorder? *Ital. J. Neurol. Sci.* **16**, 271–277.

Loong, S.C. & Ong, Y.Y. (1973): Paroxysmal kinesigenic choreoathetosis. Report of a case relieved by L-dopa. *J. Neurol. Neurosurg. Psychiatry* **36**, 921–924.

Markand, O.N., Garg, B.P. & Weaver, D.D. (1984): Familial startle disease (hyperexplexia). Electrophysiologic studies. *Arch. Neurol.* **41**, 71–74.

Matsumoto, J., Fuhr, P., Nigro, M. & Hallet, M. (1992): Physiological abnormalities in hereditary hyperekplexia. *Ann. Neurol.* **32**, 41–50.

Ryan, S.G., Sherman, S.L.,Terry, J.C., Spakers, R.S., Torres, M.C. & Mackey, R.W. (1992): Startle disease or hyperekplexia response to clonazepam and assignment of the gene (STHE) to chromosome 5q by linkage analysis. *Ann. Neurol.* **31**, 663–668.

Sacquegna,T., Andreoli, A., Baldrati, A., Lamieri, C., Guttman, S., De Carolis, P., Di Pasquale, G., Pinelli, G., Testa, C. & Lugaresi, E. (1989): Ischemic stroke in young adults: the relevance of migrainous infarction. *Cephalalgia* **9**, 255–258.

Suhren, O., Bruyn, G.W. & Tuynman, A. (1966): Hyperekplexia. A hereditary startle syndrome. *J. Neurol. Sci.* **3**, 577–605.

Stephenson, J.B.P. (1990): Fits and Faints. *Clinics in Developmental Medicine*, **109**. MacKeith Press. Oxford: Blackwell Scientific.

PART III

Chapter 10

Epileptic syndromes with drop seizures in children

Charlotte Dravet, Renzo Guerrini and Michelle Bureau

Centre Saint-Paul, 300 boulevard de Sainte-Marguerite, 13009 Marseille, France

Summary

The two best-known epileptic syndromes with fall seizures as the main seizure type which begin in childhood between 3 and 12 years are the Lennox–Gastaut syndrome (LGS), and the epilepsy with myoclonic astatic seizures (MAE), otherwise named Doose syndrome. These two syndromes have common features but they are different in clinical and electroencephalographical semeiology, aetiology, prognosis and treatment. They are fully described. However epileptic drop attacks can also occur in other types of epilepsy, which are more succinctly described here (epilepsy with myoclonic absences, epilepsy with continuous spike-waves during slow sleep, atonic collapses) or are only quoted (progressive myoclonus epilepsies, partial epilepsies) because they are discussed in other chapters. Then, the authors mention the existence of tonic seizures with multifocal abnormalities and encephalopathies with undetermined epilepsy.

Introduction

Drop seizures are frequent in childhood epilepsies and are difficult to treat. Their mechanism is not easy to determine by clinical observation, and simultaneous EEG, polygraphic and video recordings are necessary for an accurate diagnosis. They are a component of different types of epilepsies, which are generalized as well as localization-related (Table 1). These epilepsies are mainly observed between 3 and 12 years but this age-range is somewhat artificial. They may begin before and continue after. No epidemiological data concerning the drop seizure frequency in the different syndromes, particularly in partial compared to generalized epilepsies, are available. Obviously, the most known situations are those in generalized epilepsies such as Lennox–Gastaut syndrome and epilepsy with myoclonic-astatic seizures, otherwise named Doose syndrome. We first discuss these two syndromes, then we briefly approach the others, except the partial epilepsies which are treated in other chapters.

Table 1. Epileptic syndromes with fall seizures in children between 3 and 12 years

Lennox–Gastaut syndrome
Epilepsy with myoclonic-astactic seizures (Doose syndrome)

Epilepsy with myoclonic absences
Epilepsy with continuous spike-waves during slow sleep (CSWSS)
Progressive myoclonus epilepsies

Atonic collapses
Partial epilepsies
Tonic seizures with multifocal EEG
Encephalopathies with undetermined epilepsy

The Lennox–Gastaut syndrome

Among childhood epilepsies, the Lennox–Gastaut syndrome (LGS) is one of the most severe epileptic syndromes, due to the frequency of seizures, to the occurrence of sudden falls, to a marked pharmacoresistency, and to the occurrence of mental and behavioural disturbances. The physiopathogenic mechanisms of LGS are not well understood and the borderlines with other types of severe epilepsies are not easy to define. Without a precise knowledge of the clinical and electroencephalographic characteristics of the patient concerned, it may be difficult to distinguish between LGS and other childhood epilepsies such as the Doose syndrome (myoclonic-astatic epilepsy, MAE), the epilepsy with continuous spikes and waves during slow sleep, and partial epilepsies with bilateral secondary synchrony.

In the International Classification of Epilepsies and Epileptic Syndromes (Commission, 1989) LGS has been classified among the symptomatic or cryptogenic generalized epilepsies. It is defined by several criteria:

(1) polymorphous epileptic seizures, with mainly atypical absences, axial tonic, and atonic seizures;

(2) EEG patterns consisting of diffuse slow spikes and waves (SSW) and bursts of fast rhythms at 10–12 Hz during sleep;

(3) permanent psychological disturbances with psychomotor delay or personality disorders, or both.

However, other seizure types can be observed (myoclonic, partial, and generalized tonic-clonic). The seizure frequency is high and they often repeat themselves in episodes of status. Focal and multifocal abnormalities can be associated with the diffuse SSW in the EEG. These electroclinical features can occur in a previously normal child, without pathological antecedents and without signs of brain lesion, usually between 1 and 8 years (constituting the *cryptogenic* form of LGS). They also can occur in a child with prior signs of brain damage, sometimes following another type of epilepsy, such as West syndrome or a focal epilepsy (*symptomatic* form). In the latter, the age at onset can cover a wider range (between 1 and 15 years).

Aetiologic circumstances are polymorphous, ante-, peri- or postnatal (anoxo-ischaemia, vascular accident, cerebral and cerebro-meningeal infection, HHE syndrome, brain malformation and migration disorders, tuberous sclerosis, Down syndrome, hydrocephalus, head trauma, brain tumour, radiotherapy for brain tumour, etc.). Neuro-imaging studies show abnormalities related to aetiology. In some cases, in spite of a psychomotor retardation before the onset of seizures, or of cerebral atrophy demonstrated by CT scan and MRI, there is no recognizable aetiology. When epilepsy starts in the first year of life, it is often in the form of West syndrome, followed by LGS (Ohtahara et al., 1976). Otherwise the LGS can be preceded by focal seizures or can have the full-blown presentation from the very onset. It must also be stressed that the typical features of LGS can be observed only transiently in some patients (Beaumanoir, 1968). In the cryptogenic forms, there is no aetiology by definition.

The underlying mechanisms are still unknown. Even the neurophysiological pathways leading to the expression of generalized SSW on the scalp are not explained. The same processes as in the idiopathic generalized epilepsies could play a part, but in LGS it would appear to be modified by other factors, either acquired or genetic.

LGS seems to be a non-specific age-dependent condition which looks like a diffuse encephalopathy, and we do not know why it appears in either normal or brain-damaged patients (Beaumanoir & Dravet, 1992).

Clinical presentation

Boys are slightly more often affected than girls (Loubier, 1974).

The onset occurs before the age of 8, with a peak between 3 and 5 years. The mode of onset is variable and has not been specified in most series. In the cryptogenic cases (Boniver et al., 1987) the first seizures can be myoclonias, atypical absences, falls, sometimes repeated in status. Sometimes one isolated – either tonic, clonic, or tonic-clonic seizure, even a unilateral seizure – has preceded the typical seizures by several months. Nocturnal tonic attacks are usually not observed at the very onset. Psychological disturbances can be concomitant with the first seizures or can develop later, insidiously. Thus it is not easy to make the diagnosis of LGS very quickly. The EEG features at onset have not been well described. They can consist of either diffuse SSW or only more or less diffuse slow waves. One single study of nocturnal sleep at this stage has been published (Costa et al., 1992) demonstrating the presence of bursts of low-voltage rapid rhythms evoking subclinical tonic seizures. When LGS follows the West syndrome, there are two possible modalities: either infantile spasms are replaced by tonic seizures without a free interval; or infantile spasms disappear, EEG and psychomotor development improve during some length of time before the occurrence of falls, atypical absences and diffuse SSW, accompanied by a new slowing of development. When LGS complicates other types of epilepsy, the attention is drawn by the onset of falls and of behavioural changes. Several authors have reported the occurrence of LGS in adolescents and in young adults who previously had an idiopathic type of generalized epilepsy (Oller Daurella, 1967; Loubier, 1974).

Ictal symptomatology during the course of the disease

Tonic seizures are the main sign of the syndrome. They are reported in 74 per cent (Beaumanoir, 1982) to 90 per cent (Loubier, 1974) of patients. They can be axial, axorhizomelic or complete; they can occur awake or asleep. They can be symmetrical or have a marked unilateral predominance. They involve sudden flexion of the neck and of the body, raising the arms in a semiflexed or extended position, extension of the legs, contraction of the facial muscles, sometimes restricted to the lower lip, rolling of the eyes, apnoea and facial flushing. This can lead to a sudden fall. Loss of consciousness does not occur constantly and is rarely the initial symptom. Return to normal consciousness is always concomitant with the end of the EEG discharge. Enuresis can occur. The pupils are usually dilated. When these seizures are short and involve only the rolling of the eyes and respiratory changes (such as usually occurs during sleep), they can escape attention. When they last for more than 10 s, they can culminate in a tremor affecting the whole body (resulting in a 'vibratory' seizure). In the tonic-automatic seizures, described by Oller Daurella (1970), in 72 per cent of the late-onset cases there is a final phase of gestural, sometimes ambulatory, automatisms. Drowsiness and slow sleep facilitate the occurrence of tonic seizures. In the EEG, tonic seizures (Fig. 1) correspond to either a bilateral discharge of fast rhythms, predominant in the anterior areas and at the vertex, or a flattening of the background, or the combination of these two patterns, sometimes preceded by a generalized SW, followed by diffuse slow waves and SSW. No postictal silence occurs. The fast discharges are particularly common during slow-wave sleep when they can be nearly subclinical. This ictal pattern recorded during sleep was inappropriately described as the 'grand mal pattern' by Gibbs (1938).

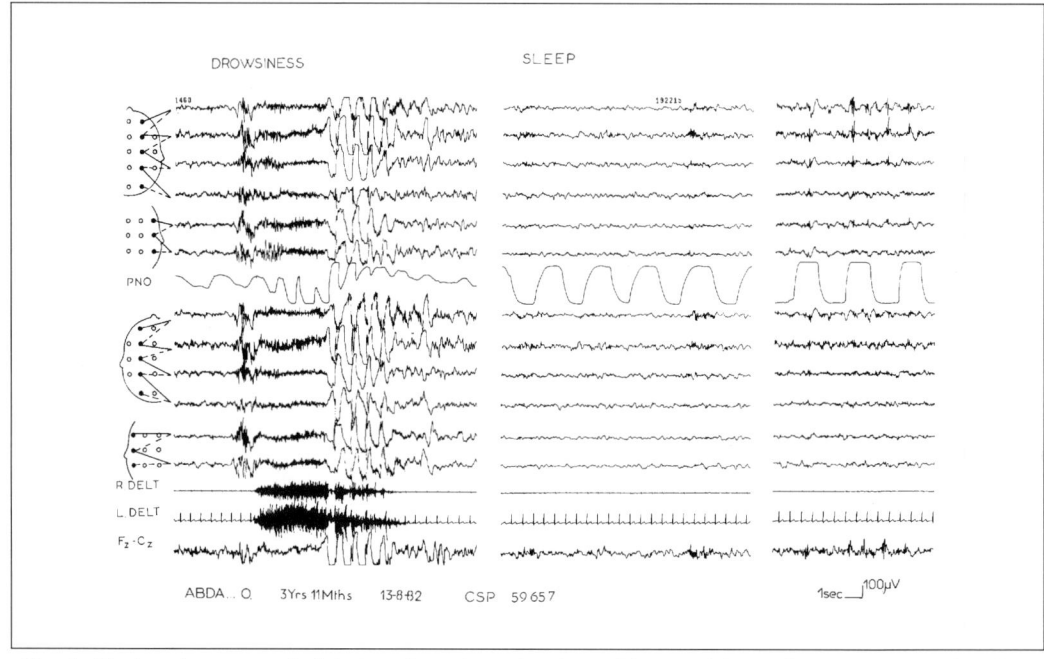

Fig. 1. Tonic seizure recorded during drowsiness in a boy of 3 years 11 months. EEG: generalized fast rhythms followed by a burst of diffuse slow SW. Polygraphy: superficial polypnoea, tonic muscular contraction sustained during the rapid rhythms, then interrupted by the slow waves. On the right part of the figure: right-hemispheric and right-frontal polyspikes and slow waves. Abbreviations: PNO = pneumogram; R. DELT. = right deltoid; L. DELT. = left deltoid.

Atypical absences are observed in a vast majority of the patients. Clinically they are often difficult to diagnose: their onset and their end are gradual; consciousness is impaired but not completely lost; a simple activity can be continued; eyelid myoclonias are not rhythmical; perioral myoclonias are frequent; a slow forward motion of the head due to loss of tone and drooling are frequent. In the EEG, atypical absences are accompanied by a discharge of diffuse SSW at 2–2.5 Hz, that is often irregular and more or less symmetrical (Fig. 2), or sometimes by a burst of rapid rhythms.

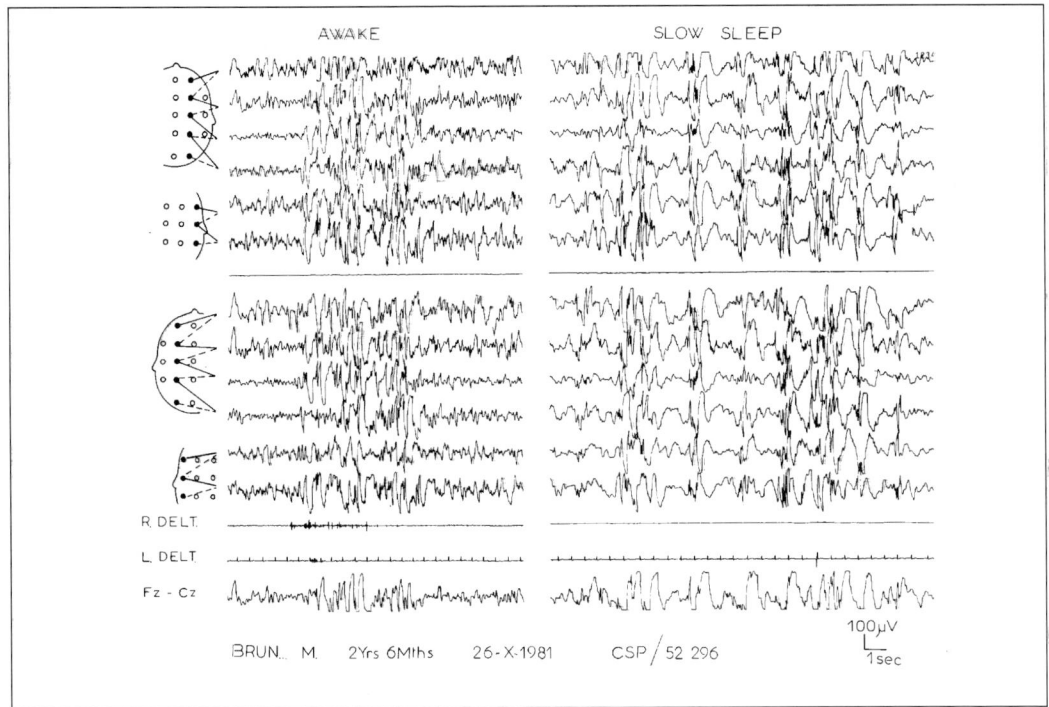

Fig. 2. On the left, one atypical absence recorded in a girl of 2 years 6 months. EEG: diffuse, irregular, slow SW during 5 s, preceded and followed by slow waves in the two anterior areas. Polygraphy: slight, arrhythmical myoclonias in the right deltoid. On the right: typical aspect of slow sleep at this age, with high-amplitude SW and polyspike-waves. R. DELT. = right deltoid; L.DELT. = left deltoid.

Massive myoclonias, atonic seizures and myoclonic-atonic seizures are uneasy to differentiate by clinical observation only. Like tonic seizures, they provoke a sudden fall, either of the head only, or of the whole body, causing injuries, followed by an immediate recovery. Their EEG correlates are polymorphous: SSW, slow poly-SW, and decremental events. The simultaneous video-EEG and polygraphic recordings allow an accurate diagnosis. They are associated in the same patient in 95 per cent of the cases. Most of the authors group these seizures with falls under the names of 'akinetic' or 'astatic' seizures (Gastaut, 1982), or 'drop attacks'. Figure 3 shows an example of head drop due to an atonic seizure.

Other seizure types that are not specific for the LGS syndrome are sometimes observed: generalized tonic clonic, generalized clonic and partial seizures.

All the seizure types can occur as status in a majority of patients (54 per cent: Loubier, 1974; 75 per cent: Beaumanoir, 1982). They consist of periods of more or less profound obtundation, even of stupor, intermixed with serial tonic attacks, sometimes with myoclonic-atonic falls. When tonic attacks are predominant, they constitute tonic status. The main characteristics of status episodes are their long duration (from days to weeks), their resistance to treatment, and their tendency to occur repetitively in the same patient. In these periods of status, the EEG becomes almost hypsarrythmic. It has been suggested they are only a temporary worsening of the usual interictal symptomatology (Beaumanoir, 1982; Dravet *et al.*, 1985).

Interictal symptomatology

Clinically two types of symptoms can be identified. The neuropsychological and psychiatric symptoms consist of an arrest or a slowing down of the psychomotor development, an apparent deterioration of the cognitive abilities, and the appearance of severe psychiatric disorders, of which the expression depends on age. The youngest children present with physical and intellectual instability, mood lability, inability to acquire new skills, and progressive fluctuations in personality. Older children present with slowness of ideation and expression, language deterioration due to motor dysfunction, particularly changes in the muscular tone of the oro-laryngo-pharyngeal area (Beaumanoir et al., 1968), aggressiveness, irritability, loss of social relationships, tendency to isolation, and sometimes psychotic outcome. Personality disorders are always present in the cryptogenic forms (Viani, 1991). Neurological signs specific to LGS do not seem to exist, apart from transient cerebellar, pyramidal or extra-pyramidal signs during prolonged status. However, in some patients the recurrent episodes of status are so long and so frequent that this semeiology can become permanent after more than 10 years of evolution. Iatrogenic factors due to heavy polytherapy might contribute to this neurological deterioration.

On the EEG, the background can be disorganized with diffuse slow waves, poor reactivity, as well as a lack of topographic differentiation. This disorganization can be constant (67 per cent of the patients) or transient, appearing only during those periods of worsening of seizures. When it is constant it is a sign of poor prognosis. Hyperventilation can elicit SSW discharges with or without clinical correlates (atypical absences), whereas intermittent photic stimulation has no effect. Paroxysmal abnormalities are constant: discharges of diffuse SSW and poly-SSW; in 75 per cent of children they are associated with focal and multifocal discharges of spikes, and slow spikes and SSW, of which the site is constant or variable, and frequently frontal or temporal. They are increased by slow sleep, when the diffuse SSW become more synchronous and more rhythmical, with prominence of the

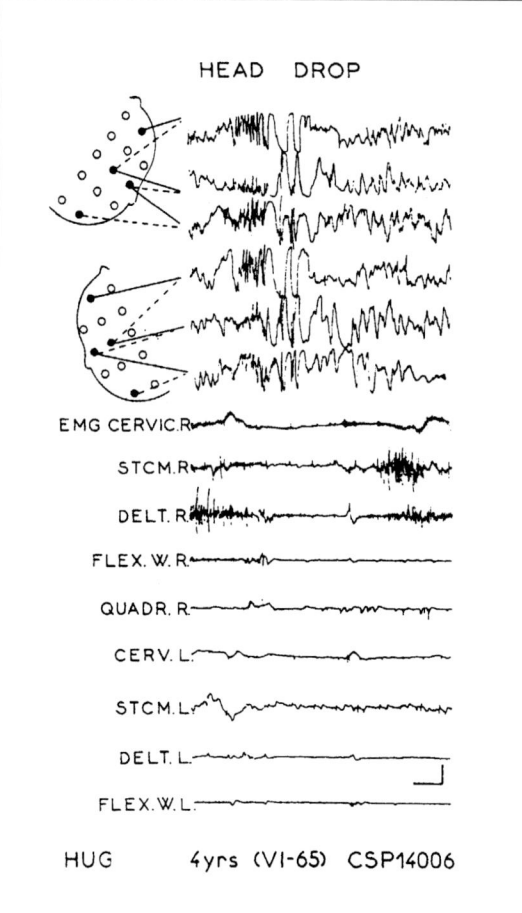

Fig. 3. Head drop recorded in a boy of 4 years. EEG: brief generalized discharge of fast rhythms, followed by a burst of two slow SW. Polygraphy: clear abolition of muscular tone of neck muscles and the right deltoid, while there is no muscular activity in the other recorded muscles. CERVIC. R. = right cervical muscle; STCM R. = right sterno-cleido-mastoideus; DELT. R. = right deltoid; FLEX. W. R. = right-wrist flexor; QUADR. R. = right quadriceps; CERV. L. = left cervical muscle; STCM L. = left sterno-cleido-mastoideus; DELT. L. = left deltoid; FLEX. W. L. = left-wrist flexor.

polyspikes. During sleep, the specific bursts of fast rhythms appear (see above). The differentiation of the sleep stages can be preserved (personal observation) or can disappear (Baldy-Moulinier et al., 1988).

Clinical forms

In the myoclonic variant of the LGS, massive myoclonias and myoclonic-atonic attacks are the prominent seizure types (18 per cent of the cases for Chevrie & Aicardi, 1972). Tonic seizures are inconstant, mainly nocturnal, and epileptic status is characterized by stupor and myoclonias. The wake-EEG is not different from the typical form but there are less runs of rapid rhythms during sleep. This myoclonic variant is cryptogenic in 64 per cent of the cases and its mental prognosis is more favourable. Probably some of the patients reported to have 'myoclonic LGS' in the literature actually had epilepsy with myoclonic-astatic seizures described by Doose (1992) and further studies should elucidate this point.

There is also an early LGS, beginning before the age of 1 year, and a late onset LGS.

Differential diagnosis

The problems are different in cryptogenic and symptomatic forms, and depend on the age at onset.

For cryptogenic LGS, the main differential diagnosis is with myoclonic-astatic epilepsy of early childhood (MAE) (Doose, 1992). This problem is discussed below in the paragraph concerning MAE. Another condition has long been confused with LGS: epilepsy with continuous spikes and waves during slow sleep (CSWSS), also discussed below. Before the description of severe myoclonic epilepsy (SME) (Dravet et al., 1982) children suffering from this syndrome were diagnosed as LGS because they had frequent and intractable seizures, often repeated in status, with a strong myoclonic component associated with severe mental deterioration. However, it seems obvious now that these two syndromes are clearly different. Sometimes in cryptogenic, but more often in symptomatic LGS, the diagnosis of partial epilepsy with secondary bilateral synchrony (SBS) must be evoked. This concept was introduced by Jasper (1949). Gastaut & Zifkin (1988), and Blume (1994) have tried to establish the differences between epilepsy with SBS and LGS. Epilepsy with SBS seems to be as severe as LGS. The mechanisms underlying SBS are not yet well elucidated.

Treatment and outcome

Treatment is disappointing. Classical anti-epileptic drugs usually do not control the seizures completely. Among them, carbamazepine, valproate and benzodiazepines are the most useful, mostly used in association. In spite of their metabolic interactions, carbamazepine and valproate give interesting results when combined. Phenytoin can be used in adolescents and adults, for the vibratory tonic and tonic-clonic attacks. Ethosuximide and diones can also help to control the atypical absences temporarily. Tonic attacks and rapid discharges during sleep are particularly resistant. One of the aims of treatment is to avoid the episodes of status. Thus it is necessary to detect them and to take the appropriate measures, sometimes using steroid treatment. Out of the periods of status, steroids should be tried in children not too late in the course of the disease, as in West syndrome. Immunotherapy and the ketogenic diet (as well as other types of diets) have also been proposed (Brett, 1988).

Among the newer drugs, vigabatrin has not proved to be very useful. However, it is worth trying and some good results have been reported in LGS associated with cortical dysplasia (Guerrini *et al.*, 1994). Some authors have claimed that lamotrigine was very efficacious (Timmings *et al.*, 1992) but these data require confirmation. As a matter of fact it seems that the only recent drug to have a specific effect on LGS seizures is felbamate. Unfortunately this drug has potentially severe side-effects and must be given very cautiously.

The course of the disease is characterized by a succession of good and bad periods. A series of tonic seizures can occur suddenly, without obvious reason, particularly in the early morning. Cognitive impairment and behavioural disturbances need special education and psychological support.

Complete seizure-free recovery is rare. Generally, the syndrome tends to persist, with some improvement in the seizures but with worsening psychological aspects. The EEG features attenuate with age. Most awake-EEGs show only a slow background without SSW discharges. The typical aspects of LGS are still recorded during sleep. SLG can disappear to be replaced by an often severe partial epilepsy. Mental deficiency is observed in 85 per cent to 92 per cent of patients. Its degree is variable, from a slight deficit to a profound deterioration. In cryptogenic cases it increases with age and repetition of seizures but it is less marked than in symptomatic cases. Frequently, but not consistently, patients become psychotic. Many patients end up being institutionalized, either in centres for epilepsy or in centres for mentally handicapped people. However, in our personal experience, some children, who were absolutely normal before the onset of their cryptogenic LGS, have relatively good social outcomes. They are able to continue normal or near-normal schooling, without obtaining diplomas, and to have more or less regular jobs in spite of persisting seizures.

The main risk factors for a bad prognosis are: the symptomatic character of the syndrome, particularly after West syndrome; early age at onset – before three years; high frequency of seizures; long duration of worsening periods; repetition of status; and presence of a constantly slow background activity and of localized abnormalities on the EEG.

The myoclonic-astatic epilepsy of early childhood

Historically, this form of epilepsy was first confused with LGS because of some common features. Kruse (1968) reported a series of 82 patients presenting with the same clinical features as the Lennox–Gastaut patients under the name of 'Myoclonic-Astatic Petit Mal'. However, he ascribed the sudden falls to myoclonus without demonstrating it by polygraphic recordings; he did not perform sleep-EEG and thus could not recognize the tonic seizures or rapid rhythms typical for LGS. Later, Doose *et al.* (1970) described an idiopathic type of epilepsy as 'Centrencephalic Myoclonic-Astatic Petit Mal', and differentiated it from the LGS which is mostly symptomatic in their opinion. But the Commission on classification of the ILAE did not retain the idiopathic character of this epilepsy and included it, wrongly, in the category of cryptogenic or symptomatic generalized epilepsies (Doose *et al.*, 1987). In recent years, several authors have tried to establish firm criteria to separate LGS from MAE on the basis of aetiology, semeiology and prognosis (Dulac *et al.*, 1990; Dravet *et al.*, 1991; Guerrini *et al.*, 1994; Maton *et al.*, 1990).

On the basis of 117 cases collected over more than 20 years, Doose described a syndrome occurring during the first five years of life, more frequently in boys (73.5 per cent) than in girls, always primary, with a high rate of positive family histories (37 per cent). Typical seizures are mainly myoclonic-astatic seizures and atypical absences, and the EEG shows a typical pattern consisting of a theta rhythm at 4–7 Hz, predominating in the parietal areas, associated with fast generalized SW. Generalized tonic-clonic seizures are also observed, but tonic seizures are rare, occurring only in the late course of the disease, almost exclusively during the night. Evolution and prognosis are variable and are less favourable with the occurrence of status of 'minor seizures'.

MAE is rare and no epidemiologic studies have been conducted for this epilepsy. Doose & Sitepu (1983) indicated that primary generalized myoclonic and myoclonic-astatic seizures occur in 1–2 per cent of all childhood epilepsies up to age 9. Of 694 patients with epilepsy onset under age 5 observed at the Centre Saint-Paul between 1986 and 1995, only twelve were classified as MAE (1.7 per cent), versus 57 (8.2 per cent) with LGS.

Opposite to LGS, acquired aetiological factors are infrequent and only 16 per cent of Doose's patients were clearly retarded before their first seizure. In contrast, genetic factors are prominent. Seizures were reported in parents, parents' siblings and/or in proband's siblings in 32 per cent of cases (febrile or afebrile generalized tonic-clonic seizures, absence seizures and myoclonic or myoclonic astatic seizures). Moreover, there was a significantly higher rate of seizures before the age of 5 in relatives. Doose & Baier (1987) demonstrated that this genetic predisposition is important in the pathogenesis of MAE, and is different from that for seizures of later onset. The frequency of electroencephalographic markers such as photosensitivity, 4–7 Hz rhythms and SW, was distinctly increased in siblings and parents. MAE is thus an example of a multifactorially determined disorder (Doose et al., 1989).

Clinical presentation

According to Doose (1992), the onset of MAE is during the first 5 years in 94 per cent of patients, during the first year in 24 per cent, with febrile and afebrile generalized tonic-clonic seizures (two-thirds of the cases) or with 'minor' seizures. The early age at onset will be commented on below.

Typical seizures are myoclonic, astatic and myoclonic-astatic seizures. Myoclonias are symmetrical, involving arms and shoulders, with a simultaneous nodding of the head of variable intensity, sometimes leading to a fall. Astatic seizures are those due to an abrupt loss of tone, rarely isolated. The most usual drop attacks are due to the combination of a symmetrical myoclonia, immediately followed by a loss of tone – this combination constituting the typical myoclonic-astatic seizure. These are associated with absences, with irregular myoclonias of the face, with a partial or total loss of tone, and with generalized tonic-clonic seizures. Tonic and focal seizures occur rarely and only in the late course of the most severe cases. The status of absences and myoclonic-astatic seizures are observed in 36 per cent of the cases. They consist of a state of apathy or stupor, irregular twitching of the facial muscles and extremities, drooling, serial drop attacks and head noddings. They may last for hours or days, with onset often after awakening.

The EEG may be normal at the onset. The most characteristic finding is the presence of 4–7 Hz theta rhythms with parietal accentuation, and of occipital 4 Hz rhythms constantly blocked by eye opening. SW can be found when minor seizures appear and are activated by sleep. Their morphology depends on the seizure type: short bursts of irregular SW and poly-SW in myoclonias; with irregular, non-rhythmical SW interrupted by high-amplitude slow waves in myoclonic astatic seizures (Fig. 4). Variable lateralization of SW can be seen; however, a consistently localized focus is unusual, found only in rare cases with previous brain damage. A photo-paroxysmal response is present in most cases. During status, the EEG shows irregular, polymorphous, hypersynchronous activity, sometimes resembling hypsarrythmia in young children. We have recorded myoclonic status with repeated fast generalized SW and SSW (Fig. 5).

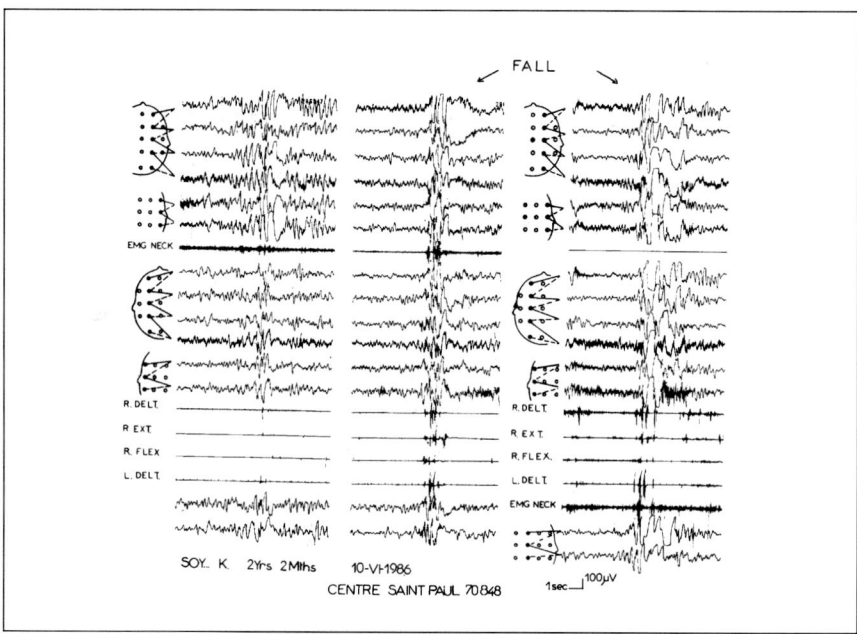

Fig. 4. Myoclonic-astatic seizures recorded in a boy of 2 years 2 months. On the left: generalized SW with only a slight myoclonia, without fall. In the middle and on the right: generalized SW with a large slow wave corresponding to the fall. Polygraphy: myoclonic jerks and post-myoclonic inhibition in all the recorded muscles.
R. DELT. = right deltoid; R. EXT. = right-wrist extensor; R. FLEX. = right-wrist flexor; L. DELT. = left deltoid.

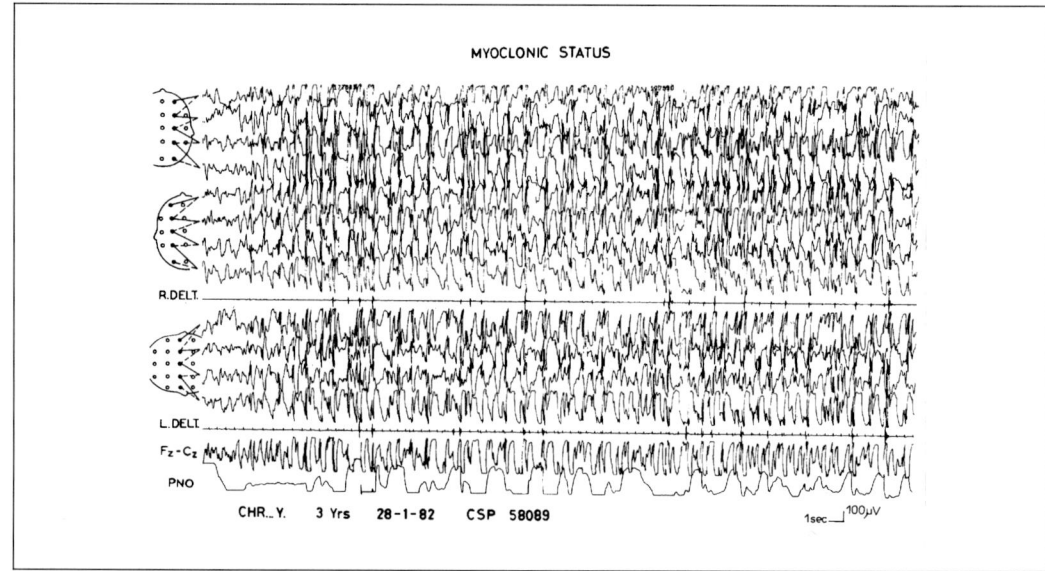

Fig. 5. Myoclonic status recorded in a boy of 3 years with MAE. EEG: continuous diffuse, irregular, high-amplitude SW and poly-SW. Polygraphy: irregular segmental myoclonic jerks, correlated with spikes in the EEG. R. DELT. = right deltoid; L. DELT. = left deltoid; PNO = pneumogram.

Diagnosis is based on clinical semeiology of the seizures and on the EEG. Children with MAE are typically normal children who repetitively fall, who have long periods of stupor, and whose EEG shows theta rhythms and irregular SW and poly-SW. Clinical examination, neuro-imaging and biological tests are normal. As in LGS, it is necessary to perform a prolonged video and polygraphic EEG in order to analyse the seizure types.

Differential diagnosis

MAE must be distinguished from benign myoclonic epilepsy (BME), SME, LGS and atypical benign partial epilepsy (Aicardi *et al.*, 1982). That is not easy. In fact, in his first description Doose seemed to include cases of SME and BME; these two syndromes being not yet well defined. However, in the last years several series of patients affected by SME and BME have been published, confirming the existence of these syndromes. Presently, it is possible to distinguish a group of patients who clearly have MAE. Following the studies by Dulac *et al.* (1990) and by Guerrini *et al.* (1994), it is possible to differentiate them by age at onset, type of initial seizures, types of other seizures, EEG features, psychological evolution and long-term outcome (Table 2).

Table 2. Distinctive features of severe childhood epilepsies

	Age at onset	First seizures	Other seizures	EEG changes	Mental status and outcome
BME	6 m – 3 yrs	myoclonias	none	generalized fast SW	N; favourable
SME	<1 yr	febrile clonic GTCS, unilateral	GTCS, unilateral, myoclonias, GTCS	generalized and focal	N → abN; unfavourable
LGS	2 – 8 yrs	variable	tonic, atypical absences, myoclonic, other	slow SW, 10 Hz rhythms during sleep	N or abN → abN; unfavourable
MAE	1 – 5 yrs	myoclonias, myoclonic-astatic, GTCS	same plus episodes of stupor	theta, generalized SW	N; variable
ABPE	3 – 8 yrs	focal	myoclonic, atypical absences, falls	focal and diffuse	N; favourable

BME = benign myoclonic epilepsy; SW = spike-waves; N = normal; SME = severe myoclonic epilepsy; GTCS = generalized tonic-clonic seizure; abN = abnormal; LGS = Lennox–Gastaut syndrome; ABPE = atypical benign partial epilepsy.

Differential diagnosis with atypical benign partial epilepsy does not raise big problems since partial seizures are the main seizure type at the onset, which is never observed in MAE.

Differential diagnosis with LGS is more difficult. However, the main seizure types are different in the two syndromes: myoclonic-atonic seizures in MAE, tonic seizures in LGS, as well as the main EEG features: only generalized SW and SSW in MAE, slow SW associated with focal spikes and slow waves, and sleep rapid rhythms in LGS. At onset, confusion is possible because tonic seizures and sleep-EEG rapid rhythms are not always present in children with LGS. But when the first seizures are repeated tonic clonic seizures, it is likely they belong to MAE and not to LGS. On the other hand, rare patients have features of both syndromes and the diagnosis remains uncertain even after several years of evolution. The existence of such intermediate types is not an argument against the concept of distinct epileptic syndromes; rather it emphasizes the complexity and the multifactorial determinants of the epilepsies.

Treatment and outcome

Therapeutic modalities depend on seizure types. The most useful anti-epileptic drugs against all the seizure types are valproate, ethosuximide, diazepines and, sometimes, phenobarbital. Lamotrigine seems also to be effective (Schlumberger, 1994). On the contrary, phenytoin, carbamazepine and vigabatrin, which are useful in LGS, must be avoided in MAE because they can increase myoclonic seizures. Acetazolamide and ACTH are indicated for status. In the most refractory cases with convulsive seizures, the German authors recommend giving bromides without delay.

Outcome is variable and factors conditioning the course of the disorder are not yet well understood. The only prognostic factor mentioned by Doose (1992) is the early repetition of prolonged status which can rapidly lead to dementia. Obviously, there are children who have many seizures of the different types at onset, apparently resistant to all anti-epileptic drugs, then progressively improve. In these patients the course of the epilepsy lasts less than three years and treatment can be withdrawn quickly. In others, epilepsy remains intractable, and tonic seizures as well as mental deterioration appear. According to Dulac *et al.* (1990), in the former group the first episode consists of stupor with massive myoclonus, tonic-clonic and atonic absence seizures; whereas in the latter stupor status is associated with hypotonia, erratic myoclonus, tonic seizures, and drooling, lasting up to one month. However, these data require confirmation by further studies. No data are available concerning the long-term prognosis because the accurate delineation of the syndrome and its two types is too recent.

Other types of epilepsies

Epilepsy with myoclonic absences

This type of epilepsy was described by Tassinari *et al.* (1969) and individualized as an epileptic syndrome in the 1989 international classification (Commission, 1985). It is a childhood epilepsy characterized by the recurrence of myoclonic absences which constitute the only or the preponderant seizure type. It is rare, affecting boys (69 per cent) more often than girls. Aetiological factors are the same as in childhood absence epilepsy. A family history of epilepsy is found in 19 per cent of the cases. Age at onset is between 1 year and 12 years (mean: 7 years). An earlier onset is possible.

Myoclonic absences (MA) have common features, with absences of the absence epilepsy. Their frequency is usually high: several a day, up to several dozens a day (pycnoleptic). The onset and end are abrupt. The impairment of consciousness varies from a complete loss to a simple obtundation; the patient feels uneasy and trys to control the jerks. They are often triggered by hyperventilation, sometimes by photic stimulation. They occur preferentially on awakening. They can occur during stage one of sleep, provoking arousal.

But they are different in symptomatology, response to drugs and outcome. The ictal motor manifestations consist of myoclonic movements, often with a tonic component, mainly involving the muscles of shoulders, arms, legs and head. The muscles of the face are less frequently involved. Head and body deviation can be observed, as well as automatic movements and autonomic manifestations such as urination and change in respiration. MA can lead to a sudden fall on the ground when myoclonic jerks are violent and involve the lower limbs, particularly in young children. A sustained tonic contraction between the myoclonias also can be responsible for a fall.

The ictal EEG is a bilateral, synchronous, symmetrical, rhythmic, spike and wave discharge at 3 Hz, similar to that recorded in the absences of childhood absence epilepsy. Polygraphic recordings allow an accurate analysis of the relationships between the EEG and the EMG ictal events (Fig. 6).

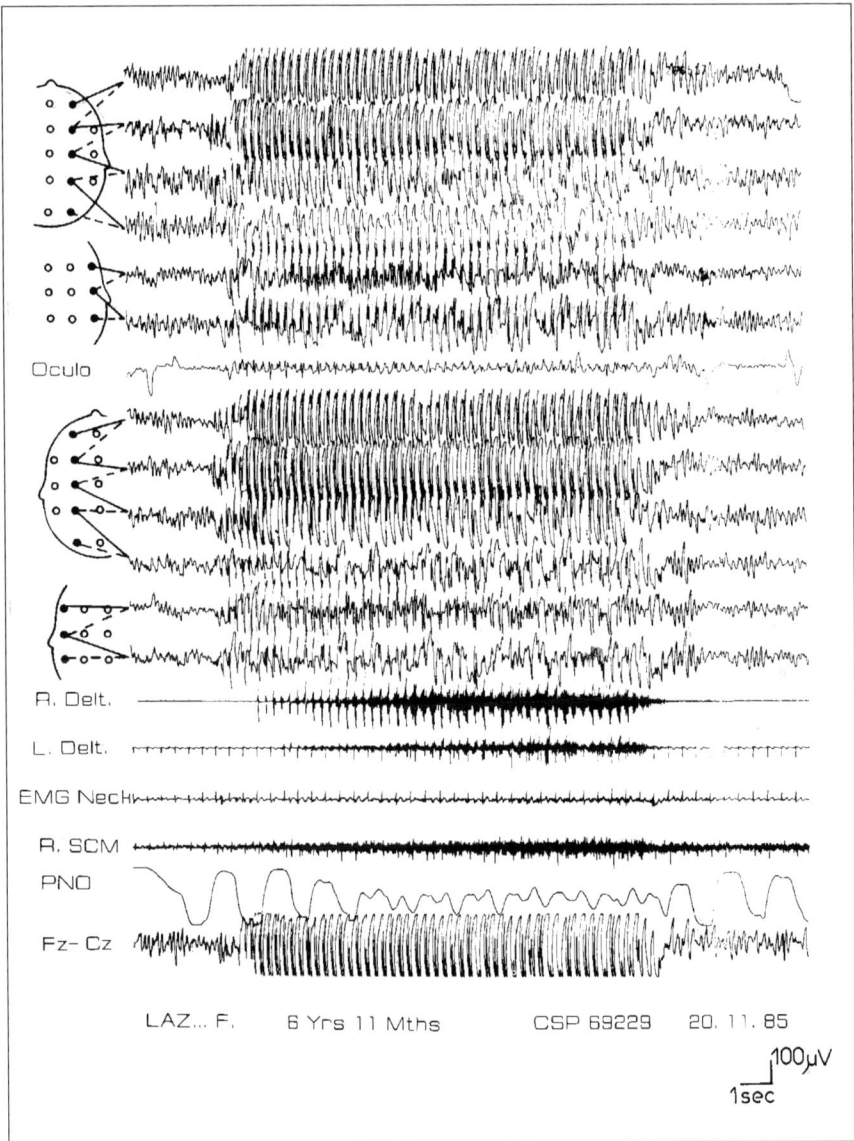

Fig. 6. Myoclonic absence recorded in a boy of 6 years 11 months. EEG: discharge of rhythmical, regular SW, at 3.5 HZ, with higher voltage in the frontal and vertex regions, during 15 s. Polygraphy: rhythmical myoclonic jerks in the two deltoids, closely related to the spikes in the EEG, progressively increased muscular tone in all the recorded segments, except the neck, and superficial polypnoea. R. DELT. = right deltoid; L. DELT. = left deltoid; R. SCM = right sterno-cleido-mastoideus; PNO = pneumogram.

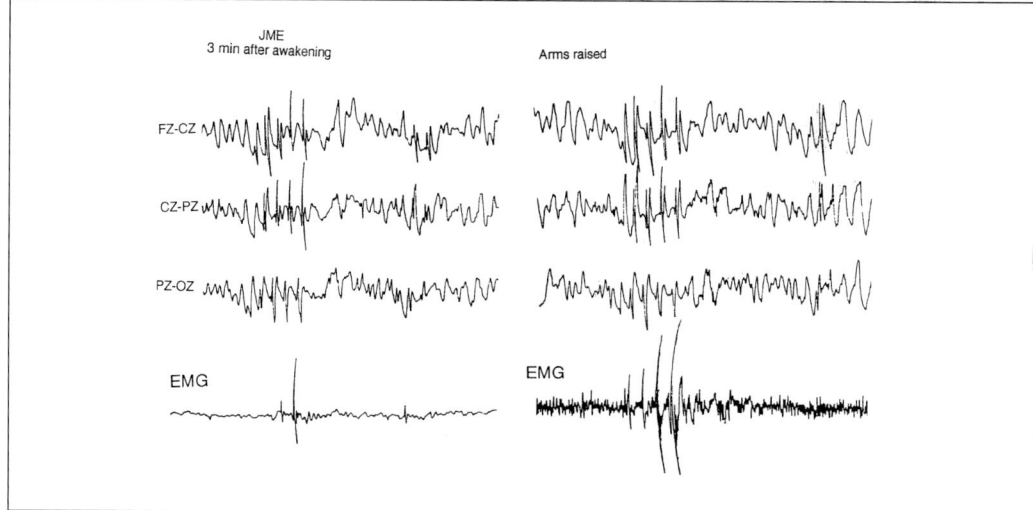

Fig. 3. Polygraphic EEG recording performed in the morning right after awakening, in a sleep-deprived JME patient. On the right, spontaneous myoclonic jerks time-locked to generalized fast spike-waves. On the left, the patient keeps his arms outstretched, demonstrating a post-myoclonic inhibition immediately following the myoclonic jerk, marked by a sudden drop of the arms and by a slight interruption of the electromyographic activity.

The existence of pure atonic seizures in JME is still being discussed. In the original paper of Janz & Christian (1957), as in the one of Asconape & Penry (1984), brief atonic seizures, sometimes associated with a very mild impairment of consciousness, were reported. In 1987, Manon-Espaillat *et al.* (1987) reported in three JME patients pure atonic seizures, occurring without impairment of consciousness independently of the characteristic myoclonic jerks. However, numerous authors (Delgado-Escueta & Enrile-Bascal, 1984; Janz, 1985; Wolf, 1992; Panayiotopoulos *et al.*, 1994) are still doubtful of the existence of these types of seizures, pointing out, as did Loiseau & Duche (1990), that no video-polygraphic recordings can actually prove their reality.

Lennox–Gastaut syndrome in adults

An epileptic fall is one of the main features of the Lennox–Gastaut syndrome (LGS), and is probably the most disabling one. It determines, with the cognitive impairment, the global prognosis of the syndrome. Various distinct types of seizures leading to brutal injurious falls are often associated in the same patient: tonic seizures, atonic seizures, myoclonic or myoclonoatonic seizures. On the contrary, a slow progressive fall on the ground after an initial phase of impaired consciousness ('amyotonic' seizure) characterizes atypical absences.

Very few authors have specifically studied LGS in adults. The most comprehensive study has been published by Roger *et al.* in 1987. These authors have studied 44 cases of LGS of late onset. The inclusion criteria were as follows: age of onset after the age of 13, no pre-existing epilepsy, presence of the characteristic triad including tonic seizures, atonic or myoclonoatonic seizures and atypical absences. Two groups could be differentiated. The first included 31 patients who presented, in addition with the typical triad, a focal symptomatology consisting in partial seizures with or without secondary generalization, and/or focal or multifocal EEG abnormalities. Sudden falls were present in 28 patients out of 31; that is, 90 per cent of these cases. Prognosis was constantly unfavourable, leading to a severe pharmacoresistent epilepsy with intellectual deterioration. The second group included thirteen idiopathic cases, with no clinical or EEG-focalized signs. Seven patients with an early onset before the age of 16 had an unfavourable evolution. Six patients had a later onset of the symptomatology, between 16 and 19 years old. In this latter subgroup, very similar on a nosological point of view of the generalized epilepsies said to be 'intermediary' (Pazzaglia et al., 1977), no tonic seizures and no fast rhythmic recruiting discharge during slow-wave sleep were noticed, and a good evolution was present in five out of six cases. In fact, rare seizures still persisted in three patients, but without any intellectual worsening, whereas recovery was apparently complete for the two others. Treatment was however maintained for all these patients.

From this study, one must remember that there is a different prognosis between cases of LGS starting before or after the age of 15: those with an early onset, 13 to 15 years old, always having an unfavourable evolution; and those with a later onset, after the age of 15, being of better prognosis.

Progressive myoclonus epilepsies of adolescence

The full-blown progressive myoclonus epilepsy (PME) syndrome is characterized by the association of the following symptoms: a myoclonus syndrome involving a combination of parcellar or segmental, arrhythmia, asynchronous, asymmetrical, myoclonias and massive myoclonias, (an epilepsy with, in most cases, generalized tonic-clonic or clonic seizures); a mental deterioration of varying degree; and a neurological syndrome almost always including cerebellar symptoms (Roger et al., 1992). PME are rare conditions. Geographic distribution is very heterogeneous. Lafora's and Unverricht–Lundborg's disease (united form of 'Baltic' and 'Mediterranean' myoclonus) are the most frequent and typical forms of PME starting around adolescence, between the age of 8 and 18. However, rarer forms, such as mitochondrial encephalomyopathy with 'ragged red fibres' (MERRF) or the juvenile form of ceroid lipofuschinosis (Spielmeyer–Vogt–Sjogren disease) can as well begin during this period of life. Physiopathology, clinical features, diagnosis and evolution of PME are not the point of this chapter and the interested reader must therefore refer to excellent review articles on this topic (Roger et al., 1992; Berkovic et al., 1993).

In most typical forms of PME, falls are frequent because of the combination of pseudocerebellar ataxia, massive bilateral myoclonic jerks and action myoclonus, which is worsened by the preparation of the movement and particularly accentuated upon wakening and when moving. As the disease progresses, standing up from a sitting position or changing direction while walking may be either problematic or impossible (Roger et al., 1992). Piracetam administered per os at very high doses (25–40 g/day) is probably the most effective means of improving the action myoclonus, and therefore to prevent the falls, in these patients (Battaglia et al., 1995).

PME patients might also exhibit, in the early course of their disease, epileptic negative myoclonus (ENM) (Fig. 4) which is a pure ictal atonic phenomenon, defined as 'an interruption of tonic muscular activity, time-locked to a spike or a spike-wave on the EEG, without evidence of an antecedent myoclonia' (Tassinari et al., 1981; 1995). Silent-period locked averaging performed on polygraphic recordings is the choice procedure to assess the neurophysiological features of ENM (Ugawa et al., 1989; Tassinari et al., 1995; Suisse et al., 1995; Rubboli et al., this volume). Depending on its intensity and its diffusion to the lower limbs, ENM can be

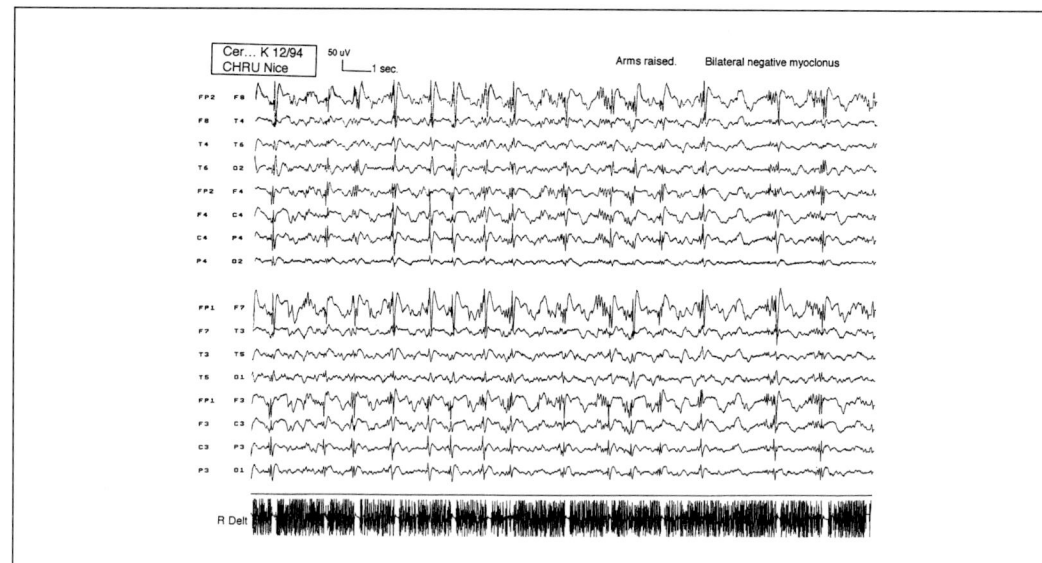

Fig. 4. Epileptic negative myoclonus organized in status epilepticus in a 16-year-old boy with progressive myoclonus epilepsy of unknown origin. At rest, there was no positive myoclonias. When the patient kept his arms outstretched, polygraphy revealed short interruptions of tonic muscular activity without evidence of antecedent myoclonias, time-locked to isolated generalized slow polyspike-waves. Silent-period locked averaging showed that there was a 28 ms delay between the top of the last spike and the onset of the negative myoclonus.

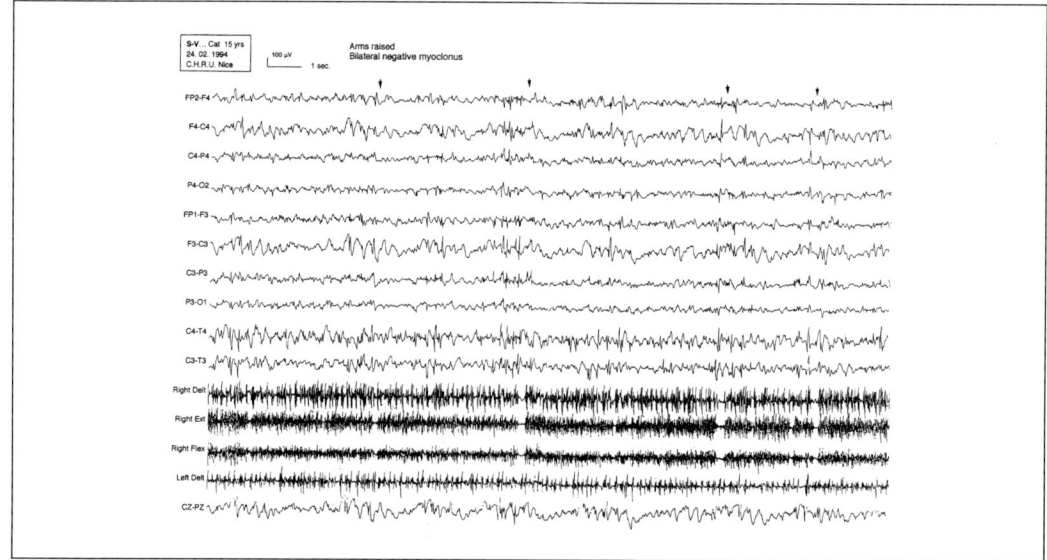

Fig. 5. Epileptic negative myoclonus revealing biopsy-proven Lafora's disease. On polygraphy, the short interruption of tonic muscular activity, lasting 50 to 250 ms (more marked on the right) were time-locked to a burst of fast diffuse high-amplitude spike-waves. Brain mapping and silent-period back averaging showed that there was a left-hemispheric dipolar organization of the 'generalized' spike-waves discharges, with a 32 ms delay between the top of the spikes and the onset of the negative myoclonus.

responsible for postural instability, dropping objects, head nodding, or falls. Some recent works (Shibasaki *et al.*, 1994; Thomas *et al.*, 1994; Tassinari *et al.*, 1995) report the presence of ENM as the revealing sign of PME, especially in Lafora's disease (Fig. 5). Moreover, two cases concerning mitochondrial diseases have been extensively published (Guerrini *et al.*, 1993; Shibasaki *et al.*, 1994). More recently, Vogt & Mothersill (1995) reported 11 patients with ENM from a personal series of 14 PME, including three patients with Lafora's diseases, seven with Unverricht–Lundborg diseases, one with MERRF and three with the adult form of ceroid-lipofuscinosis. However, ENM is probably an underestimated, aspecific sign that may be encountered in various generalized or partial epileptic conditions, classified as idiopathic, symptomatic or cryptogenic: apart from PME, benign epilepsy with centrotemporal spikes and neuronal migration disorders are probably the most frequent epileptic syndromes in which ENM is not unusual.

Focal epilepsies of adolescence

Symptomatic and/or cryptogenic focal epilepsies beginning in adolescence may also lead to severe injurious epileptic falls, most often by a direct ictal mechanism, particularly in frontal lobe epilepsies (Pazzaglia *et al.*, 1985; So, 1995). When a cardiac arrhythmia occurs in association with an epileptic seizure, mainly of temporal lobe origin, a syncope may lead the patient to fall (Howell & Blumhardt, 1989). Focal ENM has also been described in central and parietal epilepsies (Suisse *et al.*, 1995). These notions will be developed in a specific chapter (Biraben *et al.*, this volume).

Acknowledgements

We thank Dr Pierre Genton for his expert reviewing of the manuscript. We also thank Prof C. Marescaux and Dr E. Hirsch who gave us the opportunity to study their JME patients, and Dr G. Suisse who performed silent period locked averaging in some of our PME patients.

References

Andermann, F. & Tenenbaum, S. (1995): Negative motor phenomena in generalized epilepsies. A study of atonic seizures. In: *Negative motor phenomena*, eds. S. Fahn, M. Hallett, H.O. Luders, C.D. Marsden, pp. 9–26. New York: Raven Press.

Asconape, J. & Penry, J.K. (1984): Some clinical and EEG aspects of juvenile myoclonic epilepsy. *Epilepsia* **25**, 108–114.

Battaglia, D., Genton, P., Remy C., Bureau C. & Dravet C. (1995): Effet antimyoclonique du piracetam dans l'épilepsie myoclonique progressive de type Unverricht–Lundborg: observation clinique et vidéo. *Epilepsies* **7**, 387–391.

Berkovic, S.F., Cochius, J., Andermann, E. & Andermann F. (1993): Progressive myoclonus epilepsies: clinical and genetic aspects. *Epilepsia* **34**, (S3), S19–S30.

Commission on classification and terminology of the International League Against Epilepsy (1981): Proposal for revised clinical and electroencephalographic classification of epileptic seizures. *Epilepsia* **22**, 489–501.

Delgado-Escueta, A.V. & Enrile-Bascal, F. (1984). Juvenile myoclonic epilepsy of Janz. *Neurology* **34**, 285–294.

Durner, M., Sander, T., Greenberg, D.A., Johnson, K., Beck-Mannageta, G. & Janz, D. (1991): Localization of idiopathic generalized epilepsy on chromosome 6p in families of juvenile myoclonic epilepsy patients. *Neurology* **41**, 1651–1655.

Gastaut, H. (1973): *Dictionnaire de l'épilepsie*. Geneva: Organization Mondiale de la Sante.

Gastaut, H. (1984): Discussion concerning myoclonic epilepsies and the Lennox–Gastaut syndrome (summarized by O. Henricksen). In: *Epileptic syndromes of infancy childhood and adolescence*, eds. J. Roger, Ch. Dravet, M. Bureau, A. Perret & P.Wolf, pp. 100–101. London: John Libbey.

Genton, P., Salas-Puig, X., Tunon, A., Lahoz, C. & Del Socorro Gonzalez Sanchez, M. (1994): Juvenile myoclonic epilepsy and related syndromes: clinical and neurophysiological aspects. In: *Idiopathic generalized epilepsies: clinical, experimental and genetic aspects*, eds. A. Malafosse, P. Genton, E. Hirsch, C. Marescaux, D. Broglin & R. Bernasconi, pp. 229–251. London: John Libbey.

Greenberg, D.A., Delgado-Escueta, A.V., Maldonado, H.M. & Widelitz, H. (1988a): Segregation analysis of juvenile myoclonic epilepsy. *Genetic Epidemiol.* **5,** 81–94.

Greenberg, D.A., Delgado-Escueta A.V., Widelitz, H., Sparkes R.S., Treiman, L., Maldonado, H.M., Park, M.S. & Terasaki P. (1988b): Juvenile myoclonic epilepsy (JME) may be linked to the BF and HLA loci on human chromosome 6. *Am. J. Med. Genet.* **31,** 185–192.

Grunewald, R.A. & Panayiotopoulos, C.P. (1993): Juvenile myoclonic epilepsy. A review. *Arch. Neurol.* **50,** 594–598.

Guerrini, R., Dravet, C., Genton, P., Bureau, M., Roger, J., Rubboli, G. & Tassinari, C.A. (1993): Epileptic negative myoclonus. *Neurology* **43,** 1078–1083.

Herpin, T. (1867): *Des accès incomplets d'épilepsie*. Paris: Baillere.

Howell, S.J. & Blumhardt, L.D. (1989): Cardiac asystole associated with epileptic seizures: a case report with simultaneous EEG and ECG. *J. Neurol. Neurosurg. Psychiatry* **52,** 795–798.

Janz, D. & Christian, W. (1957): Impulsiv petit mal. *Dtsch Z. Nervenheilk.* **176,** 346–386.

Janz, D. (1985): Epilepsy with impulsive petit mal (juvenile myoclonic epilepsy). *Acta Neurol. Scand.* **72,** 449–459.

Janz, D. & Christian, W. (1994): Impulsive Petit Mal (translated in English by P. Genton). In: *Idiopathic generalized epilepsies: clinical, experimental and genetic aspects,*. eds. A. Malafosse, P. Genton, E. Hirsch, C. Marescaux, D. Broglin & R. Bernasconi. pp. 229–251. London: John Libbey.

Lancman, M.E., Asconape, J.J. & Penry, J.K. (1994): Clinical and EEG asymmetries in juvenile myoclonic epilepsy. *Epilepsia* **35,** 302–306.

Liu, A.W, Delgado-Escueta, A.V., Serratosa, J.M., Alonso M.E., Medina, M.T., Gee, M.N., Cordova, S., Zhao, H.Z., Spellman, J.M., Ramos Peek, J.R., Robio-Donnadiau, F.R. & Sparkes, R.S. (1995): Juvenile myoclonic epilepsy locus in chromosome 6p21.2–p11: linkage to convulsion and electroencephalographic trait. *Am. J. Hum. Genet.* **S7,** 368–381.

Loiseau, P. & Duche B. (1990): Épilepsie myoclonique juvénile. *Rev. Neurol.* **146,** 719–725.

Mai, R., Canevini, M.P., Pontrelli, V., Tassi, L., Bertin, C., Di Marco, C. & Canger, R. (1990). L'epilessia mioclonica giovanile di Janz: analisi prospettica di un campione di 57 pazienti. *Boll. Lega It. Epil.* **70/71,** 307–309.

Manon-Espaillat, R., Osorio, I., Badour, R. & Remler, B. (1987): Epileptic drop attacks in juvenile myoclonic epilepsy. *Epilepsia* **28,** S614.

Obeid T. & Panayiotopoulos, C.P. (1988): Juvenile myoclonic epilepsy: a study in Saudi Arabia. *Epilepsia* **32,** 672–676.

Oguni, H., Mukahira, K., Oguni, M., Uehara, T., Su, Y.H., Izumi T. & Fukuyama, Y. (1994): Video-polygraphic analysis of myoclonic seizures in juvenile myoclonic epilepsy. *Epilepsia* **35,** 307–316.

Panayiotopoulos, C.P., Obeid, T. & Waheed, G. (1989): Absences in juvenile myoclonic epilepsy: a clinical video-EEG study. *Ann. Neurol.* **25,** 391–397.

Panayiotopoulos, C.P., Tahan, A. R. & Obeid T. (1991): Juvenile myoclonic epilepsy: factors of error involved in the diagnosis and treatment. *Epilepsia* **32,** 672–676.

Panayiotopoulos, C.P., Obeid, T. & Tahan, A.R. (1994): Juvenile myoclonic epilepsy: a 5-year prospective study. *Epilepsia* **35,** 285–296.

Pazzaglia, P., Giovanardi-Rossi, P., Cirignotta, F., Gaudenzi, G. & Lugaresi, E. (1977): Il problema clinico e nosografico delle epilessie generalizzate. Le epilessie generalizzate intermediarie. *Riv. Neurol.* **45**, 359–391.

Pazzaglia, P., D'Alessandro, R., Ambrosetto, G., Lugaresi, E. (1985): Drop attacks: an ominous change in the evolution of partial epilepsy. *Neurology* **35**, 1725–1730.

Roger, J., Genton, P., Bureau, M. & Dravet, C. (1992): Progressive myoclonus epilepsy in children and adolescence. In: *Epileptic syndromes of infancy, childhood and adolescence,* 2nd edn, eds. J. Roger, M. Bureau, Ch. Dravet, F.E. Dreifuss, A. Perret & P. Wolf, pp. 381–400. London: John Libbey.

Roger, J., Remy, C., Bureau, M., Oller-Daurella, L., Beaumanoir, A., Favel, P. & Dravet, Ch. (1987): Le syndrome de Lennox–Gastaut chez l'adulte. *Rev. Neurol.* **143**, 401–405.

Salas-Puig, X., Camara da Silva, A.M., Dravet, C. & Roger, J. (1990). L'épilepsie myoclonique juvenile dans la population du Centre Saint-Paul. *Epilepsies* **2**, 108–113.

Tassinari, C.A. (1981): New perspectives in epileptology. In: *Trends in modern epileptology,* ed. Japanese Epilepsy Association. Proceedings of the International Public Seminar on Epileptology, pp. 42–59. Tokyo: Japanese Epilepsy Association.

Michelucci, R., Volpi, L., Passarelli, D., Meletti, S., Fontana, E., Dalla Bernardina, B., Tassinari, C.A., Rubboli, G., Parmeggiani, L., Valzania, F., Plasmati, R. & Riguzzi, P. (1995): Epileptic negative myoclonus. In: *Negative motor phenomena,* eds. S. Fahn, M. Hallett, H.O. Luders & C.D. Marsden, pp. 181–197. New York: Raven Press.

Shibasaki, H., Ikeda, A., Nagamine, Terada, K., Nishitani, N., Kanda, M., Takano, S., Hanazono, T., Kohara, N. et al., (1994): Cortical reflex negative myoclonus. *Brain* **116**, 477–486.

So, N.K. (1995): Atonic phenomena end partial seizures. A reappraisal. In: *Negative motor phenomena,* eds. S. Fahn, M. Hallett, H.O. Luders & C.D. Marsden, pp. 29–39, New York: Raven Press.

Suisse, G., Thomas P., Borg, M. & Dolisi, C. (1995). Myoclonies négatives épileptiques. Application de la technique du moyennage rétrograde. *Epilepsies* **7**, 409–417.

Thomas, P., Meneguz, C., Alchaar, H., Suisse, G. & Desnuelle, C. (1994): Pure cortical negative action myoclonus showing Lafora disease. *Epilepsia* **35**, (S7), 37–38.

Ugawa, Y., Shimpo, T. & Mannen, T. (1989): Physiological asterixis: silent period locked averaging. *J. Neurol. Neurosurg. Psychiatry* **52**, 89–92.

Vogt, H. & Mothersill, I.W. (1995): Epileptic and non-epileptic negative myoclonus in patients with progressive myoclonus epilepsies. *Epilesia* **36**, (S3), 116.

Weissbecker, K.A., Durner, M., Janz, D., Scaramelli, A., Sparkes, R.S. & Spence, M.A. (1991): Confirmation of linkage between juvenile myoclonic epilepsy locus and the HLA region of chromosome 6. *Am. J. Med. Genet.* **38**, 32–36.

Whitehouse, W.P., Pees, M., Curtis, D., Sundqvist, A., Parker, K., Chung, E., Baralle, D. & Gardiner, M. (1993): Linkage analysis of idiopathic generalized epilepsy (IGE) and marker loci on chromosome 6p in families of patients with juvenile myoclonic epilepsy: no evidence for an epilepsy locus in the HLA region. *Am. J. Hum. Genet.* **53**, 652–662.

Wolf, P. (1992): Juvenile myoclonic epilepsy. In: *Epileptic syndromes of infancy, childhood and adolescence,* 2nd edn, eds. J. Roger, M. Bureau, Ch. Dravet, F.E. Dreifuss, A. Perret & P.Wolf, pp. 313–327, London: John Libbey.

vestibular projection (Leigh, 1994; Friberg *et al.*, 1985). The fact that auditory stimulation may provoke this aura in this patient after cortectomy might reinforce this hypothesis.

Patients with paroxysmal impairment of axial tone and posture

These fourteen patients all had brief attacks in common. The falls were due to an axial hypertonic access, like the 'trunk fit' described by Jackson (1958) or the 'axial tone fit' described by Gastaut (1972). The interictal EEG showed synchronous or asynchronous spikes or polyspikes, mainly located on bi-frontal areas. An ictal EEG showed a bilateral and not localizable fast discharge during the hypertonic fit.

A depth electrode exploration was decided for these patients on the following reasons:

- the fugacious existence of clinical symptoms calling forth a more focalized origin, preceding the hypertonic attack;
- a reflex component triggering the fits in two patients;
- the existence of a unique lesion on MRI;
- stable lateralizable EEG spiking focus in addition to diffuse abnormalities.

In summary, SEEG permitted us to find:

(1) For two cases, a 'localizable' origin of the fits. In these two, during 1–2 s, there were symptoms preceding the hypertonic fit (in the first case, an undefinable feeling of strangeness during less than one second reported after the fit; in the other, a lateral inclination with a slight rotation of the head during less than 2 s). In both cases, there was a frontal lesion. A lesionectomy associated with a cortectomy was proposed and achieved on these two patients. They are both seizure free since the operation (more than two years of delay).

(2) In the two cases of reflex epilepsy, a focal origin was found; these two patients were affected by an extensive birth lesion near the central area. A cortectomy was achieved on these two patients. In one case, the cortectomy concerned the whole fronto-central convexity, including the corresponding internal cortex, and the patient has not had a new fit for the last three years. In the other case, the cortectomy was more limited to the low part of this central area because of the absence of a clear clinical deficit (cf. next example).

Patient SER...S. was 34 years old when we first saw her. When she was 2 months old, she underwent a left fronto-parietal irradiation for a cutaneous angioma of the scalp. When she was 6 months old, the diagnosis of right hemiparesis was made, and when she was 10 years old, the first fits were observed. Attacks were of various types:

- partial attack with a brutal hypertony of the right superior limb with full consciousness;
- a brutal fall of the head with hypersalivation;
- a brutal, violent and hypertonic fall as if someone had pushed her backwards and to the right. Falls happened several times a day.

All these seizures might start due to being surprised or an unexpected noise or tactile stimulus.

The clinical examination showed a right hemiparesis essentially concerning the hand, and to a

Chapter 12 Falls in epileptic seizures with partial onset

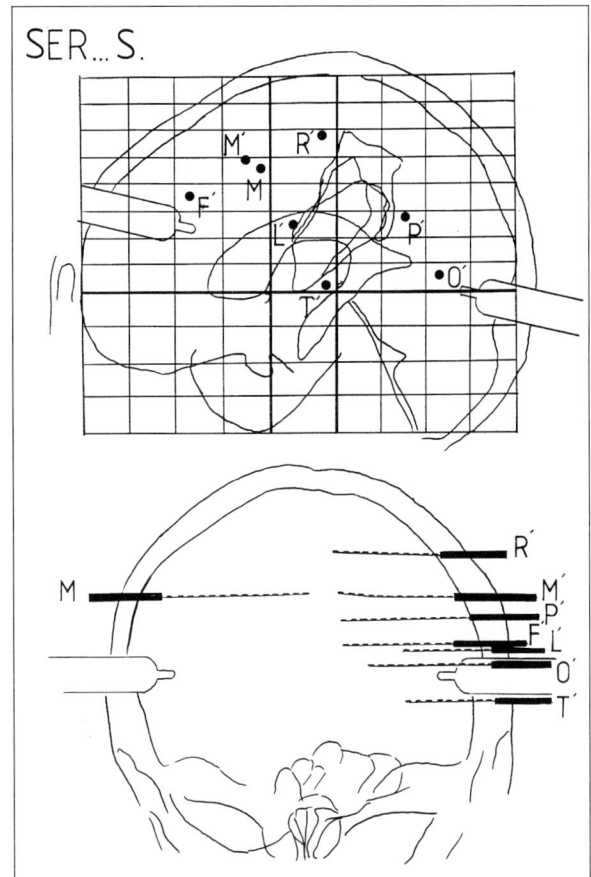

Fig. 3 (top). Patient SER...S: Schematic diagram of intracerebral electrode implantation. Seven electrodes are implanted in the left hemisphere, and one in the right hemisphere. M and M' electrodes explore the SMA (internal leads) and medial frontal gyrus (external leads). R' and L' explore the central sulcus region towards the front of the lesion; F' the prefrontal region; P' expores the temporo-parietal junction behind the lesion, and the posterior cingulate gyrus (internal leads); and O' the occipital region and T' the superior temporal gyrus.

Fig. 4 (below). Patient SER...S: Shows tonic seizure triggered by an unexpected sound. Seizure onset is marked by a spike followed by a fast discharge in L', R' spreading to M' and M.

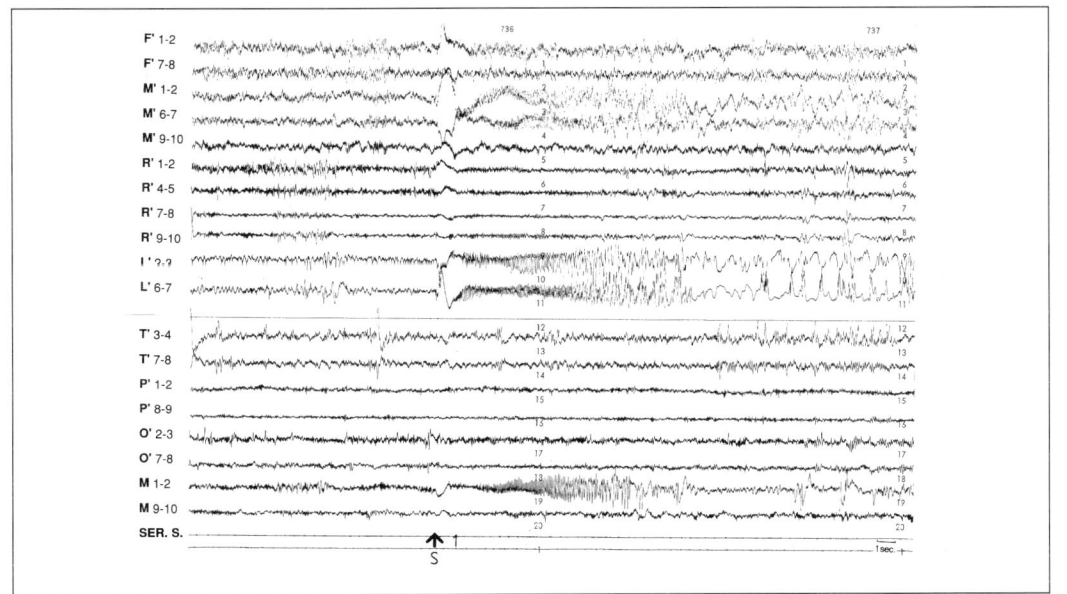

lesser extent, the rest of this superior limb, but very mildly the inferior limb. She has a normal socio-professional insertion, she is married and works as an accountant in the civil service.

The MRI showed a restricted lesion of the left low-centro-parietal area.

The interictal EEG showed either left fronto-central or bi-fronto-parietal paroxysmal anomalies.

In the ictal EEG, during the hypertonic fits, which always prevailed on the right, there was a fast bilateral fronto-centro-parietal discharge prevailing on the left.

When comparing the SEEG in Figures 3 and 4, there was a lesional activity on the outer plots of electrodes R', L'; an irritative activity (quick spikes or flushes of spike-wave) on the outer leads of electrodes R', L', spreading to inner M' and M secondarily. As for fits, they started by a fast discharge on the outer plots of electrode R' spreading to L' and, less constantly, tonically to M' and M.

In response to these facts, to the normality of the activity recorded on electrodes P, M', M, F' and T' and mostly to the patient's insistence of having no new postoperative deficit, an external left fronto-central cortectomy was achieved. Unhappily, since then she has had a few fits (1–2 a week) with falls linked to an ictal hypertony of the inferior limbs. This emphasizes the important part of the internal cortex in this kind of seizures as shown in Chauvel *et al.* (1987) where the physiopathology of startle epilepsy is detailed.

In the ten other cases of tonic seizures, the SEEG shows a very wide origin to fits which did not permit us to propose a focal cortectomy. For seven of these patients, a callosotomy was achieved – see next two examples.

Patient TRE...: She was 11 years old at the time of examination. At the age of 6 months a right hemiplegia was discovered due to a porencephalic lesion in the sylvian artery territory seen on the MRI. At the age of 6 years the first seizures appeared, clinically described as a very brief loss of consciousness with pallor; at the age of 9 years the second type of seizure appeared beginning with a loss of consciousness followed by a brief flexion of the neck, then a rotation of the head to the left with the elevation of both upper limbs and a fall backward. Seizures lasted about 10 s.

The clinical examination showed a right hemiparesia. There is no intellectual impairment; the young girl is at school.

The interictal EEG showed permanent slow activity on the left hemisphere, and synchronous rhythmic spike-wave activity 2–3 c/s predominating sometimes on the left side. Clinically, nothing is observed during these abnormalities.

In the ictal EEG, the clinical fits appear after a big, slow and sharp potential followed by a bilateral flattening.

When comparing the SEEG in Figures 5 and 6 the hypertonic seizures are contemporary with a fast discharge on the M, M' electrodes and less permanently on the P electrode. There is spike and wave activity on the other electrodes at the same time.

An anterior callosotomy was performed in this patient 28 months ago. No seizure happened since this operation.

So, for this patient, a unilateral lesion determined a dramatic improvement with a disconnection of these two precentral areas. These two regions were responsible of the hypertonic fits when fast discharging together.

Chapter 12 Falls in epileptic seizures with partial onset

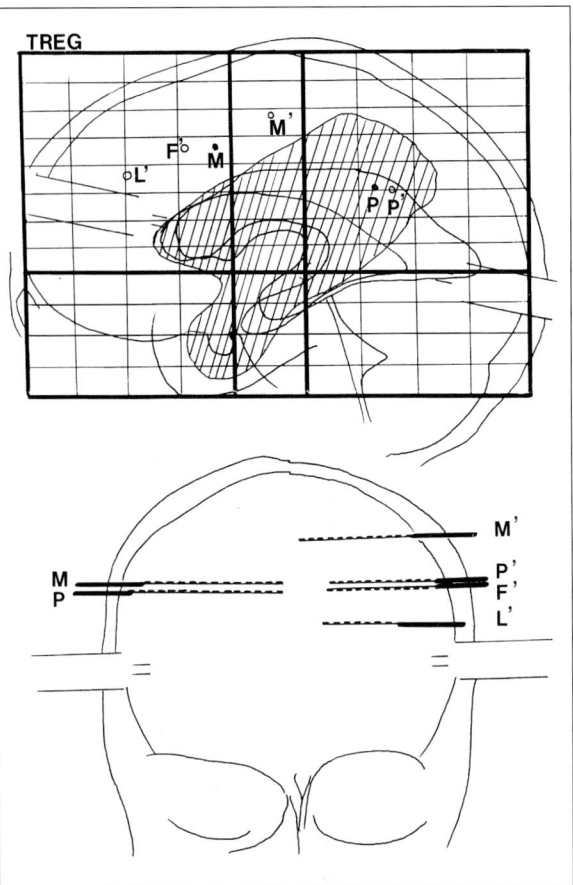

Fig. 5 (top). Patient TREG: Schematic diagram of intracerebral electrode implantation. The dashed area is the projection of the lesion. Four electrodes are implanted in the left hemisphere and two in the right one. P' explores the parietal lesion region; M' is located towards the front of the central sulcus; and F' explores the medial frontal gyrus whereas L' is more forward. M explores the SMA right side, and the medial frontal gyrus.

Fig. 6 (below). Patient TREG: Spike and wave discharge on M, M', P, P', L'. Then at the onset of the tonic flexion of the head and the trunk, a fast discharge appears on M and M' electrodes and irregular spikes on P, P', L' electrodes. The electrode F' does not seem to be involved in this seizure.

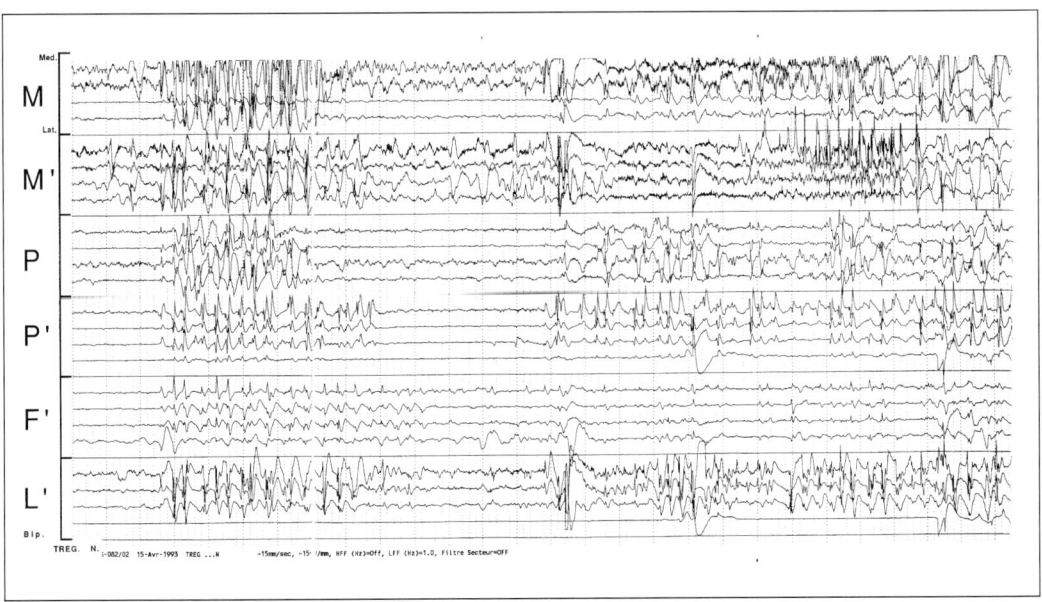

131

Patient BRIC...: is a 28-year-old women. The epilepsy began at the age of 14 by a generalized tonic-clonic seizure. With medication and until examination she presented two types of seizures:

(1) little seizures occurring only when she is seated. They begin with a sudden loss of consciousness, little movements of her eyelids – some eyes movements as if she was looking for something – then an inclination of her head occurs with some simple automatisms of her both hands;

(2) seizures occurring when she is standing up, beginning the same way, the inclination of her head is followed by a sudden traumatizing fall forwards or backwards.

She had many difficulties at school, but she passed a qualification for accountancy. Neurological examination is normal interictally.

The brain imaging is normal (TDM, IRM, interictal SPECT).

The interictal EEG shows permanent slow waves on both hemispheres, mainly on posterior regions. Many spikes are apparent, of various locations, especially on the right-anterior and on left-posterior areas spreading to the homologous region contralaterally.

For the ictal EEG, 10 s before the first clinical sign, the EEG showed a flattening in all derivations followed by a fast discharge involving all the derivations. This fast discharge slowed and stopped, lasting for about 10 s.

Depth-electrode exploration was planned to point out the antero-posterior repartition of interictal and ictal abnormalities before a possible callosotomy.

A comparison of the SEEG in Figures 7 and 8 consistently showed an altered activity in the P, T, P' and T' electrodes: the electrical activity remaining almost normal in the anterior regions. Numerous interictal paroxysms have been recorded in P, T, P' and sometimes T' electrodes. During seizures, the paroxysmal discharge onset begins in P, T, P' and T' electrodes, spreading very fast to the frontal electrodes bilaterally. In this bi-posterior epilepsy, no anterior callosotomy was proposed. One year after this exploration, seeing her handicap, and because of her insistence, an anterior callosotomy is performed in another centre in her region. Unfortunately she has almost the same amount of falls postoperatively.

The main point of interest in this report is that the SEEG predicted a poor result of a two-third anterior callosotomy, showing the onset of the seizures in the two TPO junctions a few seconds before the bi-frontal activation.

Anterior callosotomies performed

Anterior callosotomy was performed when the SEEG proved an anterior bilateral onset of the seizures. This surgical procedure was not used if the onset was generalized, or bilaterally posterior.

The results and post-surgical delays are recorded in Table 1. The number of explored and operated patients is quite low and does not allow any general conclusion to be made.

Two patients do not experience any more seizures. In these two cases, postoperative delay is more than two years: seizure onset was located close to the fronto-central area, and not the prefrontal explored areas. Is it due to the surgical procedure itself or to the disconnection of a bilateral epileptogenic zone (disconnection of a 'critical mass')?

In the only case where the anterior callosotomy did not really improve the patient (case BRA),

Chapter 12 Falls in epileptic seizures with partial onset

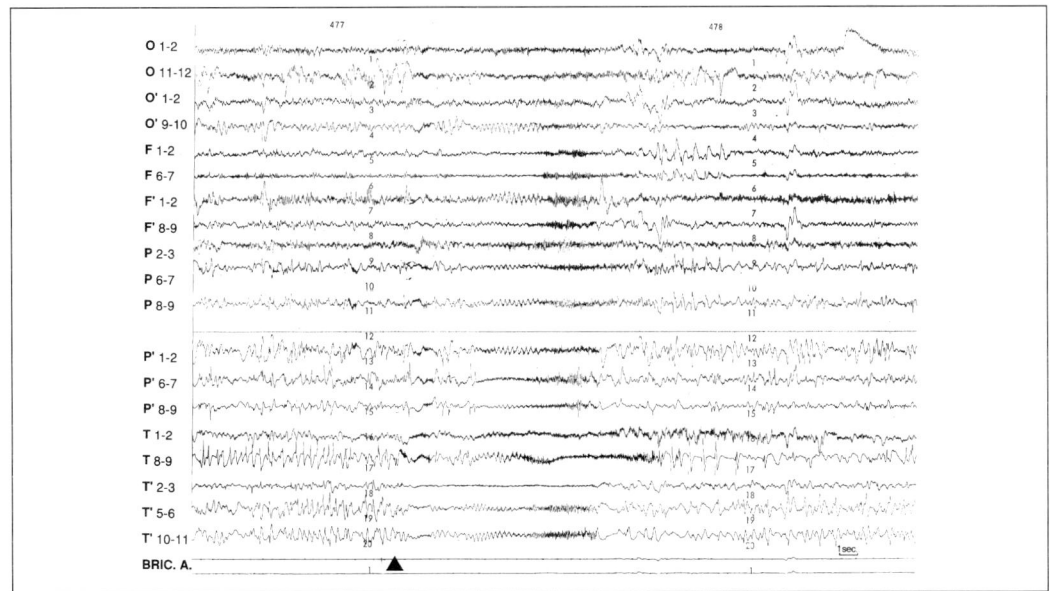

Fig. 7 (top). Patient BRIC: Schematic diagram of intracerebral electrode implantation. Four electrodes are placed in each hemisphere: T and T' in the posterior part of the temporal lobe; P and P' in the parietal lobe; F and F' in the prefrontal area; and O and O' in the orbito-frontal area.

Fig. 8 (below). Patient BRIC: At the onset of the spontaneous seizure (triangle), there is a fast discharge on T, P, then P', T' electrodes. Secondly, a rhythmic activity and a fast activity appears on every electrode. The tonic-clonic inclination of her head appears a few seconds after the discharge spreads to every electrode.

the depth-electrode exploration showed a posterior onset of the seizures. The four patients with anterior frontal onset of their seizures did improve, with the disappearance of falls during seizures. Only one patient still has a few falls occurring less than one a month instead of one a day (patient BER).

Table 1. Results of callostomy after SEEG exploration

Patient name	MRI	Postoperative result	Postoperative delay per month	Seizure onset (SEEG)
EDR	lesion	no seizures	67	bi-central
BER	lesion	improved	38	bi-frontal
BRA	normal	not improved	32	bi-TPO junction
ROB	normal	no more falls	28	bi-frontal
TRE	lesion	no seizures	28	bi-central
PEU	normal	no more falls	15	bi-frontal
VAL	normal	no more falls	12	bi-frontal

The seizure onset column shows the SEEG data: bi-central meaning that the onset of the seizures leading to a fall is located close to the central areas; bi-frontal means that it was not possible to distinguish a focal onset in the frontal lobes; bi-TPO junction means that the onset was posterior bilaterally.

Conclusions

Falls in epileptic seizures with partial onset may be seen in four main circumstances:

(1) During the generalization of a seizure with partial onset.

(2) If there is an involvement of equilibration areas, particularly some of the cortical projections of vestibular origin as seen in the first example. In this particular case, the posterior part of the insular cortex and the most internal and posterior part of the superior temporal gyrus may be involved.

(3) If there is an involvement of the postural areas, especially the mesial frontal pericentral cortex.

(4) During seizures where autonomic symptoms may be responsible for a fall. We did not explore any patient with such symptoms.

An anterior callosotomy had been performed in the patients when the SEEG proved an anterior bilateral onset of the seizures. This surgical procedure has, in this experience, a poor result if performed on patients with a bilateral posterior onset, even if there is a bilateral anterior propagation.

Further exploration of candidates for callosotomy will help in the selection of good candidates for such treatment. In our experience, some patients with clinical 'trunk fits' may have a bi-posterior onset of seizures and the anterior callosotomy will have a poor result. In our series, the best result of this surgical treatment is obtained if seizure onset is close to the central area. This series is too short to yield strong conclusions and needs more cases, but it might help in the decision of callosotomy.

References

Bancaud, J., Talairach, J., Bonis, A., Schaub, A., Szickla, G., Morel, P. & Bordas-Ferrer, M. (1965): *La stéréoélectroencéphalographie dans l'épilepsie.* Paris: Masson.

Broglin, D. & Bancaud, J. (1991): Manifestations neurovégétatives au cours des crises partielles du lobe temporal. *CP en epileptologie,* Rennes.

Chauvel, P., Vignal, J.P., Liegeois Chauvel, C., Chodkiewicz, J.P., Talairach, J. & Bancaud, J. (1987): Startle epilepsy with infantile brain damage: the clinical and neurophysiological rationale for surgical therapy. In: *Presurgical evaluation of epilepsies,* eds. H.G. Wieser & E. Elger, pp. 306–307. Springler-Verlag: Berlin, Heidelberg.

Friberg, L., Olsen, T.S., Roland, P.E. & Lassen N.A., (1985): Focal increase of blood flow in the cerebral cortex of man during vestibular stimulation. *Brain* **108,** 609–623.

Gastaut, H. & Broughton, R. (1972): *Epileptic seizures. Clinical and electrographic features, diagnosis and treatment,* pp. 41–44.

Jackson, H. (1958): *Selected writings,* ed. J. Taylor, pp. 474 and 482. London: Staples Press.

Leigh, R.J. (1994): Human vestibular cortex. *Ann. Neurol.* **35,** 383–384.

Penfield, W. & Jasper, H. (1954): *Epilepsy and the functional anatomy of the human brain.* Boston: Little, Brown.

Chapter 13

Outcome of children's epileptic falls

Pierre Loiseau*, Pierre Jallon† and Jean-Michel Pédespan‡

*Department of Neurology, University Hospital, Bordeaux, France;
†Clinical Epileptology Unit, Department of Neurology, University Hospital, Geneva, Switzerland;
‡Department of Paediatrics, University Hospital, Bordeaux, France

Summary

The study addresses the long-term outcome of childhood epilepsies with ictal falls to the ground. Eighty-three patients were followed up to adult age. To consider the group of patients as a whole was found to be extremely unrewarding because of very heterogeneous data. A syndromic approach was more rewarding. Falls occur in each syndrome with more- or less-specific characteristics, and the prognoses for the various syndromes appear to be different.

Introduction

Falls to the ground are a frequent sign observed in many types of epileptic seizures and in many of the epileptic syndromes. Therefore, a common outcome is unlikely. Falls have been reported as an ominous sign in the evolution of partial epilepsy (Pazzaglia et al., 1985) and in a severity scale (Duncan & Sander, 1991). Little research has been carried out to study the extent of this problem. Some data may be collected indirectly; that is, in studies on seizure-related injuries (Ziegler et al., 1994; Russell-Jones & Shorvon, 1989; Finelli & Cardi, 1989; Annegers et al., 1989). However, seizure types were rarely defined, most patients probably had tonic-clonic generalized seizures, and all the reported injuries were not due to falls. Nakken & Lossius (1993) found that the highest incidence of seizure-induced injuries occurred in association with atonic seizures, followed by generalized tonic-clonic seizures, while it has been said that only patients who fall stiffly, such as patients with tonic or tonic-clonic seizures, are at risk, and not those who fall with atonia (Russell-Jones & Shorvon, 1989). The present study, which is not a case-control study, tried to evaluate retrospectively the outcome of a cohort of children with epilepsy and falls to the ground.

Patients and methods

We performed a retrospective study, where paediatric outpatients seen in both private and

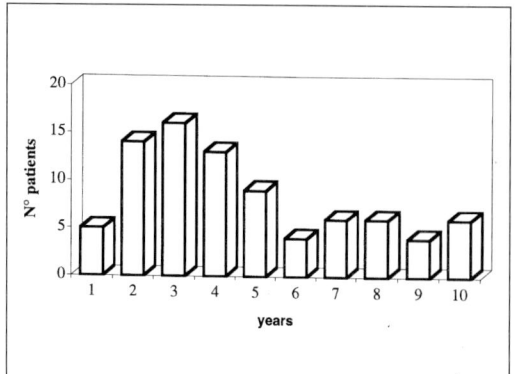

Fig. 1. Age at epilesy onset (n = 83).

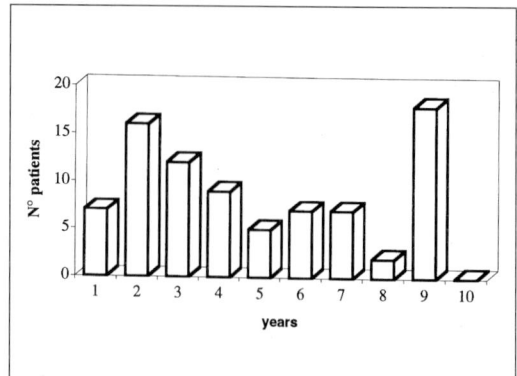

Fig. 2. Age at falls onset.

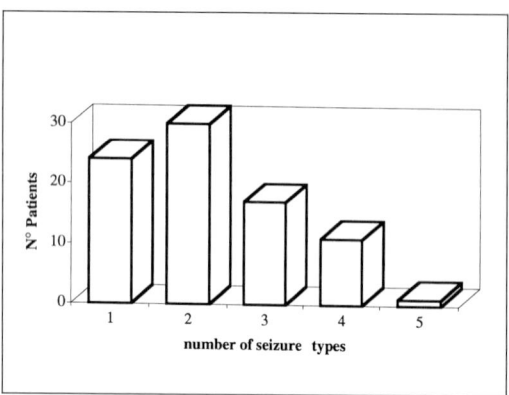

Fig. 3. Number of seizure types per patient.

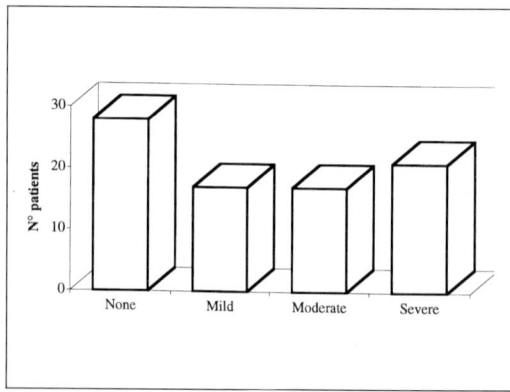

Fig. 4. Mental impairment (n = 83).

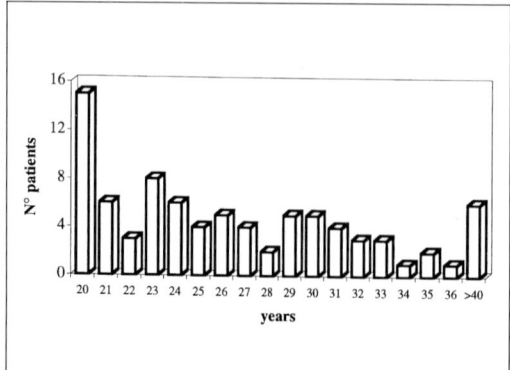

Fig. 5. Age at follow-up.

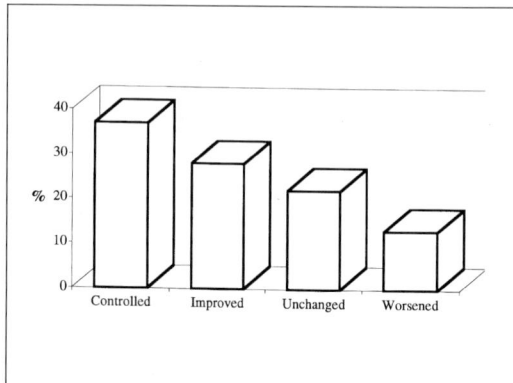

Fig. 6. Epilepsy outcome at follow-up (n = 83).

hospital practices, aged under 10 years old at first epileptic seizure and with seizures associated with falls, have been followed up to adult life (>19 years old).

Patients with falls due to primary or secondary generalized tonic-clonic seizures were excluded. Special attention has been paid to the past medical history of the patients, age at seizure onset, age at fall onset, type(s) of seizure(s) according to the International Classification of Epileptic Seizures (Commission, 1981), epileptic syndrome according to the International Classification of Epilepsies and Epileptic Syndromes (Commission, 1989), neurological and mental interictal status and the EEG records. The long-term outcome of seizures and falls was studied. Data were collected by direct consultation, mail or phone contact to their practitioners or their family.

Results

One-hundred-and-forty-two patients were studied. Five died before age 20 as a result of brain tumour (2), seizure disorder (2), and septic shock (1). Forty-nine (42 per cent) were unavailable to follow up. However, 83 patients were included in the present study. There were 48 males and 35 females.

Overall analysis

The age of epilepsy and fall onset lies, by definition, between 0.1 to 10 years. The mean and median age for epilepsy onset were 3.7 years, and 3 years, respectively. Figure 1 shows a unimodal curve, with a peak at 2–3 years. The mean and median age for fall onset were 4.8 years, and 4 years, respectively. Figure 2 shows a bimodal curve, with two peaks: at 2–3 years and 9–10 years.

Seizures were classified as partial motor seizures (33 patients), generalized tonic-clonic seizures (22 patients), myoclonic seizures (21 patients), tonic seizures (18 patients), atonic seizures (18 patients), atonic absences (17 patients), simple absences (15 patients), partial complex seizures (13 patients), myoclonic absences (8 patients), and infantile spasms (4 patients). The number of different types of seizures per patient is given in Figure 3. Of course, some types of seizures, for instance, infantile spasms or generalized tonic-clonic seizures, were not responsible for falls, due to other seizures in the same patient. On the EEG, paroxysmal activity was recorded as generalized in 29 patients, focalized in 48 and absent in six patients.

Risk factors were found in 26 patients only (31 per cent) and included perinatal anoxia (8 patients), encephalitis (7 patients), Bourneville's and Sturge-Weber's disease (2 patients each), intracerebral bleeding (1 patient), malformation (1 patient), Kern's icterus (1 patient) and progressive myoclonic epilepsy (1 patient). Eight patients had a hemiplegia or hemiparesia, three had cerebellar signs, and three bilateral pyramidal signs. Their mental status is summarized in Figure 4.

The patients' ages at follow-up ranged from 20 to 54 years: mean, 27 years; median, 25 years (see Fig. 5).

At follow-up, 31 patients were controlled, 23 had less frequent seizures, 18 were unchanged, and 11 had more frequent seizures (Fig. 6). Falls were no longer experienced by 54 patients. They had ceased before 10 years of age in 33 patients, and after age 19 in six patients (Fig. 7). Age at last fall was not available in two patients. Twenty-nine fall-free patients were controlled, sixteen were improved, six were unchanged, and three worsened (Fig. 8).

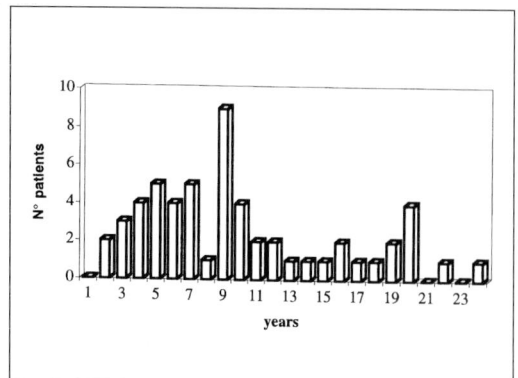

Fig. 7. Age at last fall (n = 52).

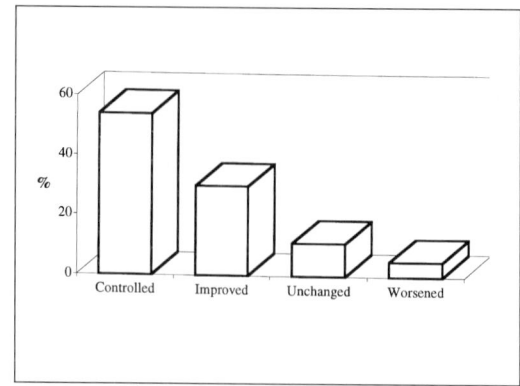

Fig. 8. Epilepsy outcome in 54 fall-free patients.

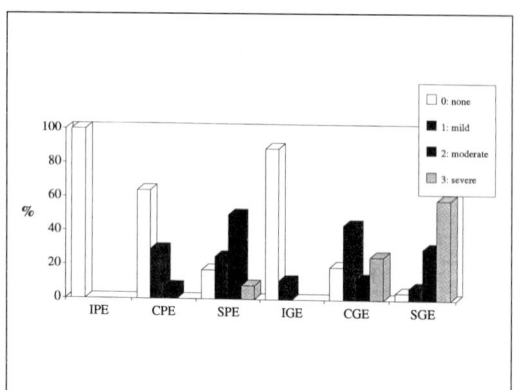

Fig. 9. Patients' mental impairment according to the syndrome (n = 83).

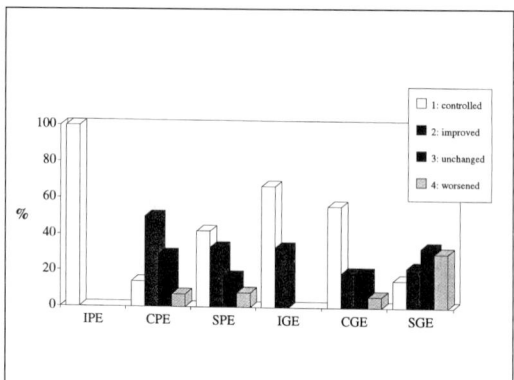

Fig. 10. Epilepsy outcome at follow-up.

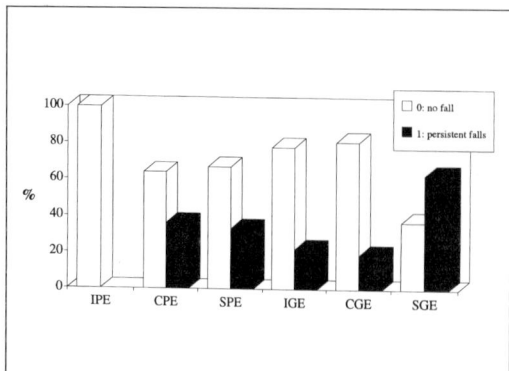

Fig. 11. Falls outcome at follow-up.

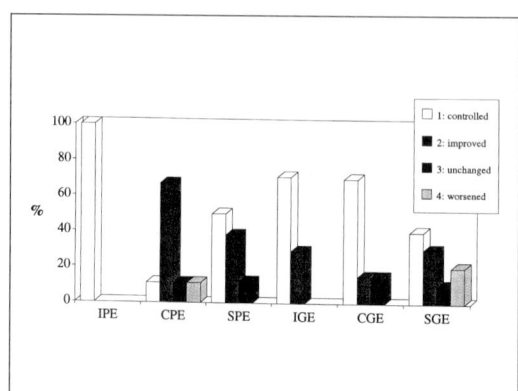

Fig. 12. Epilepsy outcome in fall-free patients.

Syndromic classification

Figures 9 to 12 compare some patients' characteristics according to the epileptic syndromes. Five patients had idiopathic localization-related epilepsies (IPE), fourteen patients had cryptogenic localization-related epilepsies (CPE), twelve had symptomatic localization-related epilepsies (SPE), nine had idiopathic generalized epilepsies (IGE), sixteen had cryptogenic generalized epilepsies (CGE), and 27 had symptomatic generalized epilepsies (SGE).

Discussion

This study allows only qualitative conclusions. Five reasons for bias are likely: (1) many biases could emerge because it is a retrospective study; (2) nearly half of the patients from the initial cohort were lost to follow-up; (3) for many patients, neuro-imaging data were not available; (4) the precise mechanism causing the falls was not known because of the lack of polygraphic records, and (5) too few patients exist in each syndrome.

To consider the group of patients as a whole was disappointing. Data only documented the following evidence: that epileptic falls correspond to various epileptic conditions. They appear at various ages and are due to numerous seizure types. Falls often occur in severe, pharmacoresistant, either partial or generalized epilepsies in severely mentally-impaired patients. Conversely, some patients are, or remain, mentally normal. Falls may disappear, and epilepsy also may be controlled. The outcome with respect to recurrences of falls does not parallel epilepsy outcome.

However, some interesting points appeared. For example, a discrepancy arose between the children's age at seizure onset, and at fall onset. In 30 children, the first fall occurred one year or more after the first seizure, with a lag time of more than three years in twelve. Epilepsy onset before walking age could not be the only explanation.

Considering each epileptic syndrome separately was more rewarding and explained the heterogeneity of our data.

Idiopathic localization-related epilepsies (*n* = 5)

Falls are rare in benign childhood epilepsy with centrotemporal sharp waves. In a personal series (unpublished) of 381 children, it occurred in ten patients. Only five of them were followed up to adult age. Two children experienced an isolated seizure, with an inhibition of muscle tone in the upper and lower limbs contralateral to the EEG focus. Another one had a bout of three cramp-like seizures limited to a leg. Two had many brief focal atonias of a lower limb during several weeks. At the same period, one had myoclonic seizures, and the other one falls due to a diffuse atonia. Their ages at onset of epilepsy and of falls were very close.

A rolandic discharge may inhibit contralateral motor control, as documented by Oguni *et al.* (1992) with a simultaneous video-polygraphic recording of unilateral focal atonia of one arm in seven patients with childhood partial epilepsy. Synchronous involvement of both motor cortices due to the spread of discharges from a unilateral focus might explain more diffuse atonic seizures (Kanazawa *et al.*, 1990; Harvey *et al.*, 1994). Drop attacks are probably unfrequent in benign childhood epilepsy with centrotemporal sharp waves because of predominant involvement of the lower part of the sensorimotor strip. Neither of the two children with frequent seizures had received carbamazepine.

The possibility of epileptic falls in children with idiopathic localization-related epilepsy is important to remember, because it does not modify the outcome of the syndrome. All the patients were mentally normal, and were cured before adult age.

Cryptogenic localization-related epilepsies (n = 14)

This diagnosis was probably over-estimated because no neuro-imaging study was available at the time. The EEG-ascertained epileptogenic area was either frontal, or parietal, or temporal. Temporal onset was documented with scalp EEG in one patient, and with stereo-EEG in an another one. As in idiopathic localization-related epilepsies, no patient experienced more than two types of seizures. Seizures were with or without loss of consciousness, and sometimes secondarily generalized. Falls were felt to be due to unilateral leg drop, movement-induced attack, secondary to a jump from the bed, when asleep, or atonic, secondary to a loss of consciousness. Except in one patient (first seizure at year 1.2, first fall at age 7.5), seizures of other types and falls began at the same time. Most of the patients were intellectually normal. Some had a mild cognitive impairment. At follow-up, only 14 per cent of patients were seizure-free. However, 64 per cent were fall-free.

Symptomatic localization-related epilepsies (n = 12)

Risk factors were present in all the cases. Seizures were mainly inhibitory motor seizures, and also myoclonic jerks, unilateral tonic seizures, and a seizure pattern similar to that found in cryptogenic epilepsies, that is, a loss of consciousness followed by an atonic fall. Different types of seizures in the same patient were more frequent than in the cryptogenic group. Similarly, mental impairment was more frequent, with only 17 per cent of normal patients. Conversely, more patients (42 per cent) were seizure-free at follow-up. The proportion of fall-free patients was the same as in the cryptogenic group. Falls often appeared several years after the first seizure. Such a delay was also noted in partial epilepsies with a later onset (Pazzaglia *et al.*, 1985). Epileptogenic areas were also frontal, parietocentral, and temporal.

Idiopathic generalized epilepsies (n = 9)

Diagnostic criteria of the ICE were strictly used; for example, runs of regular, bilateral spike-waves were mandatory. However, some cases argue for a continuum between idiopathic and other generalized epilepsies with, for instance, some mental impairment, unusual absence seizures, three to four types of seizures, and an unfavourable outcome (one-third of pharmacoresistant patients). Falls occurred rarely in myoclonic seizures, and more often in absence seizures. Some of them were definitely myoclonic or atonic absences whereas, in others, falls were due to an undetermined mechanism. The age at onset of falls was the same as that of other seizures. At follow-up, falls had ceased to exist in 78 per cent of patients, but epilepsy was controlled in only two-thirds of them.

Cryptogenic generalized epilepsies (n = 12)

As for localization-related epilepsies, and for similar reasons, this diagnosis was probably over-estimated. The majority of patients had more than one type of seizure, and mental impairment, which was severe in 25 per cent of this group. Most of the children had absence seizures with falls, and myoclonic absences. Some had tonic or myoclonic seizures. Falls never started more than two years after seizure onset. A little more than half the patients became seizure-free, and falls persisted only in 19 per cent of them.

Symptomatic generalized epilepsies (*n* = 27)

This group is, not surprisingly, the most important. It represents the epileptic syndrome where falls are the most frequently observed (Nakken & Lossius, 1993). The diagnosis of symptomatic generalized epilepsy raised important nosological problems. It was sometimes easy to document; that is, when a child had a history of diffuse cerebral injury, had had infantile spasms, had seizures of many types, showed bilateral slow spike-waves on the EEG, and a progressive mental deterioration. However, one may wonder if phacomatosis or encephalitis caused diffuse cortical lesions. Symptomatic focal and generalized epilepsies do overlap. Furthermore, the Lennox–Gastaut syndrome is not necessarily synonymous with severe epileptogenic encephalopathy of childhood. Eight patients in this series had a clear Lennox–Gastaut pattern: five multifocal, predominantly unilateral cerebral injuries; one a progressive myoclonic epilepsy; and one a non-progressive myoclonic epilepsy. Falls were due to myoclonic, tonic, and atonic seizures. Almost all the patients had several types of seizures. More than 90 per cent of the patients were severely retarded. Several years often separated epilepsy and falls onset, even in children beyond the walking age when experiencing a first seizure. Few patients became seizure-free. However, falls had disappeared in 37 per cent of adult patients, despite persistant seizures in 60 per cent of these fall-free patients.

Conclusions

Epileptic falls are often a gloomy prognostic sign, mainly in symptomatic generalized epilepsies. However, they can cease to exist, even when other types of seizures persist. These outcomes address the question of the indication and the time of a palliative surgery, such as callosotomy.

Falls also occur in less-severe epilepsies, such as cryptogenic and idiopathic generalized epilepsies, and in benign localization-related epilepsies of childhood.

References

Annegers, J.F., Melton III, L.J., Sun, Chien-an & Hauser A.W. (1989): Risk of age-related fractures in patients with unprovoked seizures. *Epilepsia* **30,** 348–355.

Commision on Classification and Terminology of the International League Against Epilepsy (1981): Proposal for revised clinical and electroencephalographic classification of epileptic seizures. *Epilepsia* **22,** 489–501.

Commission on Classification and Terminology of the International League Against Epilepsy (1989): Proposal for revised classification of epilepsies and epileptic syndromes. *Epilepsia* **30,** 389–399.

Duncan, J.S. & Sander, J.W.A.S. (1991): The Chalfont seizure severity scale. *J. Neurol. Neurosurg. Psychiatry* **54,** 873–876.

Finelli, P.F. & Cardi, J.K. (1989): Seizure as a cause of fracture. *Neurology* **39,** 858–860.

Harvey, A.S., Jayakar, P., Resnick, T.R., Duchowny, M.S., Bailey, C.A. & Shield, L.K. (1994): Rolandic drop attacks: partial-onset atonic seizures of axial musculature. *Epilepsia* **35 (suppl. 8),** 14 (abstract).

Kanazawa, O. & Kawai, I. (1990): Status epilepticus characterized by repetitive asymmetrical atonia: two cases accompanied by partial seizures. *Epilepsia* **31,** 536–543.

Nakken, K.O. & Lossius, R. (1993): Seizure-related injuries in multi-handicapped patients with therapy resistant epilepsy. *Epilepsia* **34,** 836–840.

Oguni, H.O., Sato, F., Hayashi, K., Wang, P.J. & Fukuyama, Y. (1992): A study of unilateral brief focal atonia in childhood partial epilepsy. *Epilepsia* **33,** 75–83.

Pazzaglia, P., D'Alessandro, R., Ambrosetto, G. & Lugaresi, E. (1985): Drop attacks: an ominous change in the evolution of partial epilepsy. *Neurology* **35,** 1725–1730.

Russell-Jones, D.L. & Shorvon, S.D. (1989): The frequency and consequences of head injury in epileptic seizures. *J. Neurol. Neurosurg. Psychiatry* **52,** 659–662.

Ziegler, A.L., Reinberg, O. & Deonna, T. (1994): Epilepsie et accidents: Quel risque chez l'enfant ? *Arch. Pediat.* **1,** 801–805.

PART IV

Chapter 14

The pharmacological treatment of epileptic falls

Francesco Viani, Antonino Romeo, Maurizio Viri and Elda Fabiola Gonano

Children's Epilepsy Centre, Ospedale Regina Elena, via Manfredo fanti 6, 20122, Milan, Italy

Summary

Epileptic falls, clinically defined as 'a sudden loss of postural maintenance', may be related to myoclonic, atonic or tonic seizures, or to spasms. There are few and contradictory data in the literature concerning the pharmacological treatment of falls. Our retrospective study evaluated the efficacy of anti-epileptic drugs on the various types of falls related to polygraphically documented spasms, or myoclonic, atonic or tonic seizures in a population of patients with myoclonic-astatic epilepsy (MAE) or Lennox–Gastaut syndrome (LGS).

Of the traditional drugs, sodium valproate (VPA) proved to be the most efficacious in treating myoclonic-atonic seizures in MAE patients, with an efficacy rate of more than 90 per cent whether it was administered alone or in association with clobazam. In LGS patients, VPA was fairly effective in treating tonic seizures, but had less effect on myoclonic-atonic seizures. Vigabatrin was only efficacious in cases of epileptic spasms. Lamotrigine and felbamate led to a more than 50 per cent reduction in the frequency of tonic and myoclonic-atonic seizures in the patients with LGS. Carbamazepine proved to be totally inefficacious, and is even contraindicated because of its tendency to increase the frequency of myoclonic and atonic seizures.

Introduction

For the purposes of this study, 'epileptic falls' are defined as a sudden loss of postural maintenance with a brusque flexion of the head, trunk or lower limbs, that may occur when a patient is standing or sitting (Ikeno *et al.*, 1985; Oguni *et al.*, 1992).

In the case of longer lasting attacks, the falls are associated with a probable alteration in consciousness or vigilance (Commission, 1981; Ikeno *et al.*, 1985; Oguni *et al.*, 1992; Gambardella *et al.*, 1994).

Epileptic falls occur frequently in patients with generalized myoclonic-astatic epilepsies (MAE) (Doose, 1992), as well as in those affected by Lennox–Gastaut syndrome (LGS) (Gastaut *et al.*, 1966). In the latter case, the falls are generally provoked by myoclonic, atonic or tonic seizures, or by epileptic spasms (Gastaut, 1963; Aicardi, 1994; Egli *et al.*, 1985; Ikeno *et al.*, 1985; Yaqub, 1993; Oguni *et al.*, 1992; Donat & Wright, 1991; Talwar *et al.*, 1995).

In these syndromes, the immediate cause of the fall is a sudden massive myoclonia of the lower limbs (myoclonic seizures), a brief episode of myoclony followed by the abolition of muscular tone (myoclonic-atonic seizures), a purely atonic event (atonic seizures) or a sharp increase in muscle tone (tonic seizures or epileptic spasms). These different mechanisms are difficult to distinguish without a polygraphic recording (Aicardi, 1982; Egli et al., 1985).

Epileptic falls are relatively frequent in secondary generalized partial epilepsies, and in those with foci in the central (rolandic) or mid-frontal cortical regions (Ethelberg, 1950).

In temporal lobe epilepsies, falls (or 'temporal syncope') are much rarer and occur in adults many years after the onset of complex partial seizures (Landolt, 1960). They are usually preceded by an aura and followed by alterations in consciousness that last for 1–2 min (Gambardella et al., 1994).

Epileptic falls are difficult to define clinically without the aid of polygraphic recordings. Furthermore, in those studies where they are polygraphically documented, it is difficult to find data concerning the use and efficacy of drugs in their treatment.

Epileptic falls are considered to be resistant to pharmacological therapy, although studies relating to the specific effects of anti-epileptic drugs (AEDs) are very few, dishomogeneous and poorly defined. According to the data in the literature, sodium valproate (VPA) seems to be effective in treating myoclonic and atonic seizures (Henricksen, 1982), and also seems to be fairly efficacious in treating Lennox–Gastaut syndrome (LGS) (Henricksen, 1982, Covanis, 1982).

Benzodiazepines are usually used as add-on therapy, with clonazepam (CZP) being the one that is most frequently used in LGS and related syndromes (Vassella, 1973). Particularly at the beginning, the combination of VPA and CZP seems to be fairly efficacious in treating atypical absences, myoclonic seizures and falls.

Clobazam (CLB) is as effective as CZP, but develops less tolerance and has fewer side-effects (Robertson, 1986).

Phenobarbital and phenitoin are completely inefficacious in treating epileptic falls (Bourgeois, 1995). Ethosuximide (ESM) also seems to be scarcely efficacious, although there are not many reports in the literature concerning its use.

Carbamazepine (CBZ) seems to be ineffective; furthermore, a large number of studies agree in reporting the possible onset or increased frequency of generalized seizures (absences, and myoclonic and atonic seizures) (Shields, 1983; Carter Snead, 1985), and particularly epileptic falls (Bourgeois, 1995), after its use.

The data in the literature relating to vigabatrin (GVG) vary widely, although it is certainly efficacious in the treatment of infantile spasms (Chiron et al., 1991).

A recent study (Feucht & Brantner-Inthaler, 1994) reports a more than 50 per cent reduction in seizure frequency in 85 per cent of 20 children with LGS who were treated with GVG added to VPA: in particular, this reduction was observed in 73 per cent of tonic and 72 per cent of atonic seizures, whereas the frequency of myoclonic seizures increased by 5 per cent. On the other hand, Lortie (1993) reports that vigabatrin leads to an exacerbation of epileptic falls in some LGS patients.

As far as lamotrigine (LTG) is concerned, a recent study has reported the suppression of spasms in 17 per cent of 30 children with West's syndrome (Veggiotti et al., 1994). Some studies indicate the high efficacy of this drug in the treatment of atonic seizures (Wallace, 1993; Binnie,

1993), and it has also proved to be effective in patients with LGS (Timmings & Richens, 1992; Schlumberger *et al.*, 1993), particularly in those with tonic and atonic seizures (Oller *et al.*, 1993).

Felbamate (FBM) has been shown to be effective in LGS (Felbamate Study Group, 1993; Jensen, 1994; Theodore *et al.*, 1995). The Felbamate Study Group in Lennox–Gastaut Syndrome (1993) found that it led to a 34 per cent reduction in the frequency of atonic seizures versus a 9 per cent reduction with placebo.

There are no reports concerning the treatment of epileptic falls with other drugs, such as gabapentin and piracetam.

Given the lack of uniformity of these data in comparison with the electroclinical definition of related to various types of seizure and the efficacy of anti-epileptic drugs, we retrospectively studied a hospital series of patients affected by drop attacks.

Materials and methods

From the population of patients included in the computerized archives of the Children's Epilepsy Centre at Milan's Ospedale Regina Elena since 1 March 1988, we selected a sample that satisfied the following inclusion criteria:

(1) evidence of the presence of epileptic falls;

(2) seizure frequency of more than one per day;

(3) polygraphically recorded seizures.

We retrospectively evaluated the effect of sodium valproate (VPA), carbamazepine (CBZ), vigabatrin (GVG), felbamate (FBM) and lamotrigine (LMT) on the epileptic falls related to the various types of seizure. The selected sample consisted of the following groups of patients:

(1) patients with a first diagnosis of epilepsy with myoclonic-astatic seizures (MAE) treated with VPA (19 patients);

(2) patients with a diagnosis of Lennox–Gastaut syndrome (LGS) treated consecutively or concomitantly with VPA (23 patients), CBZ (18 patients), GVG (11 patients), FBM (9 patients) and LTG (6 patients).

The falls consisted of myoclonic, myoclonic-atonic, atonic and tonic seizures, and epileptic spasms.

The efficacy of the various drugs was evaluated by comparing the number of the different types of seizure observed during the month before the beginning of each treatment with the number observed in the three months preceding the discontinuation of the treatment or the last observation.

Results

Group 1

This group consisted of nineteen patients with a first diagnosis of MAE and falls that were untreated at the time of the first observation, who were selected from a population of 66 patients with the same diagnosis. Their characteristics are shown in Table 1. Fifteen patients had cryptogenic MAE and only four were symptomatic; fifteen patients presented delayed language or psychomotor development. All of the patients suffered from myoclonic or myoclonic-atonic seizures; none of them had ever presented a tonic seizure. The patients were administered VPA alone or in association with CLB.

Of the nineteen patients, twelve responded completely to VPA alone; of the remaining seven, six achieved complete remission after the addition of CLB (Table 2). The doses of VPA ranged from 20 to 60 mg/kg/day; in the majority of the patients, doses of 20 mg/kg/day proved to be efficacious after 1–2 months of treatment.

Table 1. *Effects of sodium valproate (VPA) on epileptic falls in myoclonic-astatic epilepsy (MAE): characteristics of the patients*

Number of patients		19
Sex	Male	11
	Female	8
Age (years)	Mean	2.10 (s. d. 1.7)
	Range	0.6–7.10
	Median	2.9
Epileptic syndrome	Cryptogenic MAE	15
	Symptomatic MAE	4
Neurological examination	Normal	4
	Psychomotor/language retardation	15
Type of seizure	Myoclonic/myoclonic-atonic	19
Seizure frequency		>1 per day
Treatment duration (years)	Mean	5.4 (s. d. 3.7)
	Range	0.8–12.5
	Median	4.5

Table 2. *Effects of sodium valproate (VPA) on the myoclonic-atonic seizures in myoclonic-astatic epilepsy (MAE) (nineteen patients)*

	Complete response	No response	No. patients on VPA-MT/PT
VPA-MT*	12	7	19
VPA-PT	6**	1	7

* VPA-MT is sodium valproate monotherapy. VPA-PT is sodium valproate polytherapy.
** Six of the seven patients who failed to respond to VPA-MT achieved a complete response with a combination of VPA and clobazam (CLB).

Group 2

These patients were all affected by LGS. Twenty-three patients had received VPA, alone or in association with CLB. Their demographic and clinical characteristics are summarized in Table

Table 3. Effects of sodium valproate (VPA) on epileptic falls in Lennox–Gastaut syndrome (LGS) patients: characteristics of the patients

Number of patients		23
Sex	Male	12
	Female	11
Age (years)	Mean	7.1 (s. d. 6.4)
	Range	0.5–23.8
	Median	4.5
Epileptic syndrome	Symptomatic LGS	21
	Cryptogenic LGS	2
Type of seizure causing falls*	Tonic	7
	Myoclonic-atonic	8
	Epileptic spasms	13
Seizure frequency		>1 per day
Treatment duration (years)	Mean	4.9 (s. d. 4.5)
	Range	0.7–14.7
	Median	3.0

* More than one for each patient.

Table 4. Effects of sodium valproate (VPA) on epileptic falls in Lennox–Gastaut syndrome (LGS) patients by type of seizure (twenty-three patients)

Type of seizure	Complete response	Partial response (reduction of seizure frequency >50%)	No response, or reduction of seizure frequency <50%	Number of patients
Tonic	–	3**	4	7
Myoclonic-atonic	1*	2**	5	8
Epileptic spasms	2*	–	11	13

* Sodium valproate monotherapy (VPA-MT). ** Sodium valproate polytherapy (VPA-PT).

3, and the results of treatment in Table 4. All but two were symptomatic. The falls were caused by tonic, myoclonic or atonic seizures, or epileptic spasms.

Seven of these patients suffered from tonic seizures, and three achieved a reduction in frequency of more than 50 per cent; eight patients had myoclonic-atonic seizures, whose frequency was reduced by more than 50 per cent in three (one complete remission). Thirteen patients presented epileptic spasms, of which only two responded completely to VPA monotherapy. Subsequently, CBZ was added to the therapy of eighteen of the VPA-resistant patients, whose characteristics were similar to those described above (Table 5).

CBZ, alone or in association with other traditional drugs, did not lead to a reduction of more than 50 per cent in the frequency of any of the seizure types related to the falls. After the addition of FBM or LTG, three patients with myoclonic-atonic seizures and one with epileptic spasms experienced a more than 50 per cent reduction in seizure frequency, which probably cannot be considered a positive effect of CBZ (Table 6).

Table 5. Effects of carbamazepine (CBZ) on epileptic falls in Lennox–Gastaut syndrome (LGS) patients: characteristics of the patients

Number of patients		18
Sex	Male	8
	Female	10
Age (years)	Mean	7.2 (s. d. 6.10)
	Range	1.3–24
	Median	4.5
Epileptic syndrome	Cryptogenic LGS	1
	Symptomatic LGS	17
Type of seizure causing the falls (more than one for each patient)	Tonic	6
	Myoclonic-atonic	6
	Juvenile spasms	12
Seizure frequency		>1 per day
Treatment duration (years)	Mean	3.3 (s.d. 2.4)
	Range	0.1–9.6
	Median	2.9

Table 6. Effects of carbamazepine (CBZ) on epileptic falls in Lennox–Gastaut syndrome (LGS) patients by type of seizure (eighteen patients)

Type of seizure	Complete response	Partial response (reduction of seizure frequency >50%)	No response, or reduction of seizure frequency <50%		Number of patients
Tonic	–	–	6		6
Myoclonic-atonic	1*	2**	6	6	
Epileptic spasms	–	1***	12	12	

* One case with myoclonic-atonic seizures obtained a complete response with combined carbamazepine (CBZ) and felbamate (FBM).
** Two cases with myoclonic-atonic seizures obtained a partial response with combined carbamazepine (CBZ), lamotrigine (LTG) and felbamate (FBM).
*** One case with epileptic spasms had a partial response with combined carbamazepine (CBZ) and felbamate (FBM).

Table 7. Effects of vigabatrin (GVG) on epileptic falls in Lennox–Gastaut syndrome (LGS) patients: characteristics of the patients

Number of patients		11
Sex	Male	5
	Female	6
Age (years)	Mean	7.4 (s. d. 8.0)
	Range	1–28
	Median	4.0
Epileptic syndrome	Cryptogenic LGS	1
	Symptomatic LGS	10
Type of seizure causing the falls (more than one for each patient)	Tonic	3
	Myocolonic-atonic	2
	Epileptic spasms	8
Seizure frequency		>1 per day
Treatment duration (years)	Mean	1.4 (s.d. 1)
	Range	0.2–2.10
	Median	1.3

Eleven patients with LGS were treated with GVG (Table 7), which had no effect on the three patients suffering from tonic seizures or on the two with myoclonic-atonic seizures, although three of the eight with epileptic spasms did experience a reduction in frequency of more than 50 per cent (Table 8).

Table 8. *Effects of vigabatrin (GVG) on epileptic falls in Lennox–Gastaut syndrome (LGS) patients by type of seizure (eleven patients)*

Type of seizure	Complete response	Partial response (reduction of seizure frequency >50%)	No response, or reduction of seizure frequency <50%	Number of patients
Tonic	–	–	3	3
Myoclonic-atonic	–	–	2	2
Epileptic spasms	1*	2	5	8

* One other patient obtained a 100 per cent response with combined vigabatrin (GVG) and felbamate (FBM).

Table 9. *Effects of felbamate (FBM) on epileptic falls in Lennox–Gastaut syndrome (LGS) patients: characteristics of the patients*

Number of patients		9
Sex	Male	3
	Female	6
Age (years)	Mean	12.4 (s.d. 12.2)
	Range	3–29
	Median	8.8
Epileptic syndrome	Cryptogenic LGS	3
	Symptomatic LGS	6
Type of seizure causing the falls*	Tonic	4
	Myoclonic-atonic	3
	Epileptic spasms	4
Seizure frequency		>1 per day
Combined therapy		VPA, CBZ, GVG, CLB**
Treatment duration (years)	Mean	0.5 (s.d. 0.3)
	Range	0.1–1.0
	Median	0.5

* More than one for each patient. ** CLB means clobazam.

Table 10. *Effects of felbamate (FBM) on epileptic falls in Lennox–Gastaut syndrome (LGS) patients by type of seizure (nine patients)*

Type of seizure	Complete response	Partial response (reduction of seizure frequency >50%)	No response, or reduction of seizure frequency <50%	Number of patients
Tonic	–	3	1	4
Myoclonic-atonic	3	–	–	3
Epileptic spasms	1	1	2	4

FBM was administered to nine LGS patients (Table 9), all of whom were receiving polytherapy with VPA, CBZ, GVG and benzodiazepines. Of the four patients with tonic seizures, three responded well and achieved a frequency reduction of more than 50 per cent; all patients with myoclonic-atonic seizures achieved a complete remission. A reduction in seizure frequency of more than 50 per cent was also observed in two of the four patients with epileptic spasms, one of whom achieved a complete remission (Table 10).

Table 11. *Effects of lamotrigine (LTG) on epileptic falls in Lennox–Gastaut syndrome (LGS) patients: characteristics of the patients*

Number of patients		6
Sex	Male	3
	Female	3
Age (years)	Mean	11.5 (s.d. 9.6)
	Range	1.9–30
	Median	8.6
Epileptic syndrome	Cryptogenic LGS	3
	Symptomatic LGS	3
Type of seizure causing the falls*	Tonic	4
	Myoclonic-atonic	2
	Epileptic spasms	3
Seizure frequency		>1 per day
Combined therapy		VPA, ESM, CBZ, GVG, CLB**
Treatment duration (years)	Mean	0.8 (s.d. 0.6)
	Range	0.2–1.4
	Median	0.5

* More than one for each patient. ** CLB = clobazam; ESM = ethosuximide.

Table 12. *Effects of lamotrigine (LTG) on epileptic falls in Lennox–Gastaut syndrome patients by type of seizure (six patients)*

Type of seizure	Complete response	Partial response (reduction of seizure frequency >50%)	No response, or reduction of seizure frequency <50%	Number of patients
Tonic	–	2	2	4
Myoclonic-atonic	–	2	–	2
Epileptic spasms	1	–	2	3

LTG was given to six patients (Table 11). Of the four patients presenting tonic seizures, two achieved a reduction in frequency of more than 50 per cent; the same result was observed in both of the patients with myoclonic-atonic seizures. One of the three patients with epileptic spasms achieved a complete remission. (Table 12).

Considering the different types of seizure observed in this group of patients as a whole, we draw the following conclusions (Table 13):

– VPA was efficacious in three out of seven patients suffering from tonic seizures, whereas both CBZ and GVG proved to be ineffective; FBM was efficacious in three out of four cases, and LTG in two out of four.

– VPA had a fair effect on myoclonic-atonic seizures, even though this was observed in less than 50 per cent of the patients; FBM led to the disappearance of the seizures in all three treated patients; CBZ and GVG proved to be inefficacious.

Table 13. *Effects of anti-epileptic drugs (AEDs) on epileptic falls in Lennox–Gastaut syndrome (LGS) patients by type of seizure: number of patients who achieved a 50 per cent or more reduction in seizures*

	Sodium valproate (VPA)	Carbamazepine (CBZ)	Vigabatrin (GVG)	Felbamate (FBM)	Lamotrigine (LTG)
Tonic	3 of 7	0 of 6	0 of 3	3 of 4	2 of 4
Myoclonic-atonic	3 of 8	0 of 6	0 of 2	3 of 3	2 of 2
Epileptic spasms	2 of 13	0 of 12	3 of 8	2 of 4	1 of 3

- Finally, the small number of patients treated with LTG makes it almost impossible to express any real judgement; but two patients with seizures of this kind did achieve a more than 50 per cent reduction in their frequency.
- GVG was the only drug to have any appreciable effect on epileptic spasms.

Discussion

There are few and contradictory data in the literature concerning the pharmacological treatment of epileptic falls.

Although our study has all of the limitations generally associated with retrospective studies, it did evaluate the efficacy of various AEDs on different types of polygraphically documented seizures associated with falls in patients with two syndromes (MAE and LGS). This evaluation differs from that made in the majority of published studies where the various types of seizure were not documented or not polygraphically differentiated, as well as in those where such a differentiation was made but the results were correlated with the nosological or neurophysiological aspects, rather than with the pharmacological response of the seizures.

In the case of epileptic falls in MAE, VPA proved to be the drug of first choice (alone or in association with CLB), with an overall efficacy rate of more than 90 per cent. When administered to 23 patients with LGS, it was fairly efficacious – particularly in the case of tonic seizures – but less so in the case of myoclonic-atonic seizures.

Perhaps Covanis *et al.* (1992) reported a reduction in seizure frequency of between 50 per cent and 80 per cent in one-third of their patients with 'myoclonic-astatic epilepsy' (the term used by the authors as a synonym of LGS), complete seizure control being obtained in seven of them. Henricksen & Johannessen (1982) reported the complete control of atonic seizures in nine of their 39 patients.

In our LGS patients, CBZ proved to be inefficacious in treating any of the seizure types related to epileptic falls. This result is in line with most of the data reported in the literature, which indicate inefficacy and an increase in myoclonic and atonic seizures (Shields, 1983), but it is in disagreement with the data published by Beaumanoir & Dravet (1992), who reported that CBZ was efficacious in treating LGS patients suffering from tonic seizures.

GVG proved to be effective only in the case of patients with epileptic spasms, and has been previously reported in the literature (Chiron *et al.*, 1991). Unlike Feucht & Brantner-Inthaler (1994), we found this drug to be inefficacious in treating atonic seizures.

Various authors (Oller *et al.*, 1991; Wallace, 1993; Timmings & Richens, 1992; Schlumberger *et al.*, 1994) have reported that LTG is fairly efficacious in patients with LGS. Oller *et al.* (1991)

report that they obtained complete control in 37 per cent of their patients, and found the drug particularly successful in treating tonic and atonic seizures. Timmings & Richens (1992) obtained a reduction in seizure frequency of 50 per cent in ten out of eleven children given LTG in addition to their previous treatment. In a paper analysing the data relating to the use of LTG in a population of 120 children, Schlumberger *et al.* (1994) recognized that the best results in terms of clinical efficacy were obtained in their patients with LGS.

Although being used in only a small number of cases, our study confirms the efficacy of LTG in treating the various forms of epileptic falls encountered in LGS patients: in particular, a reduction in seizure frequency of more than 50 per cent was obtained in two out of four patients with tonic seizures, as well as in the two patients with myoclonic-atonic seizures. Complete control was obtained in one of the three patients presenting epileptic spasms.

Our data concerning the efficacy of FBM clearly confirm those already published in the literature (The Felbamate Study Group, 1993). Administered to nine patients, the drug led to the complete disappearance of the myoclonic-atonic seizures experienced by three, and a more than 50 per cent reduction in frequency in three out of four patients with tonic seizures, and in one of the four with epileptic spasms.

In conclusion, although retrospective, our data confirm the usefulness of VPA in treating the myoclonic-atonic seizures of patients with MAE, also in association with benzodiazepines. GVG proved to be efficacious in treating falls related to epileptic spasms and, although our data are not extensive, LTG seems to have an effect on the myoclonic-atonic and tonic seizures of LGS patients.

FBM proved to be certainly efficacious, particularly in treating the myoclonic-atonic and tonic seizures of LGS patients.

Prospective controlled studies, and particularly the use of polygraphic recordings, would improve the evaluation of the effect of AEDs on the various types of epileptic falls.

References

Aicardi, J. (1982): Childhood epilepsies with brief myoclonic-atonic or tonic seizures. In: *A Textbook of Epilepsy*, eds. J. Laidlaw & A.Richens, pp. 88–96. New York: Churchill, Livingstone.

Aicardi, J. (1994): Lennox–Gastaut Syndrome. In: *Epilepsy in Children*, pp. 44–66. New York: Raven Press.

Bourgeois, B. (1995): Clinical use of drugs useful in the treatment of atonic seizures. In: *Negative motor phenomena*, eds. S. Fahn, M. Hallet, H.O. Luders & C.D. Marsden, pp. 361–367. *Advances in Neurology*, vol. 67, Philadelphia: Lippincott-Raven.

Binnie, C.D. (1993): Efficacy of lamotrigine in add-on controlled studies. In: *Lamotrigine: a new advance in the treatment of epilepsy*, ed. E.H. Reynolds, pp. 25–34, Royal Society of Medicine Services International Congress and Symposium Series, no. 204, London: Royal Society of Medicine Services Limited.

Beaumanoir, A. & Dravet, C. (1992): The Lennox–Gastaut Syndrome. In: *Epileptic syndromes in infancy, childhood and adolescence*, 2nd edn, eds. J. Roger, M. Bureau, Ch. Dravet, F.E. Dreifuss, A. Perret & P. Wolf, pp. 115–132. London: John Libbey.

Carter Snead, O. & Hosey, L.C. (1985): Exacerbation of seizures in children by carbamazepine. *N. Engl. J. Med.* **313**, 916–921.

Chiron, C., Dulac, O., Beaumont, D., Palacios, L., Pajot, N. & Mumford, J. (1991): Therapeutic trial of vigabatrin in refractory infantile spasm. *J. Child. Neurol.* **6**, 52–59.

Commission on classification and terminology of the International League Against Epilepsy (1989): Proposal for revised classification of epilepsies and epileptic syndromes. *Epilepsia* **30**, (4), 389–399.

Covanis, A., Gupta, A.K. & Jeavons, P.M. (1982): Sodium valproate: monotherapy and polytherapy. *Epilepsia* **23**, 693–720.

Donat, J. & Wright, F.S. (1991): Seizures in series: similarities between seizures of the West and Lennox–Gastaut syndromes. *Epilepsia* **32**, (4), 504–509

Doose, H. (1992): Myoclonic astatic epilepsy of early children. In: *Epileptic syndromes in infancy, childhood and adolescence*, 2nd edn., eds. J. Roger, M. Bureau, Ch. Dravet, F.E. Dreifuss, A. Perret & P. Wolf, pp. 103–114. London: John Libbey.

Egli, M., Mothersill, I., O' Kane, M. & O' Kane, F. (1985): The axial spasm. The predominant type of drop seizure in patients with secondary generalized epilepsy. *Epilepsia* **26**, 401–415.

Ethelberg, S. (1950): Symptomatic 'cataplexy' or chalastic fits in cortical lesion of the frontal lobe. *Brain* **73**, 499–512.

The Felbamate Study Group in Lennox–Gastaut Syndrome (1993): Efficacy of felbamate in childhood epileptic encephalopathy (Lennox–Gastaut syndrome). *N. Engl. J. Med.* **328**, 29–33.

Feucht, M. & Brantner-Inthaler, S. (1994): Gamma-vinyl-GABA (vigabatrin) in the therapy of Lennox–Gastaut syndrome: an open study. *Epilepsia* **35**, (5), 993–998.

Gambardella, A., Reutens, D.C., Andermann, F., Cendes, F., Gloor, P., Dubeau, F. & Olivier, A. (1994): Late onset drop attacks in temporal lobe epilepsy: a reevaluation of the concept of temporal lobe syncope. *Neurology* **44**, 1074–1078.

Gastaut, H., Roger, J., Ouahchi, S., Timisit, M. & Broughton, R. (1963): An electroclinical study of generalized epileptic seizures of tonic expression. *Epilepsia* **4**, 15–44.

Gastaut, H., Roger, J., Soulayrol, *et al.*, (1966): Childhood epileptic encephalopathy with diffuse slow spike-waves (otherwise known as *petit mal variant*) or Lennox syndrome. *Epilepsia* **7**, 139–179.

Gastaut, H. & Zifkin, B. (1988): Secondary bilateral synchrony and Lennox–Gastaut syndrome. In: *The Lennox–Gastaut syndrome*, eds. E. Niedermeyer & R. Degen, pp. 221–242, New York: Alan R. Liss.

Henricksen, O. & Johannessen, S.I. (1982): Clinical and pharmacokinetic observation on sodium valproate. A five-year follow up study in 100 children with epilepsy. *Acta Neurol. Scand.* **65**, 504–523.

Ikeno, T., Shigematsu, H., Miyakoshi, M., Ohba, A., Yagi, K. & Seino, M. (1985): An analytic study of epileptic falls. *Epilepsia* **6**, 612–621.

Jensen, P.K. (1994): Felbamate in the treatment of Lennox–Gastaut syndrome. *Epilepsia* **35 (suppl. 5)**, S54–S57.

Landolt, H. (1960): *Die Temporallappenepilepsie und ihre Psychopathologie*. Ein Beitrag zur Kenntnis Psychophysischer Korrelationen bei Epilepsie und Hirnlaesionen. Basel: Karger.

Lortie, A., Chiron, C., Mumford, J. & Dulac, O. (1993): The potential for increasing seizure frequency, relapse and appearance of new seizure types with vigabatrin. *Neurology* **43 (suppl. 5)**, S24–S27.

Oguni, H., Sato, F., Hayashi, K., Wang, P.J. & Fukuyama, Y. (1992): A study of unilateral brief focal atonia in childhood partial epilepsy. *Epilepsia* **33**, 75–83.

Oller, L.F.V., Russi, A. & Oller-Daurella, L. (1991): Lamotrigine in the Lennox–Gastaut syndrome. *Epilepsia* **32 (suppl. 1), 58.**

Robertson, M.M. (1986): Current status of the 1.4 and 1.5 benzodiazepines in the treatment of epilepsy: the place of clobazam. *Epilepsia* **27**, S27–S41.

Shields, W. & Saslow, E. (1983): Myoclonic, atonic and absence seizures following institution of carbamazepine therapy in children, *Neurology* **33**, 1487–1483.

Schlumberger, E., Chavez, F., Palacios, L., Rey, E., Pajot, N. & Dulac, O. (1994): Lamotrigine in the treatment of 120 children with epilepsy. *Epilepsia* **35**, (2), 359–367.

Talwar, D., Baldwin, M.A., Hutzler, R. & Griesemer, D.A. (1995): Epileptic spasms in older children: persistence beyond infancy. *Epilepsia* **36**, (2), 151–155.

Theodore, W.H., Jensen, P.K. & Kwan, R.M.F. (1995): *Felbamate. Clinical use. Antiepileptic drugs*, eds. R. H. Levy, R. H. Mattson & B. S. Meldrum. New York: Raven Press.

Timmings, P.L. & Richens, A. (1992): Lamotrigine as an add-on drug in the management of Lennox–Gastaut syndrome. *Eur. Neurol.* **32,** 305–307.

Vassella, F., Pavlincova, E., Schneider, H.J., Rudin, H.J. & Karbowski, K. (1973): Treatment of infantile spasm and Lennox–Gastaut syndrome with clonazepam. *Epilepsia* **14**, 165–175.

Veggiotti, P.A., Ceuta, C., Rey, E. & Dulac, O. (1994): Lamotrigine in infantile spasms. *Lancet* **344,** 1375–1376.

Wallace, S.J., (1993): Lamotrigine: useful therapy for astatic seizures. *Neuropediatrics* **24,** 172.

Yaqub, B. (1993): Electroclinical seizures in Lennox–Gastaut syndrome. *Epilepsia* **34,** 120–127.

Chapter 15

Indications and results of surgical treatment (excluding callosotomy) in children with epileptic 'falls'

Claudio Munari,* Lorella Minotti,† Giorgio Lo Russo,‡ Philippe Kahane,†
Filippo Leocata,‡ Stefano Francione,* Laura Tassi,‡ Matilde Di Leo,†
Pier Paolo Quarato,† Dominique Hoffmann† and Alim Louis Benabid†

*Clinical Neurophysiology and Neurosurgery Department, University of Genova; †Neurosciences Department, INSERM U318, CHU Grenoble, France; ‡Regional Centre for Epilepsy Surgery, Niguarda Hospital, Milan, Italy

Summary

The occurrence of ictal falls strongly increases the severity of the epilepsy. Clinical information about partial seizures in studies concerning child candidates for surgical resective treatment generally does not mention the possible occurrence of falls. Conversely, falls (often called 'drop attacks' without any other precise name) appear among clinical features that can improve (or disappear) after corpus callosotomy. The aim of this study is to evaluate: (a) the possible occurrence of ictal falls in child candidates for cortical resections; and (b) the prognostic value of falls on surgical results – also considering their clinical characteristics.

The retrospective analysis concerns 58 consecutive patients who underwent presurgical evaluation for a severe drug-resistant partial epilepsy before the age of 16. Falls were anamnestically reported in 27 patients (46.5 per cent) constant in two, frequent in sixteen, rare in nine. Falling was slow and progressive in sixteen patients, sudden in seven, and both modalities were reported in four. Surgical results are similar in patients with and without falls; respectively, 72.2 per cent and 65.5 per cent of Class 1a (Engel, 1987). The best results are obtained in patients with temporal lobe epilepsy (1a: 87.5 per cent), falls were slow and progressive in seven/eight. Cortical resection is less satisfactory in patients with multilobar epilepsy, as well with (1a: 40 per cent) as without (1a: 55.5 per cent) ictal falls.

The prognostic value of ictal falls is not necessarily bad in child candidates for surgery, but it is dependent on such factors as clinical characteristics of falls, and the extent and location of the epileptogenic area(s).

Introduction

Falls are considered among ictal clinical signs with bad prognostic value in children with epilepsy (Roger *et al.*, 1981; Munari, 1984). Callosotomy is considered an effective, even if palliative, surgical treatment for children presenting seizures with falls.

After the earliest clinical report of surgical division of commissural pathways, to prevent the spread of epileptic discharge (van Wagenen & Herren, 1940), many others since the 1960s have adopted this technique in the surgical treatment of epileptic falls.

Despite 50 years' experience with this procedure, it is not completely clear, up to now, which patients should undergo and could benefit from corpus callosotomy. Difficulties for a correct understanding of the published data arise from the following considerations: (a) the sequence of surgical procedures vary among the different centres and even in the same study (Spencer *et al.*, 1988); (b) the selection criteria are inconsistent; (c) there is a lack of prospective study and control groups; (d) the seizure frequency, before and after the operation, is not appropriately assessed; and (e) the postoperative follow-up is often too short. Moreover, the wide variability of resected structures (corpus callosum, hippocampal commissures, anterior commissure, fornix) among surgeons and within individual surgical series, makes the interpretation of the results problematic.

Seizure types that will most likely benefit from a corpus callosotomy are, according to a diffuse point of view, tonic, atonic, and tonic-clonic seizures, but many authors have operated on patients suffering from 'complex partial seizures', and/or 'simple partial seizures' in addition to other seizure types (Purves *et al.*, 1988; Gates *et al.*, 1987, Spencer *et al.*, 1993). This heterogeneity of clinical characteristics of the considered population determines another bias in the outcome evaluation. Surprisingly, in most of the published series concerning surgical treatment of partial epilepsies in children, no information exists about the occurrence or absence of falls during seizures (Rasmussen, 1983; Lindsay *et al.*, 1984; Ribaric *et al.*, 1991; Morrison *et al.*, 1992; Fish *et al.*, 1993). The lack of this kind of information makes it even more difficult to appreciate the clinical criteria allowing the decision of performing a callosotomy, also remembering the selection criteria proposed by Spencer *et al.* (1988).

The aim of this study is to try to understand if and how resective surgery can contribute to cure epileptic children and adolescents presenting epileptic falls, but in whom a partial origin of seizure may be hypothesised.

Patients and methods

We have retrospectively analysed 58 patients who underwent a presurgical study for a severe, drug-resistant partial epilepsy, first evaluated before the age of 16 years (1990–1995).

Age at seizure onset varied between 1 day and 14 years (mean: 3.8 years) and mean duration of epilepsy was 6.8 years (1–16.5 years).

On the basis of neuro-imaging data (CT-scan and MRI were performed in all), epilepsy was defined as 'symptomatic' in 52 patients (89.7 per cent) and 'cryptogenic' in six (10.3 per cent). Among the 52 patients with symptomatic epilepsy, 36 (69.2 per cent) had a single and well-delimited lesion and sixteen (30.8 per cent) had either a 'not well-limited' lesion, or multiple or diffuse lesions.

Febrile convulsions were present in five patients (8.6 per cent), birth trauma in five (8.6 per cent), head trauma in four (6.8 per cent) and CNS infection in one (1.7 per cent).

Seizure frequency was daily or more in 38 patients (65.5 per cent) and weekly or monthly in 20 (34.5 per cent).

Neurological examination was normal in 40 patients (69 per cent), showed a severe sensorimotor deficit in six (10.3 per cent), a mild sensorimotor deficit in three (5.2 per cent), a visual field deficit in three (5.2 per cent), a severe psychomotor impairment in four (6.9 per cent) and in two patients (3.4 per cent) were present congenital malformations or acatisya.

At the end of the presurgical evaluation (for details, see Kahane et al. 1993; Munari & Betti, 1989; Munari et al., 1994), 52 patients (89.6 per cent) were operated on. One patient is still waiting for surgery; in three patients we proposed to 'wait and see'; in one patient seizures stopped after stereo-EEG; and one patient underwent radio-surgery for the treatment of a hypothalamic lesion (Munari et al., 1995c). The mean age at surgery was 10.9 years (2–18 years). Concerning surgical results, only patients with more than twelve-months follow-up were considered. For the purpose of this study, we separated the global population into two groups:

(1) Group A includes 27 out of 58 children (46.5 per cent) with a positive anamnestic history of seizures with falls;

(2) Group B includes the other 31 of 58 children (53.5 per cent) without anamnestic ictal falls.

Results

General characteristics of the two groups

There are not significant differences between the two groups concerning age at the different steps (Table 1), nor antecedents (Table 2). Neurological examination and psychomotor status were more frequently impaired in children with falls (Table 3). Seizure frequency was higher in Group A (Table 4): 22 of 27 (81.5 per cent) presented at least one seizure per day. Epilepsy was symptomatic of an MRI-detected lesion in 25 of 27 (92.5 per cent) of Group A patients and in 27 of 31 (87 per cent) of Group B patients.

Table 1. General characteristics (58 patients)

	Number of patients	Mean age (years)	Mean age at onset (years)	Duration (years)
Group A	27 (46.5%)	10.2 (3.5–16)	2.6 (1 day–9)	7.6 (1–14.5)
Group B	31 (53.5%)	10.5 (2–18)	4.8 (1 day–14)	6.8 (1.6–16.5)
Total	58	10.9 (2–18)	3.8 (1 day–14)	6.8 (1–16.5)

Group A: children with a positive history of seizures with falls. Group B: children without anamnestic ictal falls.

Table 2. Antecedents

	Group A (27 patients)	Group B (31 patients)	Total (58 patients)
None	22 (81.5%)	25 (80.6%)	47 (81%)
Febrile convulsions	2 (7.4%)	3 (9.7%)	5 (8.6%)
Birth trauma	2 (7.4%)	3 (9.7%)	5 (8.6%)
Head trauma	2 (7.4%)	2 (6.4%)	4 (6.8%)
Central nervous system infections	1 (3.7%)	–	1 (1.7%)

Group A: children with a positive history of seizures with falls. Group B: children without anamnestic ictal falls.

Table 3. Neurological examination

	Group A (27 patients)	Group B (31 patients)	Total (58 patients)
Normal	17 (63%)	23 (74.2%)	40 (69%)
Severe sensorimotor deficit	5 (18.6%)	1 (3.2%)	6 (10.3%)
Mild sensorimotor deficit	1 (3.7%)	2 (6.5%)	3 (5.2%)
Visual field deficit	–	3 (9.7%)	3 (5.2%)
Severe psychomotor impairment	3 (11%)	1 (3.2%)	4 (6.9%)
Other	1 (3.7%)	1 (3.2%)	2 (3.4%)

Group A: children with a positive history of seizures with falls. Group B: children without anamnestic ictal falls.

Table 4. Seizure frequency

	Group A (27 patients)	Group B (31 patients)	Total (58 patients)
1–5 per month	–	5 (16.1%)	5 (8.6%)
1–5 per week	5 (18.5%)	10 (32.3%)	15 (25.9%)
1–5 per day	17 (63%)	10 (32.3%)	27 (46.5%)
>5 per day	5 (18.5%)	6 (19.3%)	11 (19%)

Group A: children with a positive history of seizures with falls. Group B: children without anamnestic ictal falls.

Characteristics of falls

Five patients presented falls since the beginning of their seizure history. In the other 22, the delay between seizures onset and fall onset was 3 months to 1 year in eight; 1.5 to 5 years in nine; more than 7 years in five. Falls were rare in nine, frequent in sixteen and constant in two.

Falling was slow and progressive in sixteen (59.3 per cent), and sudden in seven (25.9 per cent). In four patients (14.8 per cent) both modalities were reported.

Interictal EEG

Interictal EEG was normal (both asleep and awake) in one patient, whereas abnormalities (slow and/or paroxysmal) were present in the other 57 (98.2 per cent). The patient with a normal EEG was in Group A (3.7 per cent): his seizures were characterized by a subjective sensation preceding the loss of contact. Falls were rare and late-occurring in the evolution of the seizure.

Interictal EEG abnormalities were classified as follows: Group A – focal and/or lobar in three patients (11.1 per cent); multilobar unilateral in twelve (44.4 per cent); and bilateral and/or diffuse in eleven patients (40.8 per cent). Group B – focal and/or lobar in nine patients (29 per cent); multilobar unilateral in ten (32.3 per cent); and bilateral and/or diffuse in twelve (38.7 per cent).

Ictal EEG

Spontaneous seizures were recorded in 42 patients (72.4 per cent): in 21 of 27 patients of Group A (77.7 per cent), and in 21 of 31 patients of Group B (67.7 per cent). More particularly, recorded electroclinical seizures did allow surgical decision, without any invasive presurgical investigation, in 11 of 23 of Group A patients, and 18 of 29 of Group B patients.

Stereo-EEG

Invasive presurgical evaluation (multilead intracerebral stereotactically implanted electrodes, stereo-EEG) (Bancaud et al., 1965; Munari, 1987; Munari et al., 1994) was performed in 27 patients: fourteen of the Group A (51.8 per cent), and thirteen of the Group B (42 per cent). Intracerebral electrodes were bilaterally implanted in six of fourteen (42.8 per cent) of Group A patients, and in two of thirteen (15.3 per cent) Group B patients.

Origin of seizures and type of fall

The type of fall was correlated to the type of epilepsy as follows: in the eight patients with temporal lobe epilepsy, the fall was slow and progressive in seven and sudden in one; in the seven patients with extratemporal unilobar epilepsy (six frontal and one parietal), the fall was slow and progressive in three, sudden in three and both in one; in the ten patients with multilobar epilepsy, the fall was slow and progressive in six, sudden in one and of both types in three patients. Fall was sudden in both patients with a hypothalamic hamartoma.

Type of intervention (52 patients)

The five (9.6 per cent) cryptogenic patients underwent a cortectomy (1 of 23 in Group A and 4 of 29 in Group B); eight (15.4 per cent) underwent a complete lesionectomy (2 of 23 Group A and 6 of 29 Group B); two Group A patients (3.8 per cent) underwent an incomplete lesionectomy; 23 (44.2 per cent) underwent a complete lesionectomy with an associated cortectomy (12 of 23 Group A and 11 of 29 Group B); and fourteen (27 per cent) underwent an incomplete lesionectomy with cortectomy (7 of 23 Group A and 7 of 29 Group B).

Histopathological data (52 patients)

The microscopic examination of surgically obtained specimens showed:

- six (11.5 per cent) aspecific lesion (2 of 23 Group A and 4 of 29 Group B);
- five (9.6 per cent) hamartoma (1 of 23 Group A and 4 of 29 Group B);
- fourteen (27 per cent) dysembrio-neuro-epitelial tumour (8 of 23 Group A and 6 of 29 Group B);
- eleven (21.1 per cent) low-grade glioma (2 of 23 Group A and 9 of 29 Group B);
- one (2 per cent) cavernoma (Group B);
- six (11.5 per cent) cortical dysplasia (5 of 23 Group A and 1 of 29 Group B);
- five (9.6 per cent) tuberous sclerosis (3 of 23 Group A and 2 of 29 Group B); and,
- four (7.7 per cent) Rasmussen's syndrome (2 of 23 Group A and 2 of 29 Group B).

The histopathological data are summarized in Table 5.

Table 5. Histopathological data (52 patients)

	Group A (23 patients)	Group B (29 patients)	Total (52 patients)
Aspecific	2	4	6
Hamartoma	1	4	5
Dysembrio-neuro-epitelial tumour	8	6	14
Ganglioglioma	1	7	8
Astrocytoma/Ependimoma	1	2	3
Cavernoma	–	1	1
Cortical dysplasia	5	1	6
Tuberous sclerosis	3	2	5
Rasmussen's syndrome	2	2	4

Group A: children with a positive history of seizures with falls. Group B: children without anamnestic ictal falls.

Surgery results

Effects of the intervention on seizure frequency are evaluated according to the classification proposed by Engel (1987).

Rasmussen's syndrome (4 patients)

The mean follow-up time is 37.4 months (18–65 months). Among the patients diagnosed with Rasmussen's syndrome, three are unchanged (Class 4) and one presents only subjective manifestations after the surgery (Class 1(b)).

Other 44 patients

The mean follow-up time is 33.5 months (12–66 months). Global surgery results are reported in Table 6: complete suppression of seizures (Class 1a of Engel, 1987) was obtained in 13 of 18 Group A patients (72.2 per cent) and in 17 of 26 Group B patients (65.4 per cent): there are not significant differences.

Among the Group A patients, four (15.4 per cent) only presented subjective manifestations (Class 1(b)) since the intervention. Only one Group A patient (5.6 per cent) and two (7.7 per cent) Group B patients did not benefit from surgery.

Outcome versus type of epilepsy

The best results are obtained in patients with temporal lobe epilepsy (TLE): 87.5 per cent of Class 1a in the Group A, and 78.5 per cent among the others. In multilobar epilepsy the percentage of cured patients is lower: 40 per cent in Group A, and 55.5 per cent among the others (Table 7).

Outcome versus type of fall

Surgery outcome is not clearly related to the type of fall (Table 8).

Table 6. Global results (44 patients)

	Group A	Group B	Total
Class 1(a)	13 (72.2%)	17 (65.4%)	30 (68.2%)
Class 1(b,c,d)	–	4 (15.4%)	4 (9.1%)
Class 2	3 (16.6%)	1 (3.8%)	4 (9.1%)
Class 3	1 (5.6%)	2 (7.7%)	3 (6.8%)
Class 4	1 (5.6%)	2 (7.7%)	3 (6.8%)
Total	18	26	44

Results are assessed according to Engle's classification (1987). Group A: children with a positive history of seizures with falls. Group B: children without anamnestic ictal falls.

Table 7. Outcome versus type of epilepsy (44 patients)

	Class 1(a) Total	Class 1(a) – Temporal lobe epilepsy	Class 1(a) – Unilobar exrtatemporal epilepsy	Class 1(a) – Multiobar epilepsy
Group A	13 of 18 (72.2%)	7 of 8 (87.5%)	4 of 5 (80%)	2 of 5 (40%)
Group B	17 of 26 (65.5%)	11 of 14 (78.5%)	1 of 3 (33.3%)	5 of 9 (55.5%)
Combined	30 of 44 (68.2%)	18 of 22 (81.8%)	5 of 8 (62.5%)	7 of 14 (50%)

Group A: children with a positive history of seizures with falls. Group B: children without anamnestic ictal falls.

Table 8. Outcome versus type of fall (18 patients)

Type of fall	Class 1(a): number of patients	With initial subjective manifestations	Without initial subjective manifestations
Slow and progressive	9 of 12 (75%)	5 of 8 (62.5%)	4 of 4 (100%)
Sudden	2 of 2 (100%)	–	2 of 2 (100%)
Both	2 of 4 (50%)	1 of 3 (33.3%)	1 of 1 (100%)

See also Tables 1 and 7.

The best results are obtained in patients with slow and progressive falls (75 per cent of Class 1a), but also in those with sudden falls (2 of 2 in Class 1a). Conversely, patients presenting with both types of fall had a less positive surgery outcome (50 per cent of Class 1a).

Outcome versus pre-surgical evaluation

Concerning pre-surgical strategy (Table 9), the results are discordant. In Group A, results are similar in stereo-EEG and in non-stereo-EEG investigated patients (75 per cent versus 70 per cent of Class 1a); in Group B, results are better in those patients investigated non-invasively (76.4 per cent versus 44.4 per cent of Class 1a).

Table 9. Outcome versus presurgical evaluation (44 patients)

	Group A (18 patients)		Group B (26 patients)		Total (44 patients)	
	SEEG +	SEEG –	SEEG +	SEEG –	SEEG +	SEEG –
Number of patients	8	10	9	17	17	27
Class 1(a)	6 (75%)	7 (70%)	4 (44.4%)	13 (76.4%)	10 (58.8%)	20 (74%)
Class 4	1 (12.5%)	–	2 (22.2%)	1 (5.8%)	3 (17.6%)	1 (37%)

SEEG: Stereo-electroencephalography.

Outcome versus type of surgery

Complete lesionectomy associated to a cortectomy allowed analogous results in the two groups: respectively, 66.6 per cent and 70 per cent of Class 1a. Similar results were also obtained in both groups when patients underwent a partial lesionectomy associated to a cortectomy: respectively, 60 per cent and 50 per cent of Class 1a.

For those who underwent a simple but complete lesionectomy, results are the following: 50 per cent of Class 1a in Group A, and 80 per cent of Class 1a in Group B.

Case report

A.T. is a 12-year-old boy that began experiencing seizures at the age of 2 years. Birth at term was uneventful. Neurological examination was normal. At the beginning of epilepsy, seizures lasted a few seconds and were characterized by staring and a contraction of the upper limbs. Interictal EEG demonstrated right-temporal abnormalities. The CT scan showed a right-temporal lesion. Phenobarbital and carbamazepine were introduced and achieved seizure control until the age of 4, then seizures reappeared.

At this point, seizures were characterized by staring, unresponsiveness and sometimes by groaning. Interictal EEG always demonstrated right-temporal abnormalities. A re-adaptation of phenobarbital and carbamazepine treatment induced seizure control until the age of 6, then seizures reappeared and quickly reached a daily frequency, while awake and asleep. The ictal semeiology were characterized by two types of seizures: the 'absences' with staring, unresponsiveness, and sometimes groaning; the 'seizures' with a rising epigastric sensation followed by loss of contact, unresponsiveness, pallor, anxious mimic, inconstant chewing automatisms, contraction and extension of upper limbs, screaming, head retropulsion, bilateral contraction at lip corners. Falling was sometimes present. Seizures lasted 30 s to 1 min, without postictal language disturbance. Seizure frequency remained daily despite phenobarbital, carbamazepine, valproic acid and benzodiazepines at maximum tolerated doses.

At the moment of the first observation, interictal EEG demonstrated bi-temporal slow waves, more evident on the right side and diffuse discharges of spike-waves, anteriorly predominant. Ictal EEG showed a right fronto-temporal origin of seizures. The patient was submitted to a presurgical invasive exploration by intracerebral electrodes implanted in the right frontal and temporal lobe.

Seizures originated in the right-temporal neo-cortical areas to successively involve the temporal polar region and then frontal areas (Figs. 1 and 2). A right-temporal lesionectomy associated to

Chapter 15   Indications and results of surgical treatment (excluding callosotomy)

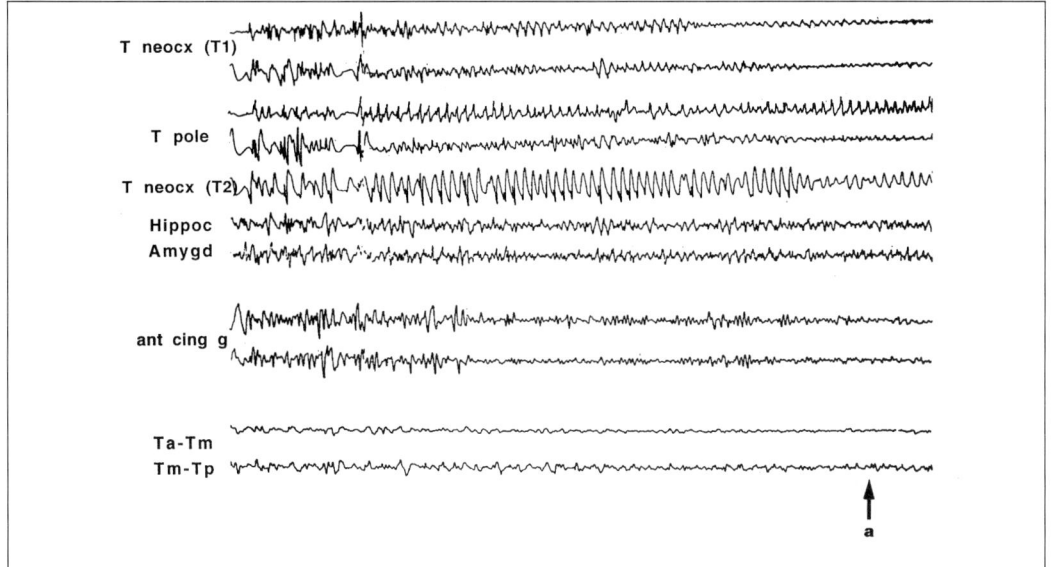

Figs. 1 and 2. T neocx (T1): neocortical areas of right first-temporal gyrus; T pole: right temporal pole; T neocx (T2): neocortical areas of right second-temporal gyrus; Hippoc: right hippocampus; Amygd: right amygdala; ant cing g: right anterior-cingulate gyrus; Ta: right anterior-temporal scalp derivation; Tm: right middle-temporal scalp derivation; Tp: right posterior-temporal scalp derivation.

Fig. 1. Low-voltage fast activity starts on the neocortical areas of the first temporal gyrus; (a) the patient open his eyes and presents eye-blinking.

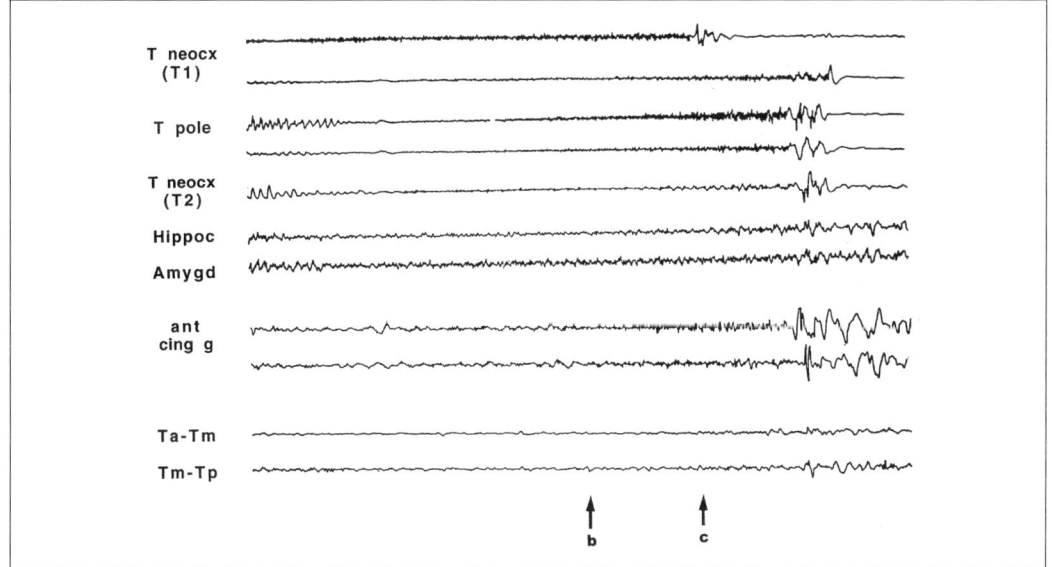

Fig. 2. Low-voltage fast activity involves (a) the temporal pole, the neocortical areas of the second temporal gyrus and then the anterior cingulate gyrus; (b) the patient presents a flexion of the head and a bilateral contraction at lip corners and then (c) a flexion of the upper limbs.

167

a cortectomy was performed in January 1995 and the patient has since been seizure-free (Class 1a of Engel, 1987). Histopathological examination demonstrated a cortical dysplasia.

Discussion

The most important function of scientific papers on 'clinical' research should be the diffusion of the data in order to improve reciprocal knowledge and comprehension of diagnostic and therapeutic strategies. Admitting that this assumption is correct, researchers are strongly puzzled when analysing papers concerning epilepsy surgery in children and/or in infancy.

The first problem to tackle is the definition of 'children': very rare are those studies only concerning children of less than 5 years of age (Duchowny et al., 1990; Chugani et al., 1990), or even under 10 years.

Most papers concern patients up to 16 years old, and even up to 20 years (Guldvog et al., 1994). We do not need to stress the possible neurobiological differences between a child of 1 year and that of another about to do his military service.

One possible critical remark raised in such papers concerns the lack of information about ictal clinical characteristics. Clinical characteristics of epileptic seizures are only rarely reported in studies concerning epilepsy surgery results, in adults as well as in children: in the best cases, one can learn that patients present with simple or complex partial seizures, sometimes secondary generalized. Aware of the poor localizing value of such definitions (Munari et al., 1982), we would like to be informed about the chronological sequence of different signs and symptoms. This request could be considered pedantic, but it is somewhat astonishing to note that studies concerning the surgical treatment of partial epilepsy are completely devoid of information about the possible occurrence of falls. Our surprise at this lack is also related to the fact that falls are considered among those symptoms that contribute to define indications for callosotomy. It is true that falls are only one argument among others, as stressed by Spencer and her co-workers in 1988, but also many children presenting ictal falls have simple or complex partial seizures, too (Geoffroy et al., 1983; Gates et al., 1987; Purves et al., 1988).

Falls occurring late during the evolution of epilepsies that are supposedly of temporal lobe origin were recently described (Gambardella et al., 1994). It is not the aim of this paper to discuss the physiopathology of falls, or of the so-called drop attacks. However, before evoking 'a spread of ictal discharge ... to the pontine reticular formation' (Gambardella et al., 1994), one must remember that bilateral fronto-temporal spreading of discharges can provoke the same 'dropping' result. It was recently demonstrated that, in patients with hypothalamic hamartoma, ictal discharges either corresponding to gelastic or dacrystic seizures are strictly localized *in* the hypothalamic hamartoma, but that, in the same patients, 'atonic' seizures with falls are related to unilateral or bilateral frontal diffuse discharges, sparing the hamartoma (Kahane et al., 1994; Munari et al., 1995c). These observations help to explain the failures found with cortical, temporal or frontal resections in this kind of patient (Cascino et al., 1993).

Moreover, it was recently shown that ictal involvement of either the orbito-frontal cortex (Munari et al., 1995a), or fronto-central cortical areas (Kahane et al., 1995), or even mesial temporal and cingulate structures (Broglin & Bancaud, 1991) could be responsible for a bradycardia with all the possible consequences.

This necessity to demonstrate if patients presenting ictal falling suffer from partial epilepsy is particularly important since it is clearly established that resective surgery does allow much more satisfactory results, in terms of total suppression of seizures, than corpus callosotomy can do.

Many early reports endorsed complete corpus callosotomy (Wilson et al., 1977; Wilson et al., 1978; Geoffroy et al., 1983), whereas interest, in the last years, has focused on a more limited callosal section (Maxwell et al., 1987; Spencer et al., 1988), usually anterior, particularly to avoid the 'disconnection syndrome'. Anterior callosotomy will be eventually completed with a resection of the posterior part, if the first step was ineffective on seizure frequency (Wilson et al., 1982). Intraoperative EEG recording is also used to guide the extent of the initial section, looking for disruption of bilateral synchrony (Gates et al., 1987; Gates 1991). No univocal agreement is reached on the real efficacy of the different type of callosal section: some authors stress better results with complete callosal section, others consider anterior corpus callosotomy (Wyler, 1991; Purves et al., 1988) as largely sufficient for a good seizure-free outcome.

Different types of outcome classification do not permit the evaluation of the real efficacy of this surgical technique, particularly referring to 'real' seizure-free patients. For example, Spencer et al. (1988) consider Class 1 as 'only simple partial seizures or no seizures at all postoperatively'; whereas Purves et al. (1988) consider an excellent result a 'more than 80 per cent reduction in frequency or severity, resulting in some improvement in functional capability'.

Although this procedure has historically been considered for patients of all ages, children constitute a major source of referrals. Selection criteria are classically represented by 'medically refractory seizures', associated with falling, in patients in whom no localised area for focal resection could be identified (Gates, 1991). Spencer et al., (1993) specify that for the studied population 'in most instances seizures classified as tonico-clonic or tonic began with [a] short-lived focal component'. For Turnel et al. (1992) the selective criteria for callosotomy in patients with frontal epilepsy are represented by SEEG recordings demonstrating bilateral synchrony in both frontal lobes or a localized onset to one frontal lobe with rapid diffusion to contra-lateral lobe and in whom no underlying pathology has been disclosed preoperatively, and in patients of a large frontal cortectomy that will determine a probable neurobehavioural sequel.

Some studies include callosotomy among the different types of performed surgical interventions, but in the seizure description, it remains unclear if seizures are associated or not with falls that we can only presume to being present (Lindsay et al., 1984; Duchowny et al., 1990; Ribaric et al., 1991; Ventureira & Higgings, 1993; Beckung et al., 1994; Guldvog et al., 1994).

The practical effect of these reflections is that it should be hoped to apply the same rigorous electroclinical methodology for studying both candidates for callosotomy, and candidates for resective surgery. And this, also remembering that well-defined partial seizures may occur (or become electroclinically more evident?) after callosotomy, clearly suggesting that, at least in some cases, epileptic seizures, also with falls, previously admitted a focal, misdiagnosed origin (Gates et al., 1987; Spencer et al., 1988; Pinard et al., 1993). The extreme consequence of these effects of callosotomies is that such an intervention is also proposed with a diagnostic aim, before hemispherectomy (Torres & French, 1973).

Hemispherectomy, with its multiple variations, is generally considered the most effective surgical procedure, but its indications are relatively limited, mostly in cases of hemimegalencephaly, Rasmussen's syndrome and infantile hemiplegia (Tinuper et al., 1988; Delalande et al., 1992). Falls are frequent in such patients, but also appear in children with multilobar cryptogenic epilepsies (Munari et al., 1995b). Individually adapted multiple stereo-

EEG investigations spare functional areas in those patients with very severe epilepsy, without severe neurological deficits.

Concluding remarks

The presented series only concerns a limited number of children, but it allows several considerations:

(1) Falls are not necessarily *per se* of bad prognostic value in child candidates for surgical treatment of their epilepsy: surgery results are not significantly different in the two studied groups. However, late occurrence of either 'complex motor seizures' (Roger *et al.*, 1981) or falls, or both, can complicate the evolution of about one-third of partial epilepsies with early onset (Munari *et al.*, 1988). Therefore, the unexpected occurrence of falls could point to an earlier presurgical evaluation, especially in temporal lobe epilepsy.

(2) Falls only occurring late during partial seizures of proved temporal lobe origin do not imply a bad outcome: 87.5 per cent of Class 1a.

(3) It seems to be illusory to pretend to explain the pathogenesis of ictal falls, as suggested by Gambardella *et al.* 1994, without both an adequate polygraphic recording (Tassinari, personal communication, 1996), and an adapted stereo-EEG investigation.

(4) Spatial and temporal organization of ictal discharges during seizures with falls appears to be often difficult to understand with only non-invasive presurgical investigations. This is indirectly confirmed by the fact that bilateral stereo-EEG was performed in 42 per cent of children with ictal falls, and in only 15 per cent of the others. But we would stress that an individually adapted strategy of stereo-EEG investigation is more important because the question's solution is more complex.

It seems clear that falls can occur, regardless of where the onset of the discharges occurs: frontal (Bancaud & Talairach, 1992), central (Olivier, 1993), parietal (Olivier, 1993; Munari *et al.*, 1996), temporal (Gambardella *et al.*, 1994), or occipital.

The role played by both the rapidity of the propagation of the discharge, and the extent of the discharge itself should be tentatively recognized in each patient. The difference seems to be in the problem of particular syndromic entities, as in the Lennox–Gastaut syndrome.

We believe that it is legitimate to propose more accurate clinical and neurophysiological observations when trying to differentiate the probable different electroclinical patterns of a phenomenon as complex as ictal falls.

References

Bancaud, J., Talairach. J., Bonis, A., Schaub, C., Szikla, G., Morel, P. & Bordas-Ferrer, M.(1965): *La Stéréo-electroencephalographie dans l'epilepsie*. Informations neurophysiopathologiques apportées par l'investigation fonctionelle stéréotaxique. Paris: Masson & Cie.

Bancaud, J. & Talairach, J. (1992): Clinical semiology of frontal lobe seizures. In: *Advances in neurology,* vol. 57, *Frontal lobe seizures and epilepsies,* eds. P. Chauvel, A.V. Delgado-Escueta, E. Halgren & J. Bancaud, pp. 3–58. New York: Raven Press.

Beckung, E., Uvebrant, P., Hedström, & Rydenhag, B. (1994): The effects of epilepsy surgery on the sensorimotor function of the children. *Dev. Med. & Child. Neurol.* **36,** 893–901.

Broglin, D., & Bancaud, J. (1991): Manifestations neurovégétatives au cours des crises partielles du lobe temporal. In: *Crises épileptiques et épilepsies du lobe temporal, tome I.* pp. 69–96. Gentilly: Documentation médicale LABAZ.

Cascino, G., Andermann, F., Berkovic, SF., Kuzniecky, R.I., Sharbrough, F.W., Keene, D.L., Bladin, P.F., Kelly, P.J., Olivier, A. & Feindel, W. (1993): Gelastic seizures and hypothalamic hamartomas: evaluation of patients undergoing chronic intracranial EEG monitoring and outcome of surgical treatment. *Neurology* **43**, 747–750.

Chugani, H.T., Shields, W.D., Shewmon, D.A., Olson, D.M., Phelps, M.E. & Peacok, W.J. (1990): Infantile spasms: I. PET identifies focal cortical dysgenesis in cryptogenic cases for surgical treatment. *Ann. Neurol.* **27**, 406–413.

Delalande, O., Pinard, J.M., Basdevant, *et al.* (1992): Hemispherotomy: a new procedure for central disconnection. *Epilepsia* **33 (suppl. 3)**, 99–100.

Duchowny, M.S., Resnick ,T.J., Alvarez, L.A. & Morrison, G. (1990): Focal resection for malignant partial seizures in infancy. *Neurology* **40**, 980–984.

Engel, J. Jr. (1987): Outcome with respect to epileptic seizures. In: *Surgical treatment of the epilepsies*, ed. J. Engel Jr., pp. 553–571. New York: Raven Press.

Fish, D.R, Smith, S.J., Quesney, L.F., Andermann. F., & Rasmussen. T. (1993): Surgical treatment of children with medically intractable frontal or temporal lobe epilepsy: results and highlights of 40 years' experience. *Epilepsia* **34**, (2), 244–247.

Gambardella, A., Reutens, D.C., Andermann, F., Cendes, F., Gloor, P., Dubeau, F. & Olivier, A. (1994): Late-onset drop attacks in temporal lobe epilepsy: a reevaluation of the concept of temporal lobe syncope. *Neurology* **44**, 1074–1078.

Gates, J.R., Rosenfeld, W.E., Maxwell, R.E. & Lyons, R.E. (1987): Response of multiple seizure types to corpus callosum section. *Epilepsia* **28**, (1), 28–34.

Gates, J.R., (1991): Candidacy for corpus callosum section. In: *Epilepsy surgery*, ed. H. Luders, pp. 119–125. New York: Raven Press.

Geoffroy, G., Lassonde, M., Delisle, F. & Décaire, M. (1983): Corpus callosotomy for control of intractable epilepsy in children. *Neurology* **33**, 891–897. Cleveland.

Guldvog, B., Loining, Y., Hauglie-Hanssen, E., Flood, S. & Biornaes, H. (1994): Surgical treatment for partial epilepsy among Norwegian children and adolescents. *Epilepsia* **35**, (3), 554–565.

Kahane, P., Di Leo, M., Francione, S., Tassi, L., Hoffmann, D., Quarato, P.P. & Munari, C. (1995): Bradycardia during fronto-central epileptic seizures in a patient having a hypothalamic hamartoma. *Epilepsia* **36 (suppl. 3)**, 239.

Kahane, P., Francione, S., Tassi, L., Hoffmann, D., Lo Russo, G., Garrel, S., Feuerstein, C., Perret, J., Benabid, A.L. & Munari, C. (1993): Traitement chirurgical des épilepsies partielles graves pharmaco-résistantes: approche diagnostique et thérapeutique (rapport préliminaire sur trois années d'activité à Grenoble). *Epilepsies* **5**, 179–204.

Kahane, P., Tassi, L., Hoffmann, D., Francione, S., Gratadou-Juery, G., Pasquier, B. & Munari, C. (1994): Crises dacrystiques et hamartome hypothalamique: à propos d'une observation vidéo-stéréo-EEG. *Epilepsies* **6**, 259–279.

Lindsay, J., Gilbertm, G., Richard, P. & Ousted, C. (1984): Developmental aspects of focal epilepsies of childhood treated by neurosurgery. *Dev. Med. & Child. Neurol.* **26**, 574–587.

Maxwell RE, Gates JR & Gummit RJ (1987): Corpus callosotomy at the University of Minnesota. In: *Surgical treatment of epilepsies*, ed. J. Engel Jr., pp. 659–666. New York: Raven Press.

Morrison, G., Duchowny, M., Resnick ,T., Alvarez, L., Jayakar, P., Prats, A.R., Dean, P. & Penate, N. (1992): Epilepsy surgery in childhood. *Pediatr. Neurosurg.* **18**, 291–297.

Munari, C., Stoffels, C., Bossi, L., Brunet, P., Bonis, A., Bancaud, J. & Talairach, J. (1982): Partial seizures with elementary or complex symptomatology: a valid classification for temporal lobe seizures? In: *Advances in epileptology, XIIIth epilepsy international symposium*, eds. H. Akimoto, H. Kazamatsuri, M. Seino & A. Ward, pp. 25–27. New York: Raven Press.

Munari, C., (1984): Discussion concernant les épilepsies partielles lésionnelles. In: *Les Syndromes épileptiques de l'enfant et de l'adolescent*, eds. J. Roger, C. Dravet, M. Bureau, F. Dreifuss & P. Wolf, pp. 310–312. London: John Libbey.

Munari, C., (1987): Depth electrode implantation at Hopital Saint Anne, Paris. In: *Surgical treatment of the épilepsies*, ed. J. Engel Jr., pp. 583–588. New York: Raven Press.

Munari, C., Marchini, M. & Bancaud, J. (1988): Aetiologic and prognostic factors in drug-resistant partial epilepsies with childhood onset. In: *Diagnostic and therapeutic problems in pediatric epileptology*, eds. C. Faienza & G.L. Prati, pp. 85–107. Amsterdam: Elsevier.

Munari, C. & Betti, O. (1989): The stereotactic biopsy of brain lesions: a critical review. In: *Excerpta medica, International congress series no. 828: Cerebral gliomas*, eds. G. Broggi & M.A. Gerosa, pp. 179–206. Amsterdam: Elsevier.

Munari, C, Hoffmann, D., Francione, S,. Kahane, P., Tassi, L., Lo Russo, G. & Benabid, A. L. (1994): Stereo-electroencephalography methodology: advantages and limits. *Acta Neurol. Scand.* **suppl. 152,** 56–67.

Munari, C., Tassi, L., Di Leo, M., Kahane, P., Hoffmann, D., Francione, S. & Quarato, P.P. (1995a): Video-stereo-electroencephalographic investigation of orbitofrontal cortex. Ictal electroclinical patterns. In: *Advances in neurology*, vol. 66, Epilepsy and the functional anatomy of the frontal lobe, eds. H.H. Jaspers, S. Riggio & P.S. Goldman-Rakic, pp. 273–295. New York: Raven Press.

Munari, C., Francione, S., Kahane, P., Hoffmann, D., Tassi, L., Lo Russo, G. & Benabid, A.L. (1995b): Multilobar resection for the control of epilepsy. In: *Operative neurosurgical techniques. Indications, methods, and results*, 3rd edn., eds. H.H. Schmidek & W.H. Sweet, pp. 1323–1339. Philadelphia: Saunders.

Munari, C., Kahane, P., Francione, S., Hoffmann, D., Tassi, L., Cusmai, R., Vigevano, F., Pasquier, B. & Betti, O.O. (1995c): Role of the hypothalamic hamartoma in the genesis of gelastic fits (a video-stereo-EEG study). *Electroenceph. Clin. Neurophysiol.* **95,** 154–160.

Olivier, A. (1993): Surgery of extratemporal epilepsy. In: *The treatment of epilepsies: principles and practices*, ed. E. Wyllie, pp. 1092–1105. Philadelphia: Lea & Febiger.

Pinard, J.M., Delalande, O., Plouin, P. & Dulac, O. (1993): Callosotomy in West syndrome suggests a cortical origin of hypsarrythmia. *Epilepsia* **34,** 780–787.

Purves, S.J., Wada, J.A., Woodhurst, W.B., Moyes, P.D., Strauss, E., Kosaka, B. & Li D. (1988): Results of anterior corpus callosum section in 24 patients with medical intractable seizures. *Neurology* **38,** 1194–1201.

Rasmussen, T. (1983): Cortical resection in children with focal epilesy. In: *Advances in epileptology*, XIVth epilepsy international symposium, eds. M. Parsonage *et al.*, pp. 249–254. New York: Raven Press.

Ribaric, I.I., Nagulic, M. & Djurovic, B. (1991): Surgical treatment of epilepsy: our experience with 34 children. *Child's. Nerv. Syst.* **7,** 402–404.

Roger, J., Dravet, C., Menendez, P. & Bureau, M. (1981): Les épilepsies partielles de l'enfant. Evolution et facteurs de prognostic. *Rev. EEG Neurophysiol.* **11,** 431–437.

Spencer, S.S., Spencer, D.D., Williamson, P.D., Sass, K., Novelly, R.A. & Mattson, R.A. (1988): Corpus callosotomy for epilepsy. I. Seizure effects. *Neurology* **38,** 19–24.

Spencer, S.S., Spencer, D.D., Sass, K., Westerweld, M., Katz, A. & Mattson, R. (1993): Anterior, total, and two-stage corpus callosum section: differential and incremental seizure responses. *Epilepsia* **34,** 561–567.

Tinuper, P., Andermann, F., Villemure, J.G., Rasmussen, T.B. & Quesney, L.F. (1988): Functional hemispherectomy for treatment of epilepsy associated with hemiplegia: rationale, indications, results, and comparison with callosotomy. *Ann. Neurol.* **24,** (1), 27–34.

Torres, F. & French, L.A . (1973): Acute section of the corpus callosum upon 'independent' epileptiform activity. *Acta Neurol. Scand.* **49,** 47–62.

Turmel, A., Giard, N., Bouvier, G., Labreque, R., Veilleux, F., Rouleau, I. & Saint-Hilaire, J.M. (1992): Frontal lobe seizures and epilepsy. Indications for cortectomies and callosotomies. In: *Advances in neurology*, vol. 57, Frontal lobe seizures and epilepsies, eds. P. Chauvel, A.V. Delgado-Escueta, E. Halgren & J. Bancaud, pp. 689–705. New York: Raven Press.

Van Wagenen, W.P. & Herren, R.Y. (1940): Surgical division of commissural pathways in the corpus callosum: relation to spread of an epileptic attack. *Arch. Neurol. Psychiatr.* **44,** 740–759.

Ventureira, E.C.G. & Higgins, M.J. (1993): Complications of epilepsy surgery in children and adolescents. *Pediatr. Neurosurg.* **19,** 40–56.

Wyler, A.R. (1991): Corpus callosotomy. In: *The treatment of epilepsies: principles and practices*, ed. E. Wyllie, pp. 1120–1125. Philadelphia: Lea & Febiger.

Wilson, D.H., Reeves, A., Gazzaniga, M. & Culver, C. (1977): Cerebral commissurotomy for control of intractable seizures. *Neurology* **27,** 708–715.

Wilson, D.H., Reeves, A. & Gazzaniga, M. (1978): Division of the corpus callosum for uncontrollable epilepsy. *Neurology* **28,** 649–653.

Wilson, D.H., Reeves, A.G. & Gazzaniga, M.S. (1982): 'Central' commissurotomy for intractable generalized epilepsy: series two. *Neurology* **32,** 687–697.

Chapter 16

Corpus callosum section for the treatment of epileptic falls or drop attacks: an effective palliative approach

Mario A. Alonso-Vanegas, Frederick Andermann and André Olivier

Department of Neurology and Neurosurgery, McGill University, and the Montreal Neurological Hospital and Institute, 3801 University Street, Montreal, Quebec H3A 2B4, Canada

Summary

Over the last 56 years, our understanding of the role of callosotomy for the treatment of intractable seizures has slowly progressed. The presence of atonic and tonic drops has emerged as the major indication, though the procedure leads to improvement of other seizure patterns as well. The complication rate has steadily diminished and appears to be inversely proportional to the surgeon's experience and meticulous approach. The procedure is now considered in individuals with normal or near normal intelligence whose seizure pattern puts them at risk for deterioration. Fortunately such patients are rare. Staged complete callosotomy may be considered, especially in individuals with low intelligence in whom the seizures represent a significantly greater handicap than the disconnection-related symptoms. In most patients, a partial section not including the splenium brings about sufficient improvement so that a second section need not be performed.

Introduction

In 1886, one of the pioneers in neurosurgery and an outstanding and creative neuroscientist, Sir Victor Horsley (1886), published a paper entitled 'Brain Surgery' in which he described three successful operations for the alleviation of epileptic 'fits'. Another giant of neurology, John Hughlings Jackson (1886), who witnessed Horsley's experimental operations, opined at that time that epilepsy surgery had a scientific basis and that its objective was the removal of the 'discharging lesion'. The first publication devoted to epilepsy surgery written by Foerster & Penfield appeared in 1930, and contained a description of post-traumatic epilepsy and the results of radical operation (Foerster & Penfield, 1930). Later, van Wagenen & Herren (1940) reported their experience with ten epileptic patients in whom they performed a surgical division of the commissural pathways, including the corpus callosum. This was devised on the basis of their personal clinical observations. They had noticed that early in the course of tumours involving the corpus callosum, the patients usually had generalized seizures, but that as the tumour grew, the patient's generalized seizures decreased in frequency and often became unilateral without loss of consciousness. Thus emerged their concept that 'if the corpus callosum is destroyed, generalized convulsive seizures become less frequent'. Since then, the general consensus has been that 'the corpus callosum is a major pathway for [the] propagation of epileptic discharges from one hemisphere to the other resulting in secondary generalized discharges' (Bogen & Vogel, 1962; Wilson et al., 1975).

From the experimental point of view, Erickson (1940) in Montreal reported his experience with epilepsy in monkeys. He studied the spread of epileptic discharges induced by electrical stimulation of the cortex and concluded that two types of procedures could be used to alter or limit the spread of these discharges; namely, 'section of the corpus callosum and transcortical section at right angles to the central sulcus of Rolando'. Based on further experimental work of Marcus & Watson (1966; 1968), and of Mutani et al. (1973), Musgrave & Gloor (1980) concluded that 'synchronization of generalized bilateral spike and wave discharges is mediated through the corpus callosum'.

In spite of encouraging initial results, callosotomy did not emerge as an acceptable and effective mode of surgery until recently. Bogen's reintroduction and demonstration of effectiveness did not lead to universal recognition of the procedure. This was most probably related to the great variability in surgical techniques used, the variable extent of the resection and the heterogeneity of the types of seizures the patients presented. These in turn produced a large amount of diverse experimental and statistical data which were not integrated into a valid and generally accepted conclusion as to the effectiveness of the procedure and indications for callosotomy. A critical change was achieved by Wilson's introduction of microsurgical technique (Wilson et al., 1975) for forebrain commissurotomy which considerably reduced the morbidity related to this procedure.

Rationale and indications

Callosal section is not a panacea for the treatment of all patients with severe medical refractory epilepsy. It is a palliative rather than a curative procedure, but is now considered a safe and effective treatment for selected patients with intractable, debilitating, generalized seizures, particularly tonic or atonic drop attacks (Olivier et al., 1988; Wyllie, 1988; Spencer & Spencer, 1989; Engel et al., 1993).

From the theoretical standpoint, the main purpose of callosotomy is to interrupt what is probably the major pathway leading to the generalization of seizure spread.

Accordingly, patients with medically intractable epilepsy with either primary or secondary generalization should have a better outcome. Certain seizure types seem to respond more favourably than others to callosotomy. Drop attacks generally have been reported to lead to a better outcome than other types of generalized seizures (Harbaugh et al., 1983; Nordgren et al., 1991a, 1991b; Oguni et al., 1994), but this does not necessarily mean that the presence of drop attacks will guarantee a successful outcome. Other forms of clinically generalized seizures such as atypical absences and tonic-clonic attacks have also been shown to improve following callosotomy (Olivier et al., 1988; Oguni et al., 1994). The control or reduction of drop seizures is usual and may be sufficient to improve the quality of life dramatically, regardless of whether other seizure types are altered. It has been reported that complex partial seizures in patients with focal pathology may also be ameliorated by section of the corpus callosum; however, in any patient with a well-defined and removable focus of epileptogenic abnormality, resective surgery should be preferred.

Patients considered for callosal disconnection procedures are thus by definition not candidates for other forms of epilepsy surgery. They are a severely disabled group with a malignant form of epilepsy. Many of them have recurrent episodes of *status epilepticus*. In such individuals, even partial control of seizures might improve the quality of life, and is thus worthwhile (Spencer & Spencer, 1989; Oguni *et al.*, 1994; Rayport *et al.*, 1985; Purves *et al.*, 1988; Cendes *et al.*, 1993). Patients with extensive bilateral polymicrogyria such as bilateral perisylvian syndrome, and those with diffuse dysplastic lesions such as a double cortex leading to drop attacks or other types of generalized seizures, may have significant improvement following section of the corpus callosum (Andermann *et al.*, 1988; Landy *et al.*, 1993; Olivier *et al.*, 1996b).

Controlling drop attacks is crucial because children and adults experiencing them often present with multiple and recurrent head and facial injuries and need to be protected by wearing helmets in order to minimize the hazards of falling.

In patients with the Lennox–Gastaut syndrome (LGS) who have medically intractable epilepsy and mental retardation, callosotomy may represent an option for the reduction or control of some seizure types associated with this severe and debilitating process (Andermann *et al.*, 1988). Dulac and N'Guyen have pointed out that in LGS, excitatory interhemispheric pathways become excessively permeable in the frontal areas at the time when these areas become mature. The synaptic reduction created by the section of the callosum could explain the efficacy of the procedure (Dulac & N'Guyen, 1993). The majority of patients who are candidates for callosotomy have, not unexpectedly, some degree of cognitive impairment, given their diffuse or multifocal disease.

A further theoretical goal is prevention of the establishment of new epileptic foci by secondary epileptogenesis. In the 1960s, Morrell (1969) proposed that transcallosally propagated discharges may be important for the development of mirror foci.

Finally, it is important to consider the patient's neurological status in the selection process, particularly for those in whom hemispherectomy is an alternative possibility. Corpus callosum section offers a surgical option for individuals with a functional hand, without particular risk of increased motor deficit (Avila *et al.*, 1980; Tinuper *et al.*, 1988; Andermann, 1992).

Definition and pathophysiology of drop attacks

A brief historical review throws light upon the difficulty of defining the so-called drop attacks. Hughlings Jackson first referred to 'sudden epileptic falls' in 1886 (Jackson, 1886). Hunt (1922) described 'sudden shock-like loss of postural control for a short duration associated with or without loss of consciousness' as an epileptic phenomenon and named such events 'static seizures' or 'drop attacks'. Later, Fisher (1958) used the term 'akinetic falling spells of the aged' to describe brief spontaneous falls not preceded or followed by convulsive movements occurring in otherwise normal elderly patients. These attacks are most likely not of an epileptic nature but illustrate the difficulty with terminology and in making an accurate diagnosis. Multiple aetiologies and pathologies have been implicated since, as causing or manifesting with 'drop attacks', so that the term has lost its specificity and is now often used in a generic sense.

The Commission on Classification and Terminology of the International League Against Epilepsy (1981) in describing atonic seizures stated that 'a sudden diminution of muscle tone occurs which may be fragmentary, leading to a head drop with slackening of the jaw, the dropping of a limb or a loss of all muscle tone leading to a slumping to the ground. When these attacks are extremely brief they are known as drop attacks'. Drop attacks can thus be defined as 'a sudden fall, with or without loss of consciousness, due either to collapse of postural tone (a negative phenomenon), or abnormal muscle contraction, a brief tonic seizure or massive epileptic myoclonus (a positive phenomenon)'. The reason for difficulty in defining the term is implicit in this definition; namely, that falling may be caused by at least two different phenomena and hence atonic seizures and drop attacks are not synonymous. Furthermore, two mechanisms could play a part in a single seizure, as when a massive myoclonic jerk immediately precedes the loss of postural tone.

In clinical practice, it may be difficult to distinguish tonic from atonic drops. Only a few studies in the literature have described the use of polygraphic recording to differentiate between these two mechanisms. Egli *et al.* (1985) recorded 239 drop seizures in 45 patients. The most frequent in 20 patients were pure tonic drop seizures or axial spasms. Nine patients showed myoclonic-atonic seizures, nine had pure atonic episodes, and seven had 'slow falls', which occurred mostly during a slowly developing tonic seizure. Ikeno *et al.* (1985) studied fifteen patients with LGS. Using a self-tracking video monitoring system, EEG, and surface EMG of ten muscle groups they described four types of epileptic falls: tonic attacks in nine patients, flexor spasms in fifteen, myoclonic atonic attacks in twelve and atonic seizures in two patients.

The range of epileptic syndromes that have been recognized to cause drop attacks has recently expanded considerably (Andermann & Tenembaum, 1995).

Atonic epileptic drop attacks can occur while sitting, standing or lying down. Generally, there is neither an aura nor postictal confusion. Patients can usually get up immediately after the fall. Daily attacks are frequent. Apparently consciousness is at least partially retained during brief atonic seizures. Contrary to the belief that atonic seizures are ushered in by one or more myoclonic jerks, Oguni *et al.* (1992) have demonstrated by their polygraphic studies that only a small minority of the atonic seizures they recorded were preceded by myoclonic jerks.

Tonic seizures may of course also occur in any posture. If tonic contractions affect the lower extremities, the patient will fall in a stiff posture like a felled tree.

From a neurophysiological point of view, generalized tonic seizures may represent a more mature form of attack, analogous to infantile spasms or periodic spasms. Egli suggested brainstem dysfunction affecting the medullopontine rather than midbrain or thalamic structures (1985). Epileptic discharge could block inhibitory extrapyramidal motor centres so that the drop attack may be considered to represent a release phenomenon that briefly eliminates all motor activity and desynchronizes the cortex. The seizure can continue in the form of a tonic seizure or as an atypical absence, depending on the spread and intensity of the discharge.

Regarding atonic seizures it has been proposed (Blume, 1995) that they involve diffuse loss of muscle tone related to inhibitory components of the synchronous spikes and waves or polyspikes and waves centred over the pre-motor and prefrontal cortices. These discharges represent bursts of action potentials in the cortex, and are probably related to corticofugal discharges to the same pontobulbar reticular regions that stimulate spinal interneurons. Such interneurons inhibit spinal motoneurons, thus inhibiting muscle tone.

Preoperative evaluation

The preliminary investigation must be detailed. As in any other type of epilepsy surgery, a complete medical history and neurological examination is mandatory. Epilepsy surgery requires a multidisciplinary approach, therefore it should be carried out within specialized comprehensive epilepsy centres with the personnel required to treat patients and their rehabilitation holistically. The staff must include a neurologist with electroencephalographic expertise, an electroencephalographer with clinical interest, a neuropsychologist, a neuropsychiatrist, a neuroradiologist and a neurosurgeon.

The following conditions should be met in patients being referred for corpus callosum section. The single most important criterion is that patients should have failed to respond to adequate trials of single or combined anticonvulsant therapy in maximum tolerated doses. Second, any well-defined resectable epileptogenic focus or lesion must be ruled out. Third, the time span between onset of intractable seizures and surgical intervention should not be delayed, if possible, for more than two years. Some authors advocate that in the paediatric age group this time span should be longer, of at least four years in order to ascertain that spontaneous remission or improved control are not likely to occur (Nordgren *et al.*, 1991b). The most challenging problem for the clinician is to identify those children whose seizures are unlikely to remit and who are prone to develop progressive neurological or neuropsychiatric dysfunction. Treatable systemic or cerebral disorders must of course be ruled out. Lindsay *et al.* (1979a; 1979b) have shown that psychotic episodes are not uncommon in patients with chronic epilepsy and are not a contraindication to surgery. Educational and social factors must be considered and the family and the patient, when applicable, must be highly motivated.

The functional investigation required to achieve optimal results includes: electroencephalography (EEG), essential for documentation of seizure activity in order to discard the possibility of a resectable epileptogenic focus. EEG video monitoring is important because it allows visualization and documentation of the type and duration of convulsive or non-convulsive phenomena. Neuropsychological testing helps document the presurgical mental and behavioural status. It is important to mention that even severe mental retardation is not a contraindication for this type of surgery (Cendes *et al.*, 1993; Geoffroy *et al.*, 1983; Oguni *et al.*, 1991). When language is suspected to be represented in the right hemisphere, an amytal speech test is advised. Sass *et al.* (1990) have reported that patients with atypical cerebral language dominance (e.g. a right-handed person who also has right-cerebral speech dominance) are at risk for post-callosotomy language impairment.

At the Montreal Neurological Institute (MNI) an arteriovenous digital angiogram (DSA) is always done with stereoscopic views (Olivier, 1985; Peters *et al.*, 1990). It allows the surgeon to delineate the shape and extent of the corpus callosum. The image can be superimposed on the midsagittal plane of the magnetic resonance imaging study (MRI) and the callosal grid is constructed (Lehman *et al.*, 1992).

The stereoscopic views of the DSA permit three-dimensional visualization. This allows the surgeon to follow the course of the ascending venous channels and their relationship to the coronal suture which is a landmark used to optimize the placement of the craniotomy.

Magnetic resonance imaging (MRI) has become one of the most important preoperative studies. It confirms the presence, shape, thickness and length of the corpus callosum and allows recognition of some focal lesions.

The improved resolution of MRI compared with CT is well documented: MR imaging has been shown to have better diagnostic sensitivity due to its higher resolution, thinness of slices which can be obtained and the possibility of reformatting images in multiple planes in order to perform volumetric analysis and measurements. Using MRI it is now possible to recognize small lesions that were undetected by other imaging methods (Watson et al., 1992; Zimmerman, 1996).

Surgical procedure

A partial section of the anterior two-thirds of the corpus callosum as an initial procedure is widely accepted. It has been the practice at the MNI to perform, when necessary, a two-stage callosotomy. Meticulous technique is essential in order to avoid most of the side-effects or complications that are not directly due to the transection of the corpus callosum itself.

The procedure is usually performed under general anaesthesia with all the usual precautions taken for epilepsy surgery (Abou-Madi, 1997). We do not perform intraoperative EEG monitoring during callosotomy. In some centres (Marino & Ragazzo, 1985; Gates et al., 1987) intraoperative recording is carried out for purposes of determining the actual length of the section: in that case appropriate anaesthetic modifications are required. Doppler and end-tidal CO_2 monitoring as well as placement of a central catheter are indicated when the incision is placed higher than the heart. Patient positioning depends on the type of craniotomy and approach desired. As a routine we use the Mayfield head holder. The anterior division of the corpus callosum is most readily accomplished through an anterior approach, via a parasagittal craniotomy centred on the coronal suture. The right-sided approach is usually chosen, unless the right hemisphere is dominant or there is pre-existing left-hemisphere damage. The patient is placed supine, with the neck in neutral position and slight flexion, particularly when there is some degree of brain atrophy (this helps to maintain the midline orientation). A lateral decubitus or thirty-degree rotation of the head toward the side of the approach can also be used (this allows gravity to separate the dependant hemisphere from the falx, reducing the need for retraction). A 'barn door' incision is performed and the skin flap is retracted out of the operative field with fish-hooks or elevation sutures. The galea is treated with special care in case it might be needed for dural reconstruction at the end of the operation. Mannitol is given at the time of craniotomy and the pCO_2 maintained in the 28–30 mmHg range. Three burr holes are made on or just off the midline and two burr holes 3–4 cm off the midline. Because adhesions are always present in the midline, the bone flap should be cautiously detached with slender elevators. It is advisable to place the burr holes in the bone for the dural elevation sutures even before opening the dura. On the bone the coronal suture serves as an orientation guide. The dura is opened by an arcuate incision and reflected toward the superior sagittal sinus. At this stage it is important to avoid any damage to the venous structures entering the sinus. The right frontal lobe is gently separated from the falx and progressively retracted. It is essential to try to preserve any draining vein, but, if an ascending vein is being considered for division or is at risk of rupture, a critical review of the venous phase of the angiogram is done to be absolutely certain that it is not draining from the central sensorimotor cortical area.

The next step is to bring the surgical microscope into the operative field or to use magnifying 3.5x wide-field loupes and illumination in order to carry out separation or microdissection of the interpial adherences formed between both cingulate gyri. Normally such adhesions exist, but they are more prominent in patients with a previous history of infection or trauma, and these conditions have often been present in patients considered for callosotomy. Once a clear plane of separation is formed, the unmistakable white corpus callosum is identified and should be approached strictly in the midline between the two pericallosal arteries. The callosal division is initiated with the ultrasonic dissector (CUSA) set at 0.2 (100–150 mmHg) for suction and 0.2 for vibration, with irrigation of 2 to 3 cm^3/min at the level of the posterior genu or anterior part of the body. This site should be chosen since it is at this level that one may fall most often into the virtual space of the cavum septi pellucidi or its remnant. Gentle anterior to posterior, lateral or circular motions should be used until the bluish colour of the ependymal lining is reached. In this way, it is possible to divide the callosal fibres and leave the ependyma intact. As the dissection progresses anteriorly through the rostrum to the level of the superior lamina terminalis, the anterior cerebral arteries may be visualized as they loop over the rostral aspect of the corpus callosum.

Then, as the dissection is carried posteriorly, the retractors are repositioned, and if necessary, the head position may be altered by a Trendelenburg manoeuvre in order to be able to perform an adequate division. The midline cleft is re-identified in order to avoid section of the callosum lateral to one pericallosal artery, which will damage the corresponding cingulate gyrus and cause disruption of perforators originating in the depth of the pericallosal sulcus, with consequent postoperative oedema. Again, with the use of the CUSA, the resection of the posterior extent of the anterior two thirds of the corpus callosum is carried out. This usually corresponds to a point 4 to 4.5 cm from the anterior part of the genu. Meticulous haemostasis must be ensured prior to dural closure.

For a posterior approach or completion of the procedure, a parietal craniotomy is performed, and a protocol similar to that used for the anterior approach can be followed. The exposure is facilitated by a deeper falx, which also provides a guide of the midline. The same attention is paid to the integrity of the ascending veins. The falx is followed to the splenium. Usually at this

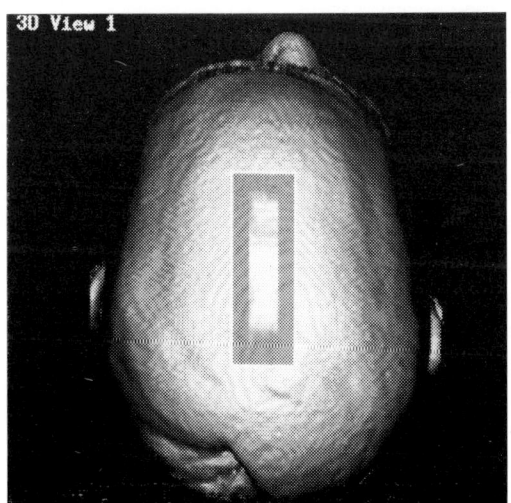

Fig. 1. A computerized head reconstruction in which an occipital depressed fracture is visualized as a dramatic effect of severe and repeated drop attacks. A 50 per cent translucent window through the scalp reconstruction permits visualization of the corpus callosum.

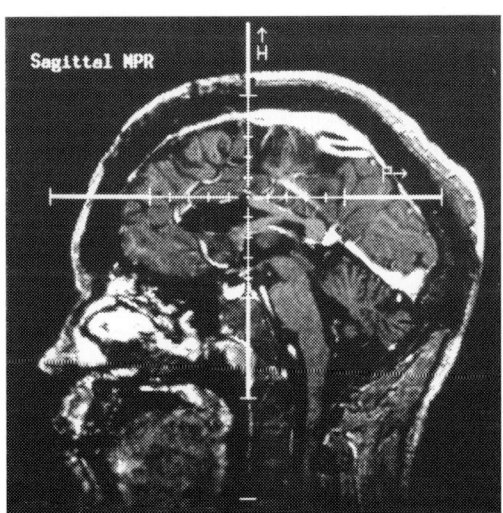

Fig. 2. A postoperative midsagittal MRI showing the extent of anterior section of the corpus callosum. The length of the corpus callosum according to the scale was 8 cm; the rostral half was sectioned.

level the interpial separation of the cingulate gyri is clear and there are usually no intercingulate adherences. In the posterior approach three anatomical features should be kept in mind. First, the isthmus of the corpus callosum is usually thinner compared with the rest of the body. Second, the course of the fornices in the ventral aspect of the most caudal part of the body is superior, anterior and medial, and should be kept in mind to avoid damaging them. Third, when the division of the splenium is achieved the dorsal leaflet of the vellum interpositum is visualized.

For the last four years we have used a frameless stereotactic system (Viewing Wand, ISG Technologies, Mississauga, Ontario, Canada) to carry out this procedure. For purposes of navigational guidance it has been very useful (Olivier et al., 1994).

The system allows planning the incision and craniotomy, permits visualization of the trajectories of draining veins and enables the surgeon to remain in the midline position, thus avoiding the risk of entering the cingulate gyrus. It is simple to operate and allows fast and reliable localization of any structure pointed at with the probe. It also permits the accurate measurement of the sectioned corpus callosum (Olivier et al., 1996a). A global gadolinium-enhanced MRI is obtained as a routine investigation in every patient who will eventually be a candidate for commissurotomy. At the same time, based on a global MRI, a three-dimensional reconstruction of the patient's face, brain and volumes of interest (VOI), such as the corpus callosum and the draining veins to the sagittal sinus is performed. Using these new technologies there is no need for an angiogram, which had previously been advocated as a useful tool to plan the craniotomy (Apuzzo et al., 1982).

Outcome

The great variability of surgical modalities employed since the first series were published, the diversity in anatomical extent of the resection, and the different and frequently electroencephalographically undocumented seizure types render a retrospective analysis of outcome difficult. This is further confounded by non-standardized postoperative evaluations, which are often difficult to assess. It cannot be overstated that the procedure is a palliative one and should not be expected to produce complete freedom from seizures. Its goal is to improve quality of life, increase social function and prevent severe injury.

Our experience and review of the literature shows that corpus callosotomy is particularly effective for the treatment of drop attacks, both atonic and tonic.

Amacher (1976) reported the complete control of atonic spells in three of four children after total callosotomy. Geoffroy et al. (1983) described the elimination of atonic attacks in two of three patients, though another patient apparently developed atonic spells after total callosotomy. Harbaugh et al. (1983) commented on the dramatic response of atonic seizures to commissurotomy when reviewing Wilson's first 20 patients and described seizure elimination in nine of them. Huck et al. (1980) and Blume (1984) described control or decrease in atonic episodes in five of eleven patients after anterior section. Spencer et al. (1988b) reported the elimination of atonic drop attacks in two out of two patients and complete control of tonic attacks in six of seven patients. Gates et al. (1987) reported statistically significant improvement in tonic or atonic drop attacks in 19 of 24 patients. Purves et al. (1988) described a significant reduction in drop attacks in five patients. Nordgren (1991a) reported complete control of atonic seizures in eleven of twelve patients and an 80 per cent reduction in the remaining one.

We (Oguni et al., 1991) reported over 75 per cent reduction in drop attack frequency in 45 per

Chapter 16 Corpus callosum section for the treatment of epileptic falls

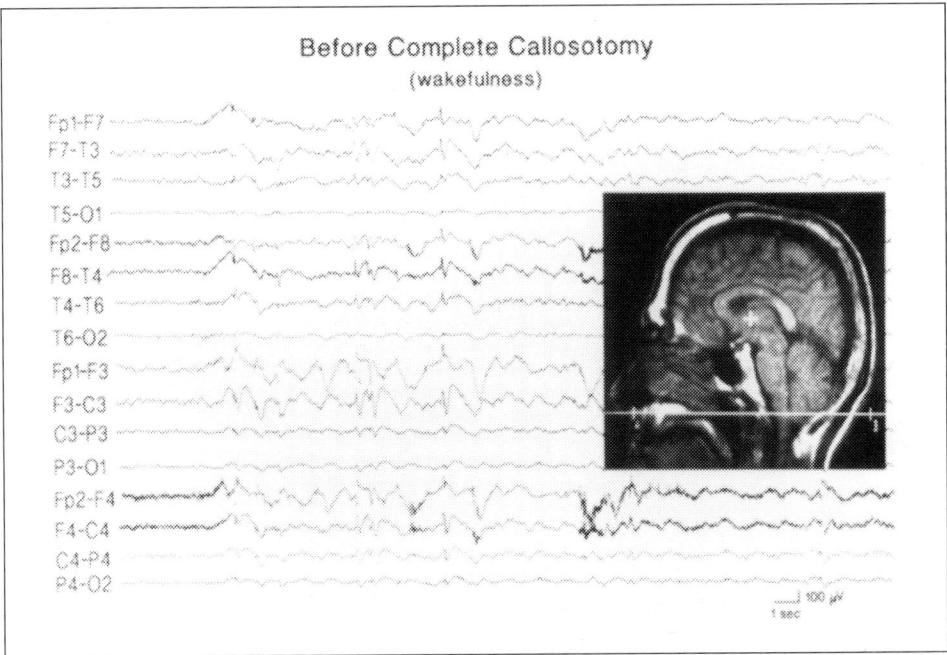

Fig. 3. Preoperative EEG showing bilateral synchronization of anterior epileptic discharges.

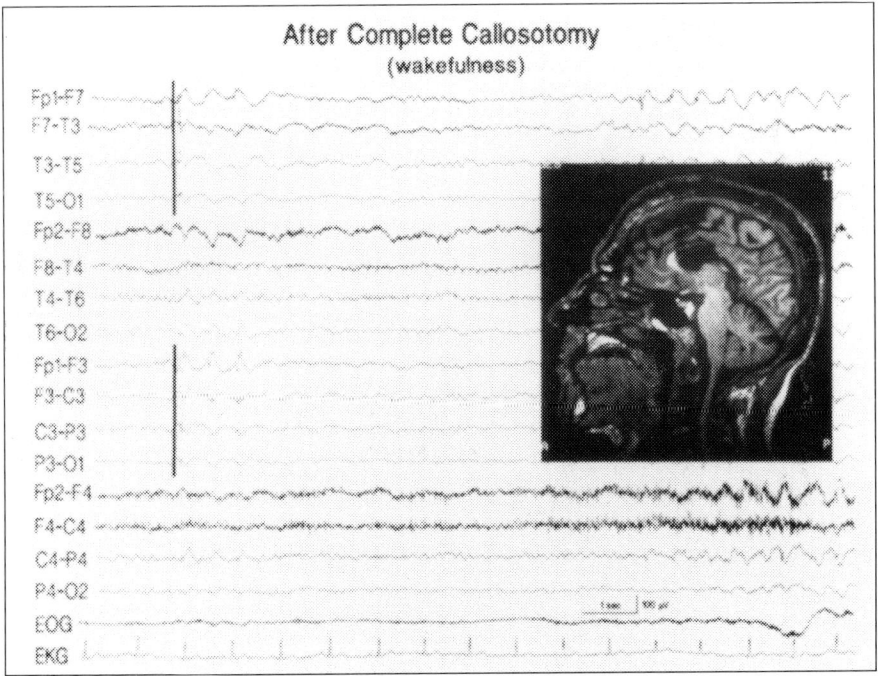

Fig. 4. Disruption of bilateral synchrony in EEG activity after complete callosotomy. The spike and wave pattern is now unilateral.

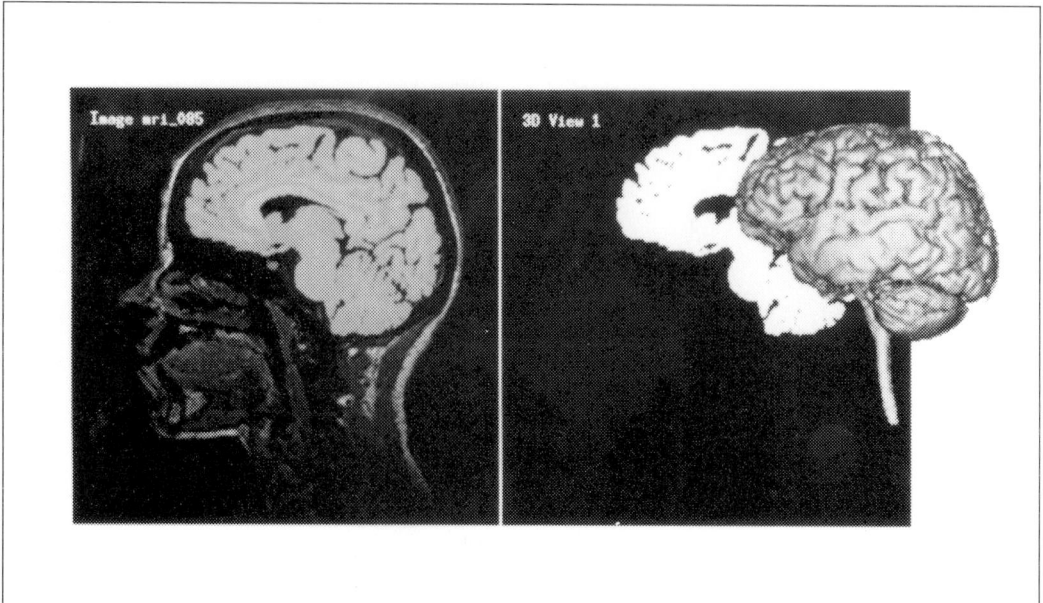

Fig. 5 Reconstructed brain images are generated using an interactive algorithm involving threshold-based segmentation and slice to slice integration allowing the creation of surface or anatomical contours.

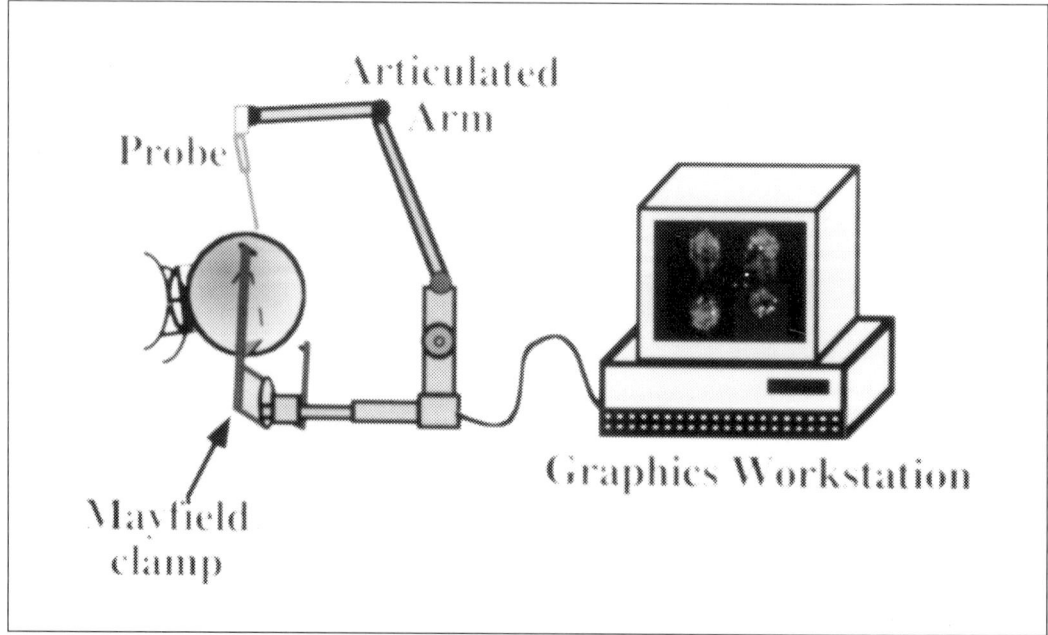

Fig. 6. Schematic representation of the Viewing Wand. The system is composed of a computer workstation, an articulated position-sensing arm attached to the head holder and a probe that is manipulated by the surgeon. This device is used to register the patient's anatomical landmarks with the three-dimensional reconstructed MR images.

cent of 31 patients and 50–75 per cent improvement in another 20 per cent. Reutens *et al.* (1993), based on the Australian co-operative study, reported over 50 per cent decrease in drop attacks (whether tonic or atonic was not specified) in 60 per cent of 47 patients. Cendes *et al.* (1993) in a study from Brazil reported a satisfactory decrease in atonic drop attacks in 90 per cent of eighteen patients and in tonic falls in 77.5 per cent of 26 patients. Four series (Stearns *et al.*, 1989; Kuzniecky *et al.*, 1990; Palmini *et al.*, 1991; Landy *et al.*, 1993) have reported results of corpus callosotomy for treatment of atonic seizures related to neuronal migration disorder, describing 80 per cent reduction in atonic seizures in one patient, 100 per cent reduction in drop attacks in five, significant improvement in head drops and atonic falls in two patients and over 80 per cent reduction in head drops and atonic falls in one each respectively. We (Alonso-Vanegas *et al.*, 1996) have reported abolition of drop attacks in 78 per cent of 44 patients after two-stage, two-thirds anterior callosotomy.

In spite of the intrinsic bias introduced by analysing all these data together it seems clear that there is a reduction of around 80 per cent in drop attack frequency after corpus callosotomy. A confounding problem encountered is that the results in most series have been reported using the 'generic' term of drop attacks. We recommend, if possible using more specific nomenclature such as atonic, tonic or myoclonic atonic drop attacks when reporting results in the future.

Regarding other seizure types, the results are much less clear. Amacher *et al.* (1976), Geoffroy *et al.* (1983), Spencer *et al.* (1988b), Gates *et al.* (1987) and Reeves & O'Leary (1985), upon reviewing the Dartmouth series, have specifically addressed the effect on tonic-clonic seizures in their series. Their experience suggests a reduction of 75 per cent after callosotomy, but the indication for attempting to treat this seizure type remains to be defined.

In the Dartmouth series (Reeves & O'Leary, 1985) seven patients with complex partial seizures had 100 per cent reduction and one of ten patients who had this form of attack had over 80 per cent reduction. Spencer *et al.* (1988b) reported a reduction of around 50 per cent, which is in accordance with our results (Oguni *et al.*, 1991) and those of Reutens *et al.* (1993). Gates (1987) reported a significant reduction in 12 of 20 patients with this type of seizure. It is clear that more standardized data have to be analysed to enable a more accurate assessment of the role of callosotomy for treatment of these seizure types.

It is important to stress that almost no patient exhibits drop attacks in isolation, and usually two or more seizure types can be identified. Thus, assessment of the effect of callosotomy on all the different seizure types is required.

Complications

The complications of callosotomy can be considered from two perspectives: those related to the operation *per se* and those related to disruption of callosal fibres and pathways.

In many of the early series (Luessenhop *et al.*, 1970) as well as in Wilson's landmark study of 1977, the complication rate was considered unacceptable (Wilson, 1977), even though the results with respect to seizure control were encouraging. Complications in three of seven patients included hydrocephalus and aseptic meningitis. As a result of this discouraging report, Wilson introduced a moratorium. When he again began to perform this type of surgery, partial or complete section of the corpus callosum alone replaced the previous practice of complete commissurotomy. The introduction of microsurgical technique reduced operative trauma to a minimum. The almost 50 per cent incidence of hydrocephalus and septic or aseptic meningitis encountered in the earlier series has greatly diminished, largely due to the practice of staying outside the ventricular lumen (Wilson *et al.*, 1982). This can be accomplished by leaving the ependymal lining intact.

Despite these improvements, morbidity and mortality from this operation were still reported to be higher than for other, resectional, procedures. The most often reported complication in this group was leg weakness from hemispheric retraction, which was usually transitory. Hydrocephalus, ventriculitis, meningitis and wound infection were also described. Intracranial swelling or venous infarction of the frontal lobe occurred when there was extensive damage to the sagittal sinus or when too many bridging veins were sacrificed. Bronchopneumonia has been reported as a systemic complication related to reduced postoperative mobility mainly associated with the transient akinetic mutism, which in our opinion is secondary to bilateral cingulum disruption (Olivier, 1991).

The incidence of these complications seems related to the experience and meticulous regard of the surgeon to nervous structures. The technological advances, particularly the use of the viewing wand and global MRI reconstruction, have largely eliminated operative complications. There is some discussion about the effect of anti-epileptic drugs, particularly valproic acid on clotting mechanisms. It has been our practice to discontinue valproate, which is often used in callosotomy candidates prior to operation.

Reduced verbal and motor activity in the immediate postoperative period has been reported to be related to the retraction of medial portions of the frontal lobe, manipulation of anterior cerebral arteries, or acute disconnection of supplementary motor areas (Roberts, 1993). Generally, this hypokinetic state is transitory and resolves completely.

The acute disconnection syndrome was described early on (Ross *et al.*, 1984), as an easily observable group of symptoms appearing, in the majority, if not in all patients, hours to days after section of the corpus callosum. It is characterized by mutism, non-dominant left-arm and leg apraxia resembling hemiparesis, inattention, bilateral Babinski sign and urinary incontinence. Other symptoms include confusion, visual or limb agnosia, bilateral grasp reflexes, apathy, infantile behaviour and alternating partial motor seizures. Not all features were seen in every patient. (Gazzaniga *et al.*, 1962; Spencer, 1988a). These symptoms were noted after a section of the callosum and were usually transitory. It was unclear whether they were related to the surgical retraction, the cortical diaschisis or the cortical disconnection (Spencer *et al.*, 1987). Nearly all patients exhibited this syndrome following single-stage total callosotomy in Wilson's early series (Jackson, 1886). Again, with time, the incidence of this type of symptomatology greatly diminished, largely due to the practice of partial or complete two-stage callosotomy.

Interhemispheric sensory disconnection occurs following section of the posterior half of the corpus callosum (McKeever *et al.*, 1985). The deficit can be demonstrated with somatosensory, auditory, and visual stimuli, suggesting that the language-dominant hemisphere does not have access to the information presented to the other hemisphere. The dissociation may not be demonstrable if the section is incomplete, whereas it is permanent with complete section. Generally, though, these symptoms are not disabling in normal daily activities. Furthermore, most patients compensate by the use of external visual cues. Through the use of specific dichotic listening tasks it has also been demonstrated that auditory disconnection can ensue after callosotomy. Using MRI and accurately defined measurements, it has been proposed that the areas responsible for the strong left-ear suppression are the splenium and possibly the part of the body of the callosum projecting to the most posterior part of the trunk (Sugishita *et al.*, 1995).

The so-called split-brain syndrome is characterized by language impairment, sensory disconnection, and non-dominant hand apraxia. The patient can not perform fine motor movements on demand, and shows impairment in attention–memory sequencing (Ferguson *et al.*, 1985). This is a long-lasting disabling syndrome, observed in a minority of patients (3–5 per cent) after total or near total callosotomy (Erickson, 1940). Recovery from the antagonistic activities of the non-dominant hand can take months, yet in a subset of patients this syndrome remains permanently disabling for daily activities. In patients with low intelligence and severe disability from their drop attacks, complete callosotomy is, however, justified, even at the cost of a disconnection syndrome which has to be carefully explained to the patients and caregivers preoperatively.

Memory deficits have been reported after a partial and complete section in a small number of patients (Zaidel & Sperry, 1974). Other authors, however, suggest that these disturbances could represent an attention disorder rather than one of memory (Beniak *et al.*, 1985). In patients with preoperative extracallosal damage, particularly to the fornix and its connections, discriminating psychometric tests have demonstrated disorders of recent memory, involving both initial encoding and retrieval of information requiring interhemispheric co-operation (Clark & Geffen, 1989).

Partial seizures, often inconspicuous before surgery, have been observed more often postoperatively by some investigators (Spencer *et al.*, 1984). Spencer *et al.* (1984) have pointed out that seizures with initially bilateral manifestations were converted to more focal patterns. Their descriptions included focal or more intense focal seizures following surgery in five of seventeen

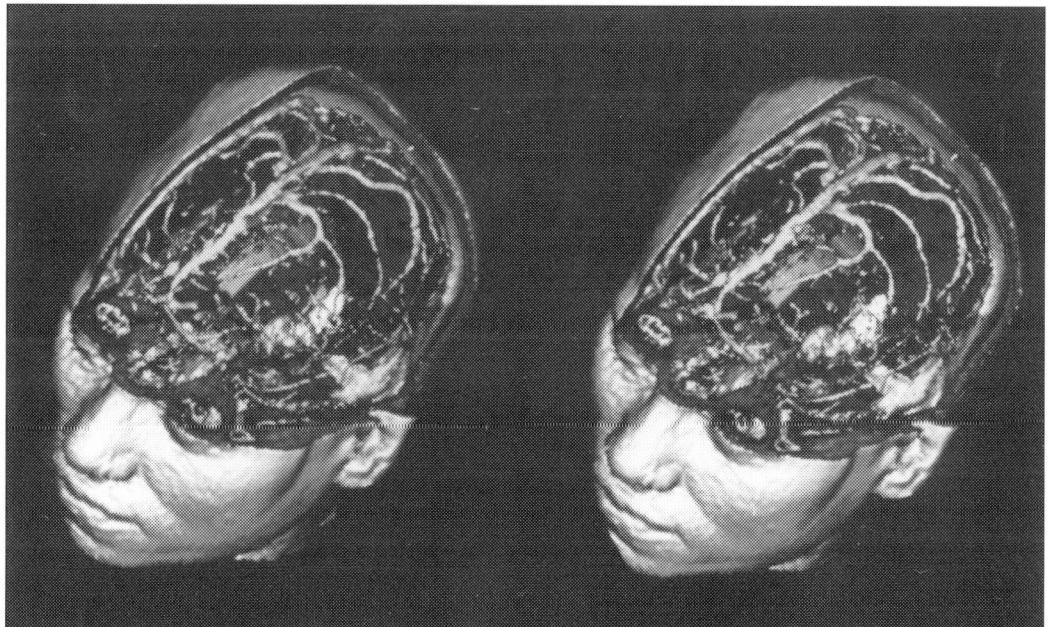

Fig. 7. Three-dimensional stereoscopic reconstruction showing the location and number of draining veins to the sagittal sinus, as well as the location and extent of the corpus callosum. Using this technique, the surgeon can select a small precoronal craniotomy and plan the angle of approach. Depth perception is appreciated in three-dimensional space.

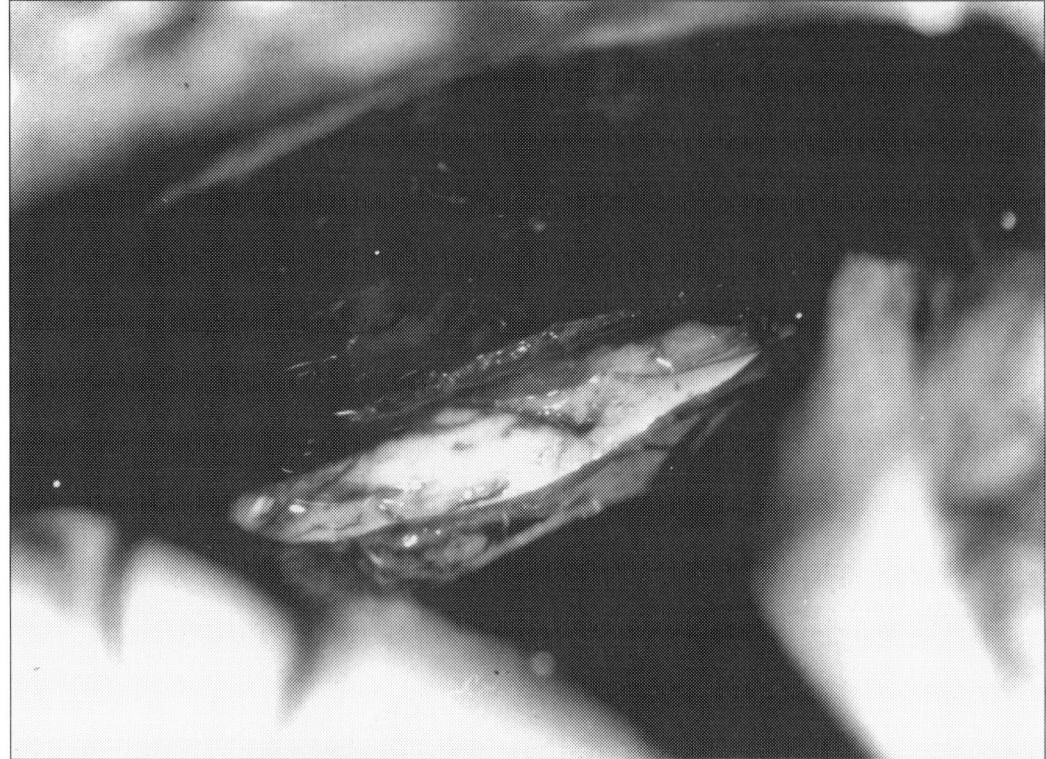

Fig. 8. Intraoperative photograph. With slight retraction on the right hemisphere, the corpus callosum and pericallosal arteries are visualized.

patients. They suggested that the procedure might disrupt an inhibitory mechanism in patients with asymmetrical frontal or bilateral synchronous frontal foci. Nordgren *et al.* (1991b) reported nine patients who developed focal seizures as a new phenomenon after surgery and another patient in whom focal manifestations were more intense than preoperatively. However, other series show different results. In a large series of over 120 patients with the Lennox–Gastaut syndrome or with drop attacks associated with other epileptic syndromes, we encountered one individual in whom preoperatively lateralization was suspected and in whom several years later an area of cortical dysplasia was found and subsequently resected. We did not find any partial seizures appearing *de novo* (Andermann *et al.*, 1988).

Conclusions

The new anti-epileptic agents, notably lamotrigine, promised better control of the seizures associated with secondary generalized epilepsy. This led to a reduction in the number of patients in whom the procedure was considered in recent years. Unfortunately, this promise was not entirely fulfilled and there is currently again an increase in the number of patients referred with a view to this form of palliative surgery. We still hope, however, that improved understanding of the seizure mechanisms and improved medical treatments will render the necessity for surgical division of the corpus callosum obsolete. In the meantime, callosotomy remains a valuable procedure for the alleviation of these most malignant forms of epileptic seizures.

References

Abou-Madi, M.N. (1997): Anesthesia considerations in epilepsy surgery. In: *Textbook of stereotactic and functional neurosurgery*, eds. P.L. Gildenberg & R.R. Tasker. McGraw-Hill, Inc.

Amacher, A.L. (1976): Midline commissurotomy for the treatment of some cases of intractable epilepsy. *Child's Brain* **2**, 54–58.

Alonso-Vanegas, M.A., Andermann, F., Lam, C.H., Preul, M.C., Dubeau, F. & Olivier, A. (1996): Callosotomy for the treatment of drop attacks (abstract). *J. Neurosurg.* **84**, 343A.

Andermann, F., Olivier, A., Gotman, J. & Sergent, J. (1988): Callosotomy for the treatment of patients with intractable epilepsy and the Lennox–Gastaut syndrome. In: *The Lennox–Gastaut syndrome*, eds. E. Niedermeyer & R. Degen, pp. 361–376. New York: Alan R Liss Inc.

Andermann, F. (1992): Clinical indications for hemispherectomy and callosotomy. *Epilepsy Research* **5**, S189–199.

Andermann, F. & Tenembaum, S. (1995): Negative motor phenomena in generalized epilepsies. In: *Negative motor phenomena*, eds. S. Fahn, M. Hallett, H.O. Lueders & C.D. Marsden, *Adv. Neurol.* **67**, 9–28.

Apuzzo, M.L.J., Chikovani, O.K. & Gott, P.S. (1982): Transcallosal interfornicial approaches for lesions affecting the third ventricle: surgical considerations and consequences. *Neurosurgery* **10**, 547–554.

Avila, J.O., Radvany, J., Huck, F.R., et al. (1980): Anterior callosotomy as a substitute for hemispherectomy. *Acta Neurochir.* **30**, 137–143.

Beniak, T.E., Gates, J.R. & Risse, G.L. (1985): Comparison of selected neuropsychological test variables pre- and postoperatively in patients subjected to corpus callosotomy. *Epilepsia* **26**, 534.

Blume, W.T. (1995): Physiology of atonic seizures. In: *Negative motor phenomena*, eds. G. Fahn, M. Hallett, H.O. Luedes & C.D. Marsden. *Adv. Neurol.* **67**, 173–179.

Blume, W.T. (1984): Corpus callosum section for seizure control: rationale and review of experimental and clinical data. *Cleveland Clinic Quarterly* **51**, (2), 319–332.

Bogen, J.E. & Vogel, P.J. (1962): Cerebral commissurotomy in man. *Bull. LA Neurol. Soc.* **27**, 169–172.

Clark, C.R. & Geffen, G.M. (1989): Corpus callosum surgery and recent memory. A review. *Brain* **112**, 165–175.

Cendes, F., Ragazzo, P.C., da Costa, V. & Martins, L.F. (1993): Corpus callosotomy in treatment of medically resistant epilepsy: preliminary results in a pediatric population. *Epilepsia* **34**, 910–917.

Commission on classification and terminology of the International League Against Epilepsy. Proposal for revised clinical and electroencephalographic classification of epileptic seizures (1981): *Epilepsia* **22**, 489–501.

Dulac, O. & N'Guyen, T. (1993): The Lennox–Gastaut syndrome. *Epilepsia* **34**, S7–17.

Fisher, C.M. (1958): The use of anticoagulants in cerebral thrombosis. *Neurology* **8**, 311–332.

Egli, M., Mothersill, J., O'Kane, M. & O'Kane, F. (1985): The axial spasm. The predominant type of drop seizure in patients with secondary generalized epilepsy. *Epilepsia* **26**, 401–415.

Engel, J. Jr, Van Ness, P.C., Rasmussen, T.B. & Ojemann, L.M. (1993): Outcome with respect to epileptic seizures. In: *Surgical treatment of the epilepsies*, 2nd edn., ed. J. Engel Jr., pp. 609–621. New York: Raven Press.

Erickson, T.C. (1940): Spread of the epileptic discharge: an experimental study of the afterdischarge induced by electrical stimulation of the cerebral cortex. *Arch. Neurol. Psychiat.* **43**, 429–452.

Ferguson, S.M., Rayport, M. & Corrie, W.S. (1985): Neuropsychiatric observations on behavioural consequences of corpus callosum section for seizure control. In: *Epilepsy and the corpus callosum*, ed. A.G. Reeves, p. 451. New York: Plenum Press.

Foerster, O. & Penfield, W. (1930): The structural basis of traumatic epilepsy and results of radical operation. *Brain* **53**, 99–119.

Gates, J.R., Rosenfeld, W.E., Maxwell, R.E. & Lyons, R.E. (1987): Response of multiple seizure types to corpus callosum section. *Epilepsia* **28**, 28–34.

Gazzaniga, M.S., Bogen, J.E. & Sperry, R.W. (1962): Some functional effects of sectioning the cerebral commissures in man. *Proc. Nat. Acad. Sci.* **48**, 1765–1769.

Geoffroy, G., Lassonde, M., Delisle, F. & Décarie, M. (1983): Corpus callosotomy for control of intractable epilepsy in children. *Neurology* **33**, 891–897.

Harbaugh, R.E., Wilson, D.H., Reeves, A.G. & Gazzaniga, M.S. (1983): Forebrain commissurotomy for epilepsy: review of 20 consecutive cases. *Acta Neurochir.* **68**, 263–275.

Horsley, Sir V. (1886): Brain surgery. *Br. Med. J.* **2**, 670–675.

Huck, F.R., Radvany, J., Avila, J.O., Pires de Camargo, C.H., Marino, R. Jr., Ragazzo, P.C., Riva, D. & Arlant, P. (1980): Anterior callosotomy in epileptics with multiform seizures and bilateral synchronous spike and wave EEG pattern. *Acta Neurochir.* **30**, S127–135.

Hunt, J.R. (1992): On the occurrence of static seizures in epilepsy. *J. Nerv. Ment. Dis.* **56**, 351–356.

Ikeno, T., Shigematsu, H., Miyakoshi, M., Ohba, A., Yagi, K. & Seino, M. (1985): An analytic study of epileptic falls. *Epilepsia* **26**, 612–621.

Jackson, J.H. (1886): A contribution to the comparative study of convulsions. In: *Selected writings of John Hughlings Jackson*, ed., J. Taylor, vol. 1. London: Hodder & Stoughton (1931), pp. 348–361.

Kuzniecky, R., Andermann, F., Fusco, L., *et al.* (1990): Corpus callosotomy in the management of the congenital bilateral perisylvian syndrome (abstract). *Epilepsia* **31**, 639.

Landy, H.J, Curless, R.G., Ramsay, R.E., Slater, J., Ajmone-Marsan, C. & Quencer, R.M. (1993): Corpus callosotomy for seizures associated with band heterotopia. *Epilepsia* **34**, 79–83.

Lehman, R.M., Olivier, A., Moreau, J.J., Tampieri, D. & Henri, C. (1992): Use of the callosal grid system for the preoperative identification of the central sulcus. *Stereotact. Funct. Neurosurg.* **58**, 178–188.

Lindsay, J., Ounsted, C. & Richards, P. (1979a): Long-term outcome in children with temporal lobe seizures. I. Social outcome and childhood factors. *Dev. Med. Child. Neurol.* **21**, 285–298.

Lindsay, J., Ounsted, C. & Richards, P. (1979b): Long-term outcome in children with temporal lobe seizures. III. Psychiatric aspects in childhood and adult life. *Dev. Med. Child. Neurol.* **21**, 630–636.

Luessenhop, A.J., de la Cruz, T.C. & Fenichel, G.M. (1970): Surgical disconnection of the cerebral hemispheres for intractable seizures. Results in infancy and childhood. *JAMA* **213**, 1630–1636.

Marcus, E.M. & Watson, C.W. (1966): Bilateral synchronous spike-wave electrographic patterns in the cat. *Arch. Neurol.* **14**, 601–610.

Marcus, E.M. & Watson, C.M. (1968): Symmetrical epileptogenic foci in monkey cerebral cortex: mechanisms of interaction and regional variations in capacity for synchronous discharges. *Arch. Neurol.* **19**, 99–116.

Marino, R. Jr. & Ragazzo, P.C. (1985): Selective criteria and results of selective partial callosotomy. In: *Epilepsy and the corpus callosum*, ed. A.G. Reeves, pp. 281–301. New York: Plenum Press.

McKeever, W., Sullivan, K., Ferguson, S., *et al.* (1985): Hemispheric disconnection effects in patients with corpus callosum section. In *Epilepsy and the corpus callosum*, ed. A.G. Reeves, p. 451. New York: Plenum Press.

Morrell, F. (1969): Physiology and histochemistry of the mirror focus. In: *Basic mechanisms of the epilepsies,* eds. H.H. Jasper, A.A. Ward & A. Pope, p. 263. Boston: Little, Brown.

Musgrave, J. & Gloor, P. (1980): The role of corpus callosum in bilateral interhemispheric synchrony of spike and wave discharge in feline generalized penicillin epilepsy. *Epilepsia* **21**, 369–378.

Mutani, R., Bergamini, L., Fariello, R., *et al.* (1973): Bilateral synchrony of epileptic discharge associated with chronic asymmetrical cortical foci. *Electroencephalogr. Clin. Neurophysiol.* **34**, 53–59.

Nordgren, R.E. (1991a): Corpus callosotomy is an underutilized procedure in children. *J. Epilepsy* **4**, 73–80.

Nordgren, R.E., Reeves, A.G., Viguera, A.C. & Roberts, D.W. (1991b): Corpus callosotomy for intractable seizures in the pediatric age group. *Arch. Neurol.* **48**, 364–372.

Oguni, H., Olivier, A., Andermann, F. & Comair, J. (1991): Anterior callosotomy in the treatment of medically intractable epilepsies: a study of 43 patients with a mean follow-up of 39 months. *Ann. Neurology* **30**, 357–364.

Oguni, H., Fukuyama, Y., Imaizumi, Y. & Uehara, T. (1992): Video-EEG analysis of drop seizures in myoclonic astatic epilepsy of early childhood (Doose syndrome). *Epilepsia* **33**, 805–813.

Oguni, H., Andermann, F., Gotman, J. & Olivier, A, (1994): Effect of anterior callosotomy on bilaterally synchronous spike and wave and other EEG discharges. *Epilepsia* **35**, 505–513.

Olivier, A., Peters, T. & Bertrand, G. (1985): Stereotaxic system and apparatus for use with MRI, CT and DSA. *Appl. Neurophysiol.* **48**, 94–96.

Olivier, A., Andermann, F. & Oguni, H. (1988): Anterior callosotomy in the treatment of intractable epilepsies. *Boll. Lega. Ital. Epil.* (**suppl.**) **64**, 81–86.

Olivier, A. (1991): Surgery of epilepsy: overall procedure. In: *Neurosurgical aspects of epilepsy*, ed. M.L.J. Apuzzo, American Association of Neurological Surgeons, pp. 117–148.

Olivier, A., Germano, I.M., Cukiert, A. & Peters, T. (1994): Frameless stereotaxy for surgery of the epilepsies: preliminary experience. *J. Neurosurg.* **81**, 629–633.

Olivier, A., Alonso-Vanegas, M.A., Comeau, R. & Peters, T.M. (1996a): Image-guided surgery of epilepsy. In: *Clinical frontiers of interactive image-guided neurosurgery*, ed. R.J. Maciunas, *Neurosurgery clinics of North America* **7**, (2), 229–243. W.B. Saunders.

Olivier, A., Andermann, F., Palmini, A. & Robitaille, Yvon (1996b): Surgical treatment of cortical dysplasias. In: *Dysplasias of cerebral cortex and epilepsy,* eds. R. Guerrini, F. Andermann, *et al.*, pp. 351–366. New York: Lippincott-Raven Healthcare.

Palmini, A., Andermann, F., *et al.* (1991): Diffuse cortical dysplasia or the 'double cortex' syndrome: the clinical and epileptic spectrum in 10 patients. *Neurology* **41**, 1656–1662.

Peters, T., Henri, C., Pike, B., Clarke, J., Collins, L. & Olivier, A. (1990): Integration of stereoscopic DSA with three-dimensional image reconstruction for stereotactic planning. *Stereotact. Funct. Neurosurg.* **54/55**, 471–476.

Purves, S.J., Wada, J.A., Woodhurst, W.B., *et al.* (1988): Results of anterior corpus callosum section in 24 patients with medically intractable seizures. *Neurology* **38**, 1194–1201.

Rayport, M., Corrie, W.S. & Ferguson, S.M. (1985): Corpus callosum section for control of clinically and electroencephalographically classified intractable seizures. In: *Epilepsy and the corpus callosum*, ed. A.G. Reeves, pp. 329–337. New York: Plenum Press.

Reeves, A.G. & O'Leary, P.M. (1985): Total corpus callosotomy for control of intractable epilepsy. In: *Epilepsy and the corpus callosum*, ed. A.G. Reeves, pp. 269–280. New York: Plenum Press.

Reutens, D., Bye, A.M., Hopkins, I.J., Danks, A., Somerville, E., Walsh, J., Bleasel, A., Ouvrier, R., MacKenzie, R.A., Manson, J.I., Bladin, P.F. & Berkovic, S.F. (1993): Corpus callosotomy for intractable epilepsy: seizure outcome and prognostic factors. *Epilepsia* **34**, (5), 904–909.

Roberts, D.W. (1993): The role of callosal section in surgical treatment of epilepsies. *Neurosurg. Clin. North Am.* **4**, 263–300.

Ross, M.K., Reeves A.G. & Roberts, D.W. (1984): Post-commissurotomy mutism. *Ann. Neurol.* **16**, 114.

Sass, K.J., Novelly, R.A., Spencer, D.D., *et al.* (1990): Post-callosotomy language impairments in patients with crossed cerebral dominance. *J. Neurosurg.* **72**, 85–90.

Spencer, S.S., Spencer, D.D., Glaser, G., Williamson, P. & Mattson, R. (1984): More intense focal seizure types after callosal section: the role of inhibition. *Ann. Neurol.* **16**, 686–693.

Spencer, S.S., Gates, J.R., Reeves, A.G., *et al.* (1987): Corpus callosum section. In: *Surgical treatment of the epilepsies*, ed. J. Engel, pp. 425–444. New York: Raven Press.

Spencer, S.S. (1988a): Corpus callosum section and other disconnection procedures for medically intractable epilepsy. *Epilepsia* **29** (**suppl. 2**), S85–99.

Spencer, S.S., Spencer, D.D., Williamson, P., Sass, K., Novelly, R.A. & Mattson, R.H. (1988b): Corpus callosotomy for epilepsy. I. Seizure effects. *Neurology* **38**, 19–24.

Spencer, D. & Spencer, S.S. (1989): Corpus callosotomy in the treatment of medically intractable secondarily generalized seizures of children. *Cleve. Clin. J. Med.* **56**, S69–78.

Stearns, M., Wolf, A.L., Barry, E., Bergey, G. & Gellard, F. (1989): Corpus callosotomy for refractory seizures in a patient with cortical heterotopia: case report. *Neurosurgery* **25,** 633–636.

Sugishita, M., Otomo, K., Yamazaki, K., Shimizu, H., Yoshiota, M. & Shinohara, A. (1995): Dichotic listening in patients with partial section of the corpus callosum. *Brain* **118,** 417–427.

Tinuper, P., Andermann, F., Villemure, J.G., Rasmussen, T.B. & Quesney, L.F. (1988): Functional hemispherectomy for treatment of epilepsy associated with hemiplegia: rationale, indications, results and comparison with callosotomy. *Ann. Neurol.* **24,** 27–34.

Van Wagenen, W.P. & Herren, R.Y. (1940): Surgical division of the commissural pathways in the corpus callosum: relation to spread of an epileptic attack. *Arch. Neurol. Psych.* **44,** 740–759.

Watson, C., Andermann, F., Gloor, P., *et al.* (1992): Anatomic basis of amygdaloid and hippocampal volume measurement by magnetic resonance imaging. *Neurology* **42,** 1743–1750.

Wilson, D.H., Culver, C., Waddington, M. & Gazzaniga, M. (1975): Disconnection of the cerebral hemispheres: an alternative to hemispherectomy for the control of intractable seizures. *Neurology* **25,** 1149–1153.

Wilson, D.H., Reeves, A., Gazzaniga, M. & Culver, C. (1977): Cerebral commissurotomy for control of intractable seizures. *Neurology* **27,** 708–715.

Wilson, D.H., Reeves, A. & Gazzaniga, M. (1982): 'Central' commissurotomy for intractable generalized epilepsy: Series 2. *Neurology* **32,** 687–697.

Wyllie, E. (1988): Corpus callosotomy for intractable generalized epilepsy. *J. Pediatr.* **113,** 255–261.

Zaidel, D. & Sperry, R.W. (1974): Memory impairment after commissurotomy in man. *Brain* **97,** 263–272.

Zimmerman, R.A. (1996): Epilepsy. *Crit. Rev. Neurosurg.* **6,** 1–5.

Chapter 17

Seizures and the risk of injury in four different clinical severity populations

Georgio Capizzi*, Piernanda Vigliano,* Maresa Perenchio,† and Giovanni Asteggiano‡

*Cattedra di Neuropsichiatria Infantile, Università di Torino, Italy;
†Servizio di Neuropsichiatria Infantile, Ivrea, Italy; ‡Servizio di Neuropsichiatria Infantile, Alba, Italy

Summary

This study examines, in groups of patients differing in the severity of epilepsy accompanied by falling, whether or not the risk of injury is related to the type and frequency of seizures, and if counselling modifies this risk. The study concerns subjects aged 3–15 years and is retrospective for the period 1 January 1992 to 31 December 1994.

Group P^1 includes 108 epileptic children who were followed by the Child Neurology Service of Ivrea; Group P^2 includes 271 patients who were followed by the University of Torino Child Neurology Institute, Epilepsy Unit; and Group P^3 includes 23 epileptic patients hospitalized in an institute for the seriously handicapped. All patients were divided into clinical groups: (1) idiopathic generalized epilepsy (IGE); (2) idiopathic partial epilepsy (IPE), (3) symptomatic generalized epilepsy (SGE), and (4) symptomatic partial epilepsy (SPE). Injury was classified as mild (A), medium (B) and serious (C) on the basis of type of injury, duration of medical treatment and severity of ensuing functional limitation. These subjects were compared with an unselected population (P^4), which included 9203 subjects aged 3–15 years who were seen a total of 17 560 times at the First Aid Department of the hospital of Ivrea.

The incidence of patients with injury is 0.9 per cent in Group P^1, 6.2 per cent in Group P^2 and 52 per cent in Group P^3. The incidence of patients with epileptic falls and/or generalized seizures accompanied by falling with ensuing injury is 32.4 per cent. The number of seizure related injury in Group P^4 is irrelevant (2/17 560 = 0.1 per cent). Thus, in subjects whose clinical condition is not serious, the risk of seizure-related injury is low, whereas in those with severe drug-resistant epilepsy, it is high but significantly lower than expected in relation to the number of seizure-related falls. We conclude that because of the increased risk, safety precautions are adopted and thus the incidence of injury in these patients declines.

Introduction

Few studies have examined whether or not patients affected by epilepsy are more exposed than normal to the risk of injury deriving from their condition. Available results of retrospective and prospective studies mostly concern adult or mixed-age subjects. This study examines four childhood- and adolescent-age populations with a different incidence of drug-resistant epilepsy with fall seizures to determine whether or not the type and frequency of seizures constitute a significant variable for the risk of injury in these subjects and whether or not the type of counselling modifies this risk.

Subjects and methods

Three retrospective case series of subjects referred from three centres during the time frame of 1 January to 31 December 1994 were examined. The subjects were aged between 3 and 15 years and differed in the incidence of severe epilepsy accompanied by falling.

Group P^1 includes 108 epileptic children followed by the Ivrea out-patient Child Neurology Service. Group P^2 includes 271 patients followed by the Epilepsy Unit of the Turin University Child Neurology Institute. Group P^3 includes 23 patients from an institute for seriously handicapped patients.

All patients were divided into the following groups: idiopathic generalized epilepsy (IGE), idiopathic partial epilepsy (IPE), symptomatic generalized epilepsy (SGE) and symptomatic partial epilepsy (SPE) (Table 1).

Table 1. Epilepsy groups

	Number of patients			
Type of epilepsy	Group P^1 (Ivrea)	Group P^2 (Torino)	Group P^3 (Alba)	TOTAL
Idiopathic partial (IPE)	29	42	0	71
Idiopathic generalized (IGE)	36	99	0	135
Total	75	141	0	206
Symptomatic partial (SPE)	30	78	5	113
Symptomatic generalized (SGE)	13	52	18	83
Total	43	130	23	196
TOTAL	108	271	23	402

Injuries consequent to falls were classified as mild (A), medium (B), and serious (C) depending on type of injury, extent of medical intervention required and functional outcome. Table 2 gives the distribution of injury in the three groups and their relationship to epilepsy.

Group P^4 includes 9203 unselected children aged 3–15 years who were seen in the above three-year period at the Ivrea Hospital First Aid Unit a total of 17 560 times.

Chapter 17 Seizures and the risk of injury in four different clinical severity populations

Table 2. Distribution of injuries in patients and their relationship to epilepsy

	Severity of illness*					
	A	B	C	Total	No. related to epilepsy	No. not related to epilepsy
Group P^1	1 (1), 0.9%	0	0	1	1	0
Group P^2	17 (4), 6.2%	5	2	24	17	7
Group P^3	12 (7), 52%	0	0	12	6	6
Total	30 (12)	5	2	37	24	13

*A = mild-severity injury, B = medium-severity injury, and C = serious-severity injury. Brackets ( ) in column A denote recurrent episodes.

Results

In Groups P^1, P^2 and P^3, type A injury, accompanied or not by seizures, was diagnosed in 0.9 per cent, 6.2 per cent and 52 per cent of subjects respectively (Table 2). Types B and C injury are only seen in Group P^2. In Groups P^2 and P^3, a significant number of patients have recurrent injury unrelated to seizures.

The severity and relation of injury to epilepsy type and seizure type are shown in Table 3. Two patients identified as 1* in Group P^2 were victims of sexual assault and their state of confusion was initially thought to be seizure related. In Group P^2, two epileptic patients had type B and one had type C injuries.

The number of occasional injuries in epileptic subjects of Group P^4 is unknown, but the number related to seizures is very small (2/17.560 = 0.1 per cent of injuries).

Table 3. Severity and relationship of injury to epilepsy and seizure type

		Epileptic seizure		GM-seizure-related injuries				Fall-seizure-related injuries				Non-seizure-related injuries				Total seizures
	Syndrome	GM	Fall	A	B	C	Total	A	B	C	Total	A	B	C	Total	
71	IPE	3	0	1	0	0	1	0	0	0	0	2	0	1	3	4
135	IGE	13 (9•)	11 (9•)	1	0	0	1	0	0	0	0	0	0	0	0	1
113	SPE	8 (1•)	15 (1•)	2	1	1	4	4	0	0	4	4	1*	0	5	11
83	SGE	3 (2•)	33 (2•)	0	0	0	0	12	2	0	14	4	1*	0	5	19
402	Total	27	59	4	1	1	6	16	2	0	18	10	2	1	13	37

* Denotes patient previously sexually assaulted. (•) denotes recurrent episodes. GM = grand mal.

Discussion

The incidence of injury in Groups P^4 and P^1 (including subjects who lead a normal life and who are mostly normal, mentally and physically) supports the data of Ziegler et al. (1994) who report four cases of injury correlated to seizures out of 3822 cases of injury examined (0.1 per cent); out of 198 epileptic patients who were physically and mentally normal and were followed by the Child Neurology Unit, six had an injury and in four cases at the first episode of seizures. The risk referred to the single patient rises to 3 per cent although the more severe cases with drug-resistant epilepsy, frequent seizures and falling, were not included. Klepel et al. (1990) investigating sports in 90 epileptic patients aged 8–18 years observed no difference with respect to controls.

Table 4. Overall risk of injury

	No. injuries related to epilepsy	No. of injuries not related to epilepsy	Total
Idiopathic epilepsies 206	2	3	5
Symptomatic epilepsies 196	22	10	32

The relatively mild risk of Group P^1 patients led us to extend the study to Groups P^2 and P^3. Table 4 reveals that risk of injury rises as clinical picture worsens, but the severity of injury does not increase. In fact, the incidence of mild injury increases progressively in Groups P^2 and P^3 with no medium-severity or serious case in Group P^3. These data might be explained by the significant limitation to movements in the patients of these groups as well as by the safety precautions adopted. In non-hospitalized patients such measures are also less efficient because they are less enforced. Three of the patients belonging to Group P^2 in this study were later hospitalized due to the difficulty of caring for them at home, particularly when in the bathroom, where, according to Lund et al. (1989) 17–60 per cent of seizure-related injury takes place. In Group P^3, except for two cases, injuries happened only in the first year of hospitalization.

In the study of Nakken et al. (1993) concerning drug-resistant seizures and rate of injury, in a series of 62 patients aged 21–82 years with physical and/or mental deficiency, it is reported that out of 6889 seizures, of which 2714 were accompanied by falling (2581 in only two patients), 73 per cent of injuries involved the head or the head and face and only six were serious. The global risk in relation to seizure is 1.5 per cent (1.2 per cent for seizures in general and 2.9 per cent for seizures accompanied by falling). Paradoxically the risk falls to 0.7 per cent in the two patients with most of the crises. Thirty per cent of patients had one or more injuries and all were after seizures with falling. In the study by Russell-Jones et al. (1989), out of 27 934 seizures in 255 hospitalized patients, 45.2 per cent were accompanied by falling which led to 766 injuries, three of which were serious. The risk of injury is thus 2.7 per cent globally and 6.1 per cent in the case of seizures with falling, and the risk of serious injury is 1/9311 and 1/4208 respectively. In the study of Russell-Jones the tonic seizures appear to mean an increased risk of injury. In our case series, 32.4 per cent of patients with epileptic falls and/or grand mal seizures have injuries (Table 5). No seizure-related death was observed.

Table 5. Summary of seizure versus injury

	No. patients with seizures	No. patients with seizure-related injuries	Percentage of injuries among patients	Overall percentage of seizure-related injuries
GM	15	4	26.6%	
Falls	47	16	34.0%	**32.4%**
GM plus falls	12	4	33%	

References

Annegers, J.F., Melton, L.J., Sun, C.A. & Hauser, W.A. (1989): Risk of age-related fractures in patients with unprovoked seizures. *Epilepsia* **30,** (3), 348–355.

Earnest, M.P., Thomas, G.E., Eden, R.A. & Hossack, K.F. (1992): The sudden unexplained death syndrome in epilepsy: demographic, clinical, and postmortem features. *Epilepsia* **33,** (2), 310–316.

Harvey, A.S., Nolan, T. & Carlin, J.B. (1993): Community-based study of mortality in children with epilepsy. *Epilepsia* **34,** (4), 597–603.

Holzgraefe, M. (1992): May an epileptic patient participate in sports? *Versicherungsmedizin* **44,** (4), 130–133.

Kirby, S. & Sadler, R.M., (1995): Injury and death as a result of seizures. *Epilepsia* **36,** (1), 25–28.

Klepel, H., Gloch, V. & Weinhold, A. (1990): Accident risk of epileptic children and adolescents in the area of school sports and leisure activities. *Z. Arztl. Fortbild. Jena.* **84,** (15), 779–782.

Nakken, K.O. & Lossius, R. (1993a): Injuries in epileptic sizures. *Tidsskr. Nor. Laegeforen* **113,** (21), 2690–2692.

Nakken, K.O. & Lossius, R. (1993b): Seizure related injuries in multihandicapped patients with therapy-resistant epilepsy. *Epilepsia* **34,** (5), 836–840.

Quan, L., Gore, E.J., Wentz, K., Allen, J. & Novack, A.H. (1989): Ten-year study of pediatric drownings in King County, Washington: lesson in injury prevention. *Pediatrics* **83,** (6), 1035–1040.

Ritter, G. & Buller, T. (1993): Accident risk in epilepsy. *Versicherungsmedizin* **45,** (3), 99–101.

Russell-Jones, D.L. & Shorvon S.D. (1989): The frequency and consequences of head injury in epileptic seizures. *J. Neurosurg. Psychiatry* **52,** (5), 659–662.

Wiese, J. & Schneider, V. (1990): Death in an epileptic seizure. *Versicherungsmedizin* **42,** (4), 113–115.

Ziegler, A., Reinberg O. & Deonna T. (1994): Épilepsie et accidents: quel risque chez l'enfant? *Arch. Pédiatr.* **1,** 801–805.

Chapter 18

The social life of the epileptic child presenting falls

Laura Mira, Bona Oxilia and Carlo Zerbi

Servizio di Neurologia, Ospedale dei Bambini 'Vittore Buzzi', via Castelvetro 32, Milan, Italy

Introduction

In recent years, considerable progress has been achieved to modify and to improve the social life of epileptics, yet old problems remain unsolved and new ones emerge. The analysis of the current life condition of the epileptic child with falling seizures points out the persisting difficulties and provides the opportunity to work out proposals and projects for interventions aimed at bringing about further improvements.

Since it would not be feasible to deal here with the whole problem of the social life of the epileptic child, we focused our study on the analysis of the social interactions caused by the epileptic child's fall.

In fact, falling constitutes an event which triggers social interaction. By social interaction we mean a relationship between two or more subjects, individual or collective, in the course of which each subject repeatedly modifies his/her behaviour in reference to the other's behaviour or action. This can happen either after the other's action has already taken place, or anticipating and predicting what action the other will take in response to one's own.

Repeated and unpredictable falls of the epileptic child with falling seizures imply a peculiar social interaction, characterized by psycho-social features which very often take on negative attributes for the child and are best envisaged within the wider framework of the social representation of epilepsy.

Considering then the social interaction initiated by the fall event of the epileptic child, we must approach the problem of the consequent modification of the behaviour of the child himself, of the individuals close to him, of groups and of institutions. The aim of the present study is to attempt to analyse each of these possible modifications and to try to understand their social significance.

Social issues concerning the falling epileptic child

The event of falling affects the social role of the falling epileptic child, whose status has already been modified with reference to the dichotomy illness/health by his being epileptic.

Social rules constrain a person's behaviour from outside and tend to impose a predetermined role. The main effect of the social role is to adjust behaviours, to make the subject's behaviour predictable by others (individuals or institutions) and suitable to integration. The social role is characterized by external objectiveness, a kind of obligation that the subject cannot avoid without risking sanctions. In extreme terms, one could say that the subject is forced into the role to avoid self-destruction.

What new rules does the falling child impose to himself, constrained by his perception of the social interaction triggered by his own falling? In fact, he loses his status as a child; that is, as an individual who falls more frequently than the adult but who must and can learn not to fall, and takes on the status of epileptic who falls not only unpredictably, but also unavoidably (Revol, 1988; Soulayrol, 1991).

Therefore, in learning the role prescriptions, the falling child feels that his behaviour must be adjusted in such a way as to be liable to prediction and integration (liable to prediction = reassuring; liable to integration = syntonic). Role prescriptions then influence a new and different balance between rights and duties. The right to new experiences, the right to pursue new motor abilities, maybe being reckless, and the right to find wider and wider autonomy, come into conflict with the duty not to raise anxiety because his falling (in contrast with his peers') evokes painful images of his disease and because his autonomy contrasts with the prescription to be always under control 'waiting' for an unpredictable and unavoidable fall.

Falling, then, easily implies restriction of potentiality rank, too: the social role, with its prescriptions, imposes, or tries to impose, behaviours aimed at avoiding the unpredictable and, specifically, the event of falling. The risk involved in every experience, exercise, search or exploration – a risk that in a sense is assumed by children and by people close to them – becomes instead the unexpected to be avoided. The falling epileptic child is thus diminished from his potentiality rank.

In his attempt to develop his own model of social behaviour in response to the behavioural messages from others (either individuals or informal groups or institutional groups) the falling epileptic child can assume a role behaviour of the adapted and syntonic type; or, alternatively, a reactive one, a bearer of sanctions. Role behaviours are unplanned and unintentional and are tuned by the interference of important emotional variables: the variety of role behaviours is in fact very wide.

The adapted child, driven by these emotional variables, accepts role prescriptions: he can reasonably and adequately adapt to reassuring requests by the environment, but he could possibly interpret these requests by using his falls for secondary advantage. Finally, the social interactions sometimes urge the child to emphasize social behaviour of the regressive type and, occasionally, to give up any initiative to the point of debility (Soulayrol, 1990).

As an alternative to the adapted behaviour, the child who reacts with rebellion could undertake provocative and non-adapted role behaviours, presenting to his social environment in unpredictable and non-integrative ways. He can emphasize overtly contrasting and daring behaviours to the point of carrying the 'falling risk' into a blackmailing spiral, related either to overprotection or refusal. A social interaction is then triggered in which the surrounding environment puts into action new defences against his disrupting behaviours, ending with new sanctions to the rebel. Thus, the necessary dialectics between the predicted and the unpredicted and between risk and safety, a common feature of everybody's life, is destroyed and becomes unacceptable for the falling epileptic child.

Therefore, depending on social environment (family, school, neighbourhood), the child with falling seizures finds himself exposed in turn to contrasting reactions and behavioural models. These can be characterized by overprotection or, on the contrary, by denial of some aspects of his being. The former models are present in environments that are well aware of the occurrence of seizures, always feared and expected; the latter ones are found in environments where the occurrence of seizures and falls has been removed. Mechanisms of refusal, isolation, even disparagement of the child's abilities are then initiated, up to the surfacing of new forms of demonization. It even happens that the teenagers falling in the street are easily suspected of drug addiction, modern repository of demonizing social thrusts: the drug addict, too, is harbinger of death and loss of rational control.

Moreover, the ignorance of the relative frequency of child epilepsy has produced inattention and indifference to this issue in large parts of the society, preventing the development of cultural and emotional tools to face falling seizures adequately.

What kind of positive social interaction, then, should we offer to the falling epileptic child to lead him back to a predictable and adequately integrated role? The best social response is of course to acknowledge and to emphasize the integrity of sound abilities, but also to accept the objective and subjective unexpected event and to discriminate between emotional symbolic meanings and the real nature of the event itself.

The new status of the child can thus be envisaged as an adequate balance between rights to equality and rights to diversity, in the course of what is a disease and not a shameful event.

Social issues in the family of the falling epileptic child

The social interactions among family members, as individuals and as a group, are multifarious: we will outline only some aspects to give an idea of the problem in all its complexity.

Considerable drives to effect role modification are felt within the family: the social interaction favours adapted behaviours which preferably burden the family with the unpredictability of the fall event, while at the same time relieve the other social contexts. An example of family adapted role behaviour becomes available when the child is at school (Zanelli Quarantini et al., 1992; Diebold et al., 1986).

The mother finds great difficulties in delegating some of her duties, is urged by feelings of exclusive responsibility, is forced to several renouncements, must re-adjust her relationship with the other children and is increasingly exasperated by conflicts with her own job requirements. Within the family and the society the mother is subjected to pressure to restrict outside access to the family, while the social interaction requires that she give up emancipation and accepts the limited and regressive role of housewife, guardian of the risks of her child's unpredictable fall (Mittan, 1990; Muratori et al., 1992).

The father, too, feels the urge for role modification, either in the direction to take upon himself greater responsibility for the ill child and even for the other children, or in the direction to entrust his wife with more and more responsibility and duties.

Siblings are also subjected to a social interaction triggered by the problem of falls, and roles in the family are modified. In particular, those proper to one's rank are affected, disrupting the balance of rights/duties and expectancies/demands among siblings, between parents and children and vice versa. In particular, protection–admiration and dependence–autonomy among siblings are modified and do not correspond any more to age ranks. Demands and expectancies from parents to children and from children to parents are also modified, especially with reference to requested and desired levels of responsibility and autonomy.

It might happen that the younger, healthy brother would take upon himself the behaviour role of his older brother, 'ill' because of falling, and the latter, in turn, would become object of 'protection' rather than admiration. It might also be that the older, healthy brother would confront himself with a falling little brother, who for this reason always remains very little and in need of so much maternal care. Envy could rise for parental care, feelings of disdain for the 'ill' brother could emerge and somebody, the 'ill' or the healthy one, could choose to humble himself because he can't find his own rights (Soulayrol, 1991).

Role restrictions occur for all the members of the family, affected by a problem which is still featured socially as shameful (adding to its being psychologically distressful), and interactions between families change (Mittan, 1990; Belvedere *et al.*, 1993). The processes of keeping away from 'different' (i.e. without illness) families develop: it is believed that 'different' families can't understand, that lack of knowledge implies indifference and inattention and thus the falling epileptic child becomes the family's shameful secret (Bianchini *et al.*, 1993).

The attempt to aggregate 'homogeneous' (i.e. with epileptic children) families means a thrust to the isolation of self-marginalization. It is indeed possible to oppose this marginalizing and self-marginalizing thrust to maintain the status of a normal family (Sallou & Beauchesne, 1988). This would imply a large investment of energy in a new sociocultural endeavour to act on social mechanisms without denying the problem, but setting it in a balance which favours the 'healthy parts', while, at the same time, integrating the 'unhealthy parts'.

Social issues in social environments: school, neighbourhood, play and sport activities

We have already discussed the significance of some social interactions, analysing the child and family role with reference to different social contexts, where the social environment leads to role and role behaviour modifications. School attendance of an epileptic child at risk for falling seizures represents the crucial point of confrontation of complex and likely conflicting social interactions between three institutions: family, school and the health system. Actually, it gives rise to the problem of whether the family should inform others about the risk of the child's possible falling seizures. In case this information is provided, it is likely to arouse negative alarm reactions with behaviours of overt or hardly concealed refusal by the teachers in charge of the child. On the other hand the principle of honesty and co-operation among institutions is preserved.

In the opposite case, when the information is not provided, the family finds itself in the objective situation of keeping a secret in which the child is also involved, with the physicians' silent or explicit consent. The pupil will then be not only bearer of possible seizures, so fearful for him as well, but also of a secret which assumes the meaning of a shameful and blameful event (Borgatti *et al.*, 1988; Sallou & Viellard-Baron, 1986). Whenever a falling seizure occurs in such a difficult context, the school–family relationship irremediably deteriorates. The teachers will experience feelings of betrayal and disloyalty towards the family behaviour (Soulayrol, 1991).

These objective problems, characterized by a highly conflicting significance, could also arise in the family–physician relationship, with reference either to the question of whether to inform the school or to the question of who is to undertake this task.

Certainly the family represents the weakest link in the chain and often finds itself in a condition of decisional isolation. Moreover, when the child falls at school or in the playground or in the street or during a sport or game activity, often the consequent emotional reaction is to point immediately to the adult in charge of the child as the responsible or even the guilty person. Society defends itself and initiates a social interaction with the aim to displace and change responsibility, which then shifts among institutions and individuals and tends to weigh heavily on the family rather than being attributed to the disease features (Belvedere et al., 1993).

Social issues of the medical world related to the falling epileptic child

In the current historical time of rapid scientific progress and incessant flow of information, more than ever the social role deceptively assigned to the medical world is to cure, to wipe out disease signs: a duty of omnipotence, where the limits of omnipotence are censored as mistakes. The epileptic child who repeatedly falls in spite of pharmacological or surgical treatment triggers a social interaction that sometimes even gets to wish sanctions against the person who did not comply with his/her role: curing.

The medical world that accepts to inform, to found the culture necessary to establish a therapeutic alliance, responds to the sanctioning provocation of the social interaction.

Widespread knowledge allows to accept the risk of falls as an event integrated in the disease reality, removing the anguish of guilt. Further cultural awareness, rooted in the rational, could substitute for ignorance and for misleading emotional contents which fill in the so-called gap of ignorance.

Thus, within the medical world, new relationships of burden-sharing can develop among general and speciality practitioners, and school physicians and sport physicians (Feuerstein, 1988; Tridon & Weber, 1988). New relationships with families come about, endowed with greater awareness, participation and co-operation.

Discussion

Role prescriptions and social behaviours, with their interactive complexity, should also be analysed in the framework of the social representation of epilepsy. This representation, which has radically changed in the last 30 years, in turn changes interaction processes. Epilepsy does not constitute any more a demoniac, unavoidable, unpredictable and uncontrollable event, to be reacted to only by exorcization or concealment. Nowadays, thanks to new scientific information and spread of medical culture, epilepsy is regarded as a disease among others, i.e. an event characteristic of the human condition within the dichotomy of health and illness. It is thus referred to predictable, though undesired, events which can occur in the course of single, individual vicissitudes – predictable, but also controllable events, thanks to the identification of a wide and varied set of therapeutic interventions. This produced a fairly good cultural awareness of chance for cure and/or control of seizures, which, however, can even lead to ignoring the fact that intractable epilepsy still exists: many but not all epilepsies are curable.

The new representation gave rise to two phenomena: disease trivialization and normalization. Trivialization brings as a consequence a tendency to deny the seizure event and the fall event, with concomitant removal of the unbearable anguish which it arouses in the actor and in the witness of the event. Normalization implies acknowledgement that epilepsy is not necessarily linked to a condition of global and permanent infirmity. These new cultural convictions led to the assertion of the epileptic child's right to enjoy the same education opportunities as all children. The realization of this right by political enactment brought to the shutdown of special schools for epileptics, who now can attend everybody's schools. Social integration in educational structures has given the epileptic child the same status as his healthy peers, with acknowledgement and appreciation of similar competences in learning.

Ahead of such a positive evolution, one must face new contradictions related to the problematic and conflicting nature of the symptomatic manifestation. Falling seizures, objectively unpredictable and socially removed, seem twice as disgraceful. They represent lack of control and loss of regulating rationality, and at a symbolic level, they evoke death and sexuality. New social taboos are broken in a society that neither thinks about nor accepts death, a society that gives pre-eminence to rationality and does not integrate emotions, denied and instrumentalized publicly, but dramatically present privately (Broussaud, 1988; Diebold et al., 1986).

Conclusions

Within a few years the epileptic child's life has radically changed, in parallel with changes in our social thought. Marginalization in schools for epileptics has been overcome, coming in some cases to the opposite extreme of denying the existence of an epilepsy problem.

Recent changing processes in the cultural, scientific and institutional domains have allowed them to overcome marginalizing circuits within the social body, but at the same time have opened new and still alive contradictions when facing the fall event, unpredictable and ill-suited to integration.

The child feels that he must become predictable and is in difficulty with the fall event, uncontrollable and evocative of unbearable emotions. Despite the effort to integrate this event culturally and socially, several social components have yet not developed the ability to integrate the emotions evoked by epileptic seizures, and in particular by falling seizures. The discrimination between the intrinsic seizure significance and its symbolic representation is still lacking: the society acknowledges and integrates the diversity of disease, but is unable to bear the emotions triggered by the fall. The falling risk is not perceived as a necessary feature of the disease, but instead it still evokes guilt and leads to a search for a scapegoat.

The richness of social interactions increasingly initiates changing processes; it helps to activate further development of knowledge about epilepsy and seizures and improves the ability to integrate otherwise unbearable and misleading emotions. Considerable problems have been solved – we are beginning to recognize that many childhood epilepsies are only transient conditions which will disappear completely and a show a diversity that will not keep up with time. Nonetheless, in the meanwhile, new contradictions play a role essentially on the emotional side and are supported by the pressure of badly integrated emotions.

A paradox still exists between tolerant and integrated positions at the rational level, while lack of control at the emotional level still provokes refusal. Our society is able to use up-to-date scientific culture to establish the rules that set diseases and their symptoms in their common meaning of obstacles to preservation and search for health, but it is also a society that still perceives as different those who evoke unbearable unconscious phantasies. Much has yet to be done to modify the current social feeling, shaping it according to the principle of legitimization of diversity and claim to equality in diversity as the first stage in the process of full integration.

References

Belvedere, D., Minotti, L. & Canger, R. (1993): Problematiche sociali delle epilessie. In: *Le epilessie oggi*, ed. R. Canger, pp. 205–215. Milan, Paris, Barcelona & Bonn: Masson.

Bianchini, L., Veggiotti, P. & Lanzi, G. (1993): L'approccio al nucleo familiare dei bambini affetti da epilessia. *Giorn. Neuropsich. Età Evol.* **13,** 187–199.

Borgatti, R., Comelli, D., Tassini, M. & Costa, P. (1988): Importanza della modalità di presa in carico e della comunicazione della diagnosi sull'evoluzione dell'epilessia. *Boll. Lega It. Epil.* **62/63,** 335–336.

Broussaud, G. (1988): Résultats et analyse de l'enquête menée auprès d'épileptiques et de médecin épileptologues sur les risques des épileptiques. In: *Épilepsie et risques,* ed. C. Sallou, pp. 19–27. London: John Libbey.

Diebold, G., Maillefaud, T. & Beauchesne, H. (1986): Épilepsies, deuils et psychothérapies. *Psychiatrie de l'enfant* **29,** 61–124.

Feuerstein, J. (1988): Risques pour la descendance des patients épileptiques (hérédité exclue). In: *Épilepsie et risques,* ed. C. Sallou, pp. 45–50. London: John Libbey.

Mittan, R.I. (1990): Psychosocial considerations in difficult epilepsy. In: *Recent advances and controversies in epilepsy,* pp. 83–94. Miami: AAN.

Muratori, F., Masi, G., Passani, G. & Patarnello, M.G. (1992): Il diario tra memoria e razionalizzazione: a proposito di una adolescente con epilessia parziale sintomatica. *Giorn. Neuropsich. Età Evol.* **12,** 245–259.

Revol, M. (1988): Accidents inhérents aux crises d'épilepsie et aspects cliniques des crises. In: *Épilepsie et risques,* ed. C. Sallou, pp. 3–10. London: John Libbey.

Sallou, C. & Vieillard-Baron, J.M. (1986): L'adolescent épileptique: étude à partir d'une population de 100 adolescents. *Boll. Lega It. Epil.* **54/55,** 27–33.

Sallou, C. & Beauchesne, H. (1988): Psycho-dynamique de la famille de l'épileptique. *Boll. Lega It. Epil.* **62/63,** 295–298.

Soulayrol, R. (1990): L'indépendance impossible de l'enfant épileptique. *Neuropsychiatrie de l'Enfance* **38,** 314–317.

Soulayrol, R. (1991): Épilepsie et psychodynamique de la personne. *Neuropsychiatrie de l'Enfance* **39,** 55–66.

Tridon, P. & Weber, M. (1988): Influence du facteur 'risque' sur l'acte médical. In: *Épilepsie et risques,* ed. C. Sallou, pp. 133–139. London: John Libbey.

Zanelli Quarantini, A., Grioni, D., Neri, F., Peretti, A. & Bertolini, M. (1992): Riflessioni cliniche su un caso di epilessia psicosomatica. *Giorn. Neuropsich. Età Evol.* **12,** 291–302.

Chapter 19

The fall in epileptic children: psychopathological and humanistic aspects

René Soulayrol

Head of Paedopsychiatry, CHU Ste Marguerite, 270 boulevard de Ste Marguerite, 13009 Marseille, France

I have often seen my teacher Henri Gastaut, his beard bristling with anger, explode over the term *aura epileptica*; a term which he labelled 'improper' in his dictionary of epilepsy because the term 'aura' seemed to him to correspond already to critical, rather than precritical, symptoms. Nevertheless the term is attractive and deserves to be maintained not only for the delicacy of its etymology of 'subtle emanation', but as well for the furor of its mythology which relates that a nymph of the same name killed her child in a moment of madness.

Thus, in order to give a new breath-of-life to this term, I ask myself if aura could not signify broadly all that encompasses the epileptic and epilepsy, both from the subjective aspect concerning how the epileptic himself feels and the objective and social aspect regarding what epilepsy generates among others. Thus the epileptic aura would embrace everything from the psychopathology and the dynamic psychology of the epileptic to the mythology, history and sociology of epilepsy.

To put it briefly, all this is what we should talk about today with regard to the fall in the seizures of the epileptic child.

This fall, to employ the terms of a well-constructed De Gaulle speech, has both an appearance and a reality; a reality where the brutality of a certain tonic spasm, astatic falls, causes injuries or trauma evidenced by scarred faces, stitched-up scalps or heads protected by bicycle racers' crash helmets. But other less brutal falls can have equally catastrophic consequences if the epileptic falls in the street, in a fire, in deep water, through an open window or on cutting machines. The fear of falling is therefore a reality that no one, not even psychiatrists, has the nerve to deny. (One of our patients, feeling a fall coming on and not succeeding in opening the door of her room to call for help opened, in her confusion, the latch on her window and fell out, hurting herself severely.)

But the fall also has an appearance which draws us to reflect with caution. The fall itself underlines the gravity of the crisis and of epilepsy itself. And this falling sickness (as it is called since it makes one fall) is stamped with an ancestral and mythical horror that has been transmitted intact down to our days.

In O. Temkin's book, appropriately titled *The falling sickness*, the author relates that the Assyrians recognized 'the illness that causes one to fall to the ground' thus underlining the fact that the fall is the primal aspect above all others of the illness. Hippocrates in his treatise *On sacred illness* strikes out against the claimed divine origin of the illness and explains the fall as a neurological failure caused by a flux of phlegm which blocks the 'veins' of the brain and hinders the free flow of air. And it is well known that the spectacular fall of a person afflicted by epilepsy was considered such a dire omen that it interrupted the Roman peoples' assemblies with the result that the falling sickness was Romanized into 'assembly sickness'. In the African societies that I was able to visit in Senegal, people even today avoid walking on the ground where an epileptic has fallen, and it must be purified by fire.

We must therefore examine the horror of the fall beyond the context of epilepsy, viewing it as an insult to the verticality of man who, supported by his anti-gravitational muscles, launches a challenge to gravity or as a blasphemy to the sacred equilibrium of worlds which keep on tumbling down – without ever even touching – upon one another.

Michel Tournier, in a recent essay entitled 'The mirror of ideas', calling upon the the Kantian notions of thought, opposes a certain number of key concepts like existence and nothingness, space and time, right and left; however, aside from a chapter which deals with the differences between the cellar and the attic, he makes no reference to the opposition between the high and the low or the earth and the sky, while in his first novel *Friday or the limbs of the Pacific* he dissertated magnificently on the contrast between the Aeolian character of Friday and the telluric character of Robinson. We must therefore ourselves endeavour to penetrate into the feeling of high and low in order to understand the fear of falling in general and in epilepsy in particular.

The first words of the first chapter of Genesis are 'In the beginning God created heaven and earth'; the first task of God is to give a verticality to chaos and to draw a line between heaven and earth, the high and the low. When the religions of cosmogony, such as they were, became anthropomorphic, we see that the actions of the gods take place between heaven and earth and that falls and ascendances were the resulting unhappy or happy events.

Whether it is a question of Eurynome in the Pelasgian myth of creation or the incestuous Uranus in the Olympian myth, high represents the absolute, perfection, power, the fecundatory principle whose function is always threatened by fall.

The divine recompense granted to the demi-gods, even to mortals, is the power to have access to the Olympic heaven, or to be transformed into constellations whose perfect equilibrium protects against fall forever.

It is from on high that the God of Abraham and Moses spoke to them, even if the latter took a small walk to meet Him on Mount Sinai.

The vertical journey of Christ should also be interpreted first as a descent through the incarnation of a human person towards suffering, the Passion and death on a standing cross which prefigures the elevation of the Ascension from where, transfigured into the Holy body, He tells his disciples that He is rising to heaven as the son of God to sit at his right hand. Just as the Assumption of the Virgin Mary is an anticipation of the body and soul resurrection of a human body prior to its ascension towards the glory of heaven.

Chapter 19 The fall in epileptic children: psychopathological and humanistic aspects

Finally, from the strict anthropological point of view, the slow process of our ancestors' standing up on their hind feet has enabled the men that we are to free their thumbs to become dextrous and to allow their brains to develop and become homo sapiens. This uprightness as a source of pride is celebrated by our human society in our monuments (menhirs, obelisks, cathedrals or World Trade Centre towers) and in the individual intimacy of our bodies when a man's tumescent penis erects proudly towards the sky. But this arrogance sets up the groundwork for the anguish of the fall when one knows that an attack can shatter these erected walls or that impotency can put our flaccid banner at half mast.

But then will you ask if high is so prestigious, so phallic, so honourable, so divine in some ways, does that mean that low is just the opposite and thus an inferior condition? Certainly not, low is the domain of Mother Earth which every evening offers its plowed, moist fields to the sperm of Uranus, out of which issue the vegetable, animal and human kingdoms. Low is the domain of the real, of the organic, as well as of the tangible material, the domain of raw material, of concrete work and industry, the domain of the pain of childbirth and that of tears, but also that of nursing. Low is the matrix of all gestation and the base on which all elevation stands. Low is in fact necessary to it, and we know that we shall all return to earth without this necessarily being a decline. It is true that there is always a lower than low and that the dungeons, the Tartarus regions, the Underworld or Hell are places fed by the anguish of falling.

No, what creates the horror of falling is the unexpected, non-consented and incongruous return to earth; it is this infringement of the prestige of equilibrium that throws one down and makes one bite the dust – the lot of the defeated. The fall is much more than a descent; it is brutal, violent, uncontrolled and seems to evade the victim itself. It represents a sudden and unforeseeable change of condition; 'the worse the fall' or 'the Tarpeian rock is close to the Capitol' are expressions which reflect the precariousness of all elevation which can be applied to societies (the fall of the Roman Empire, the fall of an institution, the fall of the Usher House) as well as to a human being, and all the more so to an epileptic who passes in one instant from the status of living to that of death.

Thus in the case of the epileptic the fall can lend itself to many interpretations.

First of all as a fall in itself for those who tell us that they felt themselves falling. But there is still more: any crisis can be perceived as a fall including as well as partial or absence epilepsies where, even if the individual remains on his feet he can tell us: 'I felt myself fall, it was like a black hole and then nothing; I felt myself drawn into a big void; I felt dizzy; it was nothingness; I had no landmarks'. Here we find something like an indication that the loss of spatial landmarks precedes the dissolution of the conscience of being.

The fall, especially of the child but why not of the adult as well, can be seen as a regression, as a return to Mother Earth; this is one of the themes among others of the Icarus myth. A return to the supine, bedridden, clinical position of the ill, to the passive status of the patient subjected to the all-powerful doctor or of the analysand subjected to the violence of the interpretations of his analyst.

The fall, due to the brutal privation of corporeal integrity and to its aggressive character can assume the importance of castration, precipitation of the rival Cyclopes by the Titans into the Tartar chasm, the successful castration by Chronos of his father Uranus whose genitals were thrown into the sea, the overthrowing in turn of Chronos by his son Zeus, the punishment of Icarus who, wishing to rise above his father, saw the wax attachments of his wings melt under the sun, the frantic dismantling of the statues of the great dictators during revolutions. The fall is such a loss of arrogance, such a clobbering that the silent cinema take-offs or circus clowns turn them into comedy. Even the restrained otherwise Bergson notes that the fall of an elderly lady in the street can cause laughter.

The fall, or rather the fear of it, can enter into the framework of phobias. Wallon rightfully made of it a form of agoraphobia if one considers that empty space, repulsive and alluring at the same time, can usually be more phobogenic when it is vertical. And many people are acquainted with the fear of heights that seizes you with its ambivalence on the top of a cliff or on a skyscraper and which has been magnificently exploited by Hitchcock in his films. In the epileptic child this fear is less his own than that of his parents who, in order to fight against it, often resort to means of protection which can approach contraphobic rituals and which contribute to making dependency tighter and more constraining.

In this regard one can, in the case of adolescents for example, interpret the use of the fall as a dangerous conduct which would be an opportunity to take up a challenge to oneself and to the parents to stand up against the prohibitions that the illness accumulates as a number of provoking obstacles.

It is true that in these cases what is involved is less the fear of the fall than the repetition of the unbearable spectacle of life and death that it prompts. Every epileptic fall is in effect a fatal fall. It is the prelude, the mime or the sign of the death which remains the major theme of the epileptic tragedy. Repetition, annihilation, division, traumatic dreams, unfulfilled bereavements, phantom-like doubles and aggressive phantasmal are the sly witnesses of the insidious undermining and drive of death that is especially active in the epileptic child and his parents. But the fall in itself because of its suddenness, its surprise, its violence, its injury has nothing sly about it; it is the most public, shameless and brutal manifestation of an aggressive drive, destructive angel, which assaults the subject and terrifies the onlooker.

Nevertheless the epileptic fall can hold its share of pleasure. In effect, this interpretation which can seem shocking or insane is suggested to us by Dostoevsky's literary descriptions of the crises of prince Mychkin or of those of the 'Gambler' where one could think that they are nothing but the transposition of what he may have felt himself. It would appear that the aura of a crisis, however unbearable it may be, provides the subject with an ineffable feeling of transition between life and death up to the point where it can make him envisage what could be the Nirvana, unless it amounts to a 'disturbing strangeness'. He would feel something like a 'radical metamorphosis which is invading the whole of his existence'. In short, the epileptic crisis can become an existential crisis where the foreboded transformations end up either as a 'transfiguration', as we shall see later, or a total 'dissolution'. This brings to mind the 'flashes' of drug addicts. (One of our patients, a difficult adolescent at odds with his family and his anti-epileptic treatment, had chosen as a profession that of a swimming teacher and as a sport that of high-board diving because he experienced during the time of his long dive which separated him from the water a pleasure comparable to the one that the fall of his crisis gave him.)

It is therefore almost impossible to talk about the fall without immediately evoking a symbolic meaning. A meaning which leads downwards, to destruction, to catastrophe, to unhappiness, to the instinct of evil and to death. And if the fall characterizes epilepsy to such an extent, *mutatis mutandis*, epilepsy and the subject which it invades will be permeated with this same tragic sense.

Consequently, we should be particularly attentive to and grateful for an article by Dieter Janz, which appeared in 1986 in *Epilepsia* and which, through an analysis of a painting by Raphael in the Vatican Gallery called *Transfiguration*, offers us, by means of the gospels, a metaphysical interpretation of epilepsy. This article is so useful for our discussion that I urge you to contemplate this painting giving it a new title which could be *The Redemption of the fall of the epileptic child*.

The painting is cut in two by a horizontal line in the upper third. The upper part contains the light, the light of heaven in which the celestial beings bathe, Jesus in full ascension, Moses bearer of the Law and Elijah who announces the resurrection. Below, in the lower two-thirds, all is black, humans struggle in full confusion, among them an epileptic child in crisis is being held by his father who is protecting him from his fall. Between the dark and the light, Peter, James and John are lying prone, overcome by what they are seeing and hearing.

Below, among the terrestial people, no one is looking up except the child in crisis, who is undergoing a crossed tonic crisis, his upper right leg extended straight forward, his left leg tensed in internal rotation, while his eyeballs are diverging, one looking at Jesus and the other at his father. He who is holding his son is staring fixedly in front of him with an expression of painful perplexity. One notes that the only oblique line that connects the upper part of the painting to the lower part is the virtual line of visual exchange between Christ and the child, while none of the eyes of the other 27 people meet. Janz points out that the divergence in the look of the child is voluntary on Raphael's part, since in a preliminary study that he used as a model, the artist sketched from life the same epileptic child in crisis whose two eyes rolled backwards to look at the father.

It now remains for us to interpret why Raphael joined together in the same painting called *Transfiguration* two episodes of the gospels. First of all that of the majestic Ascension of Christ at Mount Tabor, telling His disciples that He has undergone the Passion on this earth, that He is dead but that He is resuscitated because He is the son of God, just as they too will suffer, be sacrificed but resuscitated in turn to sit like Him, with Him, at the right of God. And on the other hand that of the epileptic child of the Gospel of Saint Mark where Jesus, in front of the lifeless body of an epileptic child, whom the crowd said was dead, ordered the deaf and blind spirit 'to leave the child and never return'. Now what seems important in this testimony is not that the child rises and stands up on his feet, but that Christ sets out to prophesy in front of His disciples 'who did not understand well what He was saying' that He Himself would die and would be resuscitated. Thus Raphael by joining together these two scenes in the same space clarifies the symbolic meaning by an after-the-event phenomenon. He shows that the sufferings, the falls and the little 'dyings' of the epileptic child have been shouldered by Christ Himself during His passion, His three falls during the climbing of Golgotha and His crucifixion. In the complicity of the glances in this painting there is an analogy between the destiny of Christ and that of the epileptic child who can live, he as well, in the hope of a rehabilitation from his fall by means of an accession, or even an ascension, to a recovery. A recovery, possibly a material one, but surely a spiritual one since his earthly sufferings rehabilitated by Christ's sympathy are the image of those of the son of God. Thus the Christian message perpetuates, by reinterpreting it, the holy sense of the epileptic illness if the epileptic child, at the time of each of his crises, reminds us of the Passion, death and resurrection of Christ just as Mass reactuates the remembrance of the Last Supper.

I am particularly grateful to the organizers of this eminently scientific congress to have reserved a symbolic place for the analysis of a symptom which could at first glance appear secondary since it is only the consequence of the loss of consciousness which characterizes epilepsy. In fact epileptology, like any speciality, establishes its pedigree when, aside from its clinical and immediate physiopathological concerns, it encompasses historical, sociological, even geopolitical, dimensions. But it enriches itself even further when, centring itself again on the individual, it endeavours, by studying him as well as the origin and uniqueness of his life history as intimately as possible, to understand to what extent the illness has shaped his way of being and his thinking in both conscious and unconscious dimensions. But once again detached from the individual, it achieves its real heights if the men who suffer and those who are responsible for taking care of them can integrate the meaning of this suffering into a philosophy which since Plato has become part of the invisible world of knowledge. The epileptologists should have no shame in going beyond the more and more visible world (that their ever-more-scientific works disclose in order for them to enter it), for it becomes more and more enigmatic of humanistic – and why not spiritual – understanding. There should be nothing against embracing the beyond-visible world just as one embraces the hope of achieving by other paths that which we are searching for in our laboratories, which are at times caught up in deadlock.

References

Bergson, H. (1947): *Le rire* (The laughter). Paris: Alcan-PUF.

Danjou, A. (1987): Si je tombe donc je suis (If I fall I must therefore exist). (Essay illustrating the epileptic crisis generalized by the Icarus myth.) In: *Psychopathologie de l'épilepsie. Doc. Med.* Paris: Labaz.

Dostoevsky, F. (1953): L'idiot (The Idiot). In: *La pléiade III*. Paris: Gallimard.

Dostoevsky, F. (1956): Le joueur (The Gambler). *La pléiade V. NRF*. Paris: Gallimard.

Graves, R. (1967): *Les mythes grecs* (The Greek Myths), 2nd edn. Paris: Fayard.

Hippocrates: *De morbo sacro*. Loeb Classics.

Janz, D. (1986): Epilepsy viewed metaphysically: an interpretation of the biblical story of the epileptic boy and of Raphael's *Transfiguration*. *Epilesia* **274,** 317–322.

Temkin, O. (1945): The falling sickness. In: *A history of epilepsies from the Greeks to the beginning of modern neurology*, Baltimore: J. Hopkins.

Tournier, M. (1967): *Vendredi ou les limbes du Pacifique*. (Friday or the limbs of the Pacific), *NRF*. Gallimard: Paris.

Tournier, M. (1994): Le Miroir des idées. In: *Mercure de France*, Paris.

Synopsis

Giuliano Avanzini

Istituto Nazionale Neurologico C. Besta, Milan, Italy

The Colloquium was opened in the name of Henri Gastaut (to whom it was dedicated) by his pupil and friend Annette Beaumanoir, who paid a warm and moving tribute to his scientific and human personality and acknowledged the invaluable contribution of this outstanding scholar to modern epileptology. Echoes of Gastaut's scientific work could be heard in the presentations of all of the speakers, one-third of whom had been either his pupils or his collaborators.

As Frederick Andermann put it during the Colloquium, if Henri Gastaut had been sitting somewhere and looking down, he would probably have been smiling at hearing the ideas that he first put forward many years ago still being passionately debated today. A few months after the Colloquium, the epileptology community suffered another great loss with the death of Francesco Viani on 1 March 1996. Francesco brought to the discussion of epileptic falls the enormous contribution of his great experience and scientific soundness that we had all learned to value so much during many years of friendship and collaboration. We will sadly miss his gentle and lively intelligence that contributed so significantly to the development of epileptology in Italy.

The general programme of the Colloquium is to be found in Annette Beaumanoir's introductory chapter and it is faithfully reflected in this book. Epileptic falls can be primarily determined by myoclonic, tonic or atonic seizures that are usually considered to be part of the symptomatology of generalized epilepsies; however, falls can also be due to locally originated discharges whose rapid generalization makes it sometimes difficult to identify their precise site of origin. The basic mechanisms responsible for epileptic falls involve epileptogenic changes in cell excitability and the effects of epileptic discharges on the mechanisms responsible for the control of tone and posture. The characteristics of the falls depend upon the interaction of these two elements, as is discussed in the first section of the book. A prerequisite for an effective therapeutic approach to epileptic falls is their careful semeiological definition within the context of the clinical pictures of the epileptic syndromes of which they are a part. This is dealt with in the second and third sections of the book, in which the prognostic factors relevant to clinical, psychological and social aspects are also extensively discussed. Finally, a special section is devoted to the therapeutic strategies aimed at alleviating, if not controlling, epileptic falls.

The contributions of Jean Massion, Giorgio Innocenti, Paolo Rossini, Guido Rubboli and Giuliano Avanzini in the first part of the book allow the following conclusions to be drawn. Falling occurs when there is a failure of antigravity posture, which may depend on the projection of the centre of gravity outside the supporting area, or a loss of anti-gravity muscle activity. The maintenance of an anti-gravity posture is a dynamic process that requires the continuous adjustment of agonist–antagonist contractions: the effect of an epileptic discharge can transiently disrupt this delicate balance at various levels of its integration in the central nervous system, from the cortex to the spinal motor neurons. The combination of recording (e.g. video polygraphy) and stimulation procedures (e.g. transcranial magnetic stimulation) makes it possible to analyse in great detail the characteristics of falling seizures and negative myoclonus, and to investigate the putative cortical mechanisms underlying the different types of fall and their topographic representation. In addition to providing specific information on the suppressory–inhibitory effects of transcranial stimulation and on negative myoclonus-related EEG potentials, the presented data stress the potential value of the advanced neurophysiological methodologies now available in every well-equipped neurophysiological unit to pathophysiological studies in humans.

The effect of the maturational processes of the central nervous system on the generation and expression of epileptic falls needs to be considered with respect to two aspects: on the one hand, it should take into account the age-dependent anatomo-functional development of the structures responsible for anti-gravity postures; on the other, the maturation of the physiological properties and connectivity patterns relating to the generation and propagation of epileptic discharges. During the first two years of post-natal life, the passive and active properties responsible for the excitability of cortical neurons undergo significant changes regarding both the subject's susceptibility to epileptogenic agents and the phenomenological expression of the seizures. During the same period, postural control evolves from its initially very primitive organization to the ability to stand up and walk. Parallel analysis of the maturation of the motor system and cortical excitability accounts for the age-dependent changes in the expression of seizures impairing anti-gravity posture control, such as spasms, tonic and atonic seizures and negative myoclonus. An important point is the peculiar development profile of commissural callosal fibres, which are over-represented during the early post-natal period and undergo significant reshaping during development, with the elimination of exuberant axonal structures. Since the development of neural connectivity and synaptogenesis are greatly affected by the functional activity present in a neuronal network, it can be reasonably expected that the excessive activity of an epileptogenic focus during critical developmental stages may interfere with the normal reshaping process, thus leading to permanent abnormal connectivity. The extent to which this theoretical possibility actually occurs in early onset epilepsies is a very important question that needs to be approached from both basic and clinical points of view. Should an early epileptogenic focus be found to prevent the elimination of the supranumerary callosal axons in a given area, this may provide the still lacking rational basis for the claimed result of callosotomy on epileptic falls. In general, our understanding of the possible interference of an epileptogenic process that takes place at a given maturational stage, with the further development of the central nervous system, is limited and needs to be extended further.

The next two sections, which are dedicated to the semeiological and clinical aspects of epileptic falls, constitute the core of the book.

Electroclinical semeiology is extensively dealt with in the chapters prepared by Michelle Bureau, Henri Régis, Silvana Franceschetti, Giuseppe Gobbi and their associates, Charlotte Dravet,

Synopsis

Pierre Thomas, Arnaud Biraben, Pierre Jallon and Pierre Loiseau provide detailed clinical accounts of the partial and generalized syndromes presenting with epileptic falls including their prognostic aspects.

The first message that can be drawn concerns the need for a reliable methodology. Polygraphic and video-EEG recordings should be individually designed on the basis of the information obtained from a cerebral clinical examination of the phenomenon. The EMG surface electrodes should be placed along the axis of the muscle fibres, with their topography depending on the anatomy of the muscle group involved in the falling seizures. Collodion-attached scalp EEG electrodes must be placed according to the complete 10–20 system array in order to provide a simultaneous recording of all of the relevant EEG correlates. As a rule, polygraphic EEG–EMG recordings should be combined with a video recording and any type of transducer that allows the optimal monitoring of the motor phenomena to be explored.

The anti-gravity position of the patient, as well as the motor patterns and stimulations explored during the video polygraphic examination should be carefully monitored.

These guidelines, which are systematically set forth in the chapter by Bureau & Régis, also come out in all of the other contributions. As trivial as they might seem, they need to be particularly stressed in view of the growing everyday use of computerized systems in neurophysiology laboratories. Useful though they may be, the sophisticated elaborations of the signals that such equipment makes feasible become meaningless if the reliability of the original signal cannot be strictly taken for granted and the resulting picture is nothing but garbage in a fancy coloured display.

When using polygraphy in infants, it is particularly important to be able to detect erratic non-obvious failures of postural activity involving only limited groups of axial (e.g. neck) and limb muscles.

The information derived from a detailed analysis of motor phenomenology and of its EEG correlates may be relevant in making a pathophysiological interpretation, a point that clearly comes out from the discussion on the cortical versus the brainstem origin of the discharge responsible for infantile spasms. In the first instance, the spasm-associated slow-wave EEG transient should be seen as the electrographic correlate of the primary cortical discharge, which spreads secondarily to the brainstem structures responsible for the motor effect; in the second case, it would simply represent a cortical response evoked from the primary activation of the brainstem generator. This debate applies to some general concepts concerning epileptic seizures because it raises the possibility that seizure symptoms are not necessarily a functional representation of the site of origin, but may depend on the secondary activation of a rather stereotyped subcortical effector (such as the brainstem tonogenic structures). In this case, the differentiation of generalized and partial seizures becomes clearly academic: the spasm can be considered generalized in that it generally involves both sides globally, but it can also be considered partial in the sense that its brainstem generator is triggered by a focal cortical discharge. In general, the classification criteria of both seizures and epilepsy were repeatedly challenged by the examples shown during the video sessions which underlined the great inter- and intra-individual variability of the characteristics of seizures.

If they exist at all, pure atonic seizures should be considered very rare since, in most cases, the loss of anti-gravity muscle activity is associated with myoclonic or tonic components that should be carefully investigated by means of polygraphic recordings. It must be admitted that, in the past, we sometimes tended to force observations into the framework of our theoretical

215

conceptions (or preconceptions); this is no longer possible now that everybody can present convincing documentation of the exceptions. If this were to lead us to revise the classifications of seizures and epilepsies in order to reflect the reality better, this would certainly improve their alignment with the need to define homogeneous forms that putatively correspond to specific pathophysiological and causative (namely genetic) mechanisms, and deserve further investigation. Moreover, a precise definition of the type of epilepsy in which the epileptic falls occur is crucial to the prediction of individual prognoses.

Evaluations of the consequences of falling seizures on social life and patients' feelings can be found in the reports by Giorgio Capizzi, Laura Mira, René Soulayrol and their associates. The catastrophic consequences of brutal falls account for patient fear and negative environmental reactions that need to be borne in mind by all of the physicians, psychologists, nurses and social workers involved in patient care.

The points mentioned above give only an incomplete picture of the book's comprehensive treatment of the semeiological and clinical aspects of epilepsies with falling seizures, and suffer from obvious limitations due to the subjectivity of the present reviewer. Detailed information can be found in the specific chapters. However, what the reader will certainly miss is the high-quality video documentation that was provided during the meeting by many speakers and especially by Federico Vigevano, Perrine Plouin and their associates in the two sessions devoted to video.

The last section is devoted to the therapeutic problems; and 'problem' is the right word when considering seizure/epilepsy types such as those dealt within this book, which are particularly difficult to treat. The first chapter by Francesco Viani and his collaborators, Antonio Romeo and Maurizio Viri, provides a comprehensive account of the effectiveness and limitations of anti-epileptic drugs based on published results and wide-ranging personal experience. Valproic acid is the most effective of the traditional drugs on the myoclonic, myoclonic-atonic and tonic seizures occurring in myoclonic-astatic epilepsies and Lennox–Gastaut syndromes, especially when it is associated with the benzodiazepines. The percentage of good results varies considerably in different case series because of differences in the definition criteria; but according to the available data, lamotrigine, felbamate and vigabatrin (especially for spasms) seem to be promising. However, there was general consensus concerning the limited effectiveness of drugs, which means that a considerable number of patients with epileptic falls are poorly controlled. The extent to which surgery may be beneficial in such cases is discussed in the two chapters on surgical treatment based on the experiences of the Genova-Grenoble-Milano centres (by Claudio Munari and co-workers) and the Montreal Institute (by Frederick Andermann).

Sudden or slowly progressive ictal falls occur in almost half of the patients who undergo presurgical evaluation for severe drug-resistant partial epilepsies. The main message here is that epileptic falls occurring in partial epilepsies do not necessarily predict a bad outcome from the surgical resection of the epileptogenic area, provided that the surgical indication is based on rigorously rational criteria. However, this population of patients only accounts for a limited number of the pharmacoresistant cases that could potentially benefit from appropriate surgical treatment. For those who are not candidates for resective surgery because of the multifocal or undefined origin of the epileptogenic discharge, callosotomy might be considered: this procedure has undergone considerable technical improvements that have led to a marked reduction in complications and functional defects that occurred in the past (split brain syndrome).

Both the personal experience of the authors and the data from the literature suggest that callosotomy may decrease the number of seizures with postural failure in a certain number of patients. However, predictive efficacy criteria cannot be assessed in most series since the types of seizure (tonic versus atonic or myoclonic), the site(s) of origin of the discharges, and even the type(s) of epilepsy in improved versus unchanged patients, were unevenly specified. During the discussion, Claudio Munari also stressed the need for a careful presurgical study in order to be able to rule out the possibility of a non-obvious monolocalized origin of the epileptogenic discharges, which would indicate resective surgery rather than callosotomy. In general, the selection criteria for callosotomy in patients with epileptic falls need to be further investigated before the procedure can be proposed as a definite therapeutic alternative. In my opinion, particular caution is required when dealing with situations such as epilepsies with falling seizures which are so burdened with anguish that they could sometimes lead the involved physician to be less selective toward treatments of doubtful effectiveness.

In closing these remarks, I would like to thank the Fondazione Mariani which once again made it possible for us to enjoy a meeting of high scientific quality, as is testified by this valuable book. We all particularly appreciated the warm and productive atmosphere created by our exquisite hostess Maria Majno, who took the main weight of the organization on herself.

I would also like to thank the University of Milan, whose distinguished representative, my friend Luciano Martini, was with us during the meeting.

My special gratitude is due to Laura Mira who made it possible for me to sit on the scientific committee by compensating for all of my delays and defaults; and in praising the beautiful job she did, I would like to associate the name of David Zerbi, who made a discreet but important contribution to the organization of the meeting.

Everybody also appreciated the active and productive participation of Frederick Andermann throughout the meeting, which significantly contributed to its success.

Last but not least, we would all like to warmly praise Annette Beaumanoir, the inspiration behind the Colloquium whose 'sprighthly and fashinating' personality imprinted the entire meeting. Annette is one of the most distinguished representatives of the French School to which we owe many of the ideas that were debated: it is no accident that a French cadence was so often listened to during the meeting, something which might also have brought a pleased smile to the face of Henri Gastaut.

Index

A

acute disconnection syndrome, 186–187
adolescence, falling attacks during 113–121
age, and expression of, epilepsy
    34–37, 55, 76, 95–97, 106, 114
akinetic seizures 38–39, 58, 98, 114
anti-epileptic drugs 147–156, 188, 216
antigravity function, of posture 12–13
astatic seizures 3, 29, 30, 38–39, 98, 114
atonic seizures
    classification 1
    collapse seizures 109
    drop attacks 3, 113–114, 147–148
    EEG pattern 70, 72, 73
    electroclinical features 58, 59
    EMG pattern 69, 73
    in juvenile myoclonic epilepsy 118
    in Lennox–Gastaut syndrome 98, 118
    pathogenesis 3–4
    pathophysiology 178–179
    pharmacological treatment of 148, 150
    rarity of 215
    relation to cerebral maturation 38–39
    response to callosotomy 176, 185, 188
aura 207
axonal geometry 20, 20–22

B

balance
    contrasted with posture 13–14
    loss of 5
    sources of disequilibrium 11–12, 12
basal ganglia epilepsy 89

benign myoclonic epilepsy 35, 141–142
benzodiazepines 148, 153, 156, 216
bilateral perisylvian syndrome 177
brain transcranial stimulation *see*
    transcranial stimulation
breath-holding spells 85–86

C

callosal axons
    abnormal development of, and epilepsy 25–26
    axonal geometry 20, 20–22
    corpus callosum of the cat 19–21, 20
    differentiation of 22–25, 23
    elimination of exuberant axonal
        structures 25
    functional implications 21–22
    growth 23, 23–25, 26
    morphology 21–22
callosotomy 175–188
    as a palliative treatment 159
    cases of 'trunk fit' 130, 132
    complications 185–188
    history 175–176
    outcome 182–185
    preoperative evaluation 179–181, *184–184*, *187*
    rationale and indications for
        134, 160, 176–178, 216–217
    surgical procedure 181–184, *188*
    versus resective surgery 168–169
    see also callosal axons
carbamazepine 148–149, 151–155
cataplexy 89
CBZ *see* carbamazepine

219

cerebral maturation
    epileptic postural lapses   37–39
    maturation of cortical and
        thalamic neurons   31–33, *32*
children, long-term outcomes for
    137, *138*, 139, *140–141*, 141–143
clobazam   148
clonazepam   148
convulsive syncope   84
corpus callosum   19–21, *20*, 175–176
    see also callosotomy
cortectomy   128, 163, 166, 168
cortical neurons
    connectivity   19–26
    maturation of   31–33, *32*, 214
    possible cortical origin of
        falling seizures   60–61, 75, 77–79
cortical resection   159–170
craniotomy   181–184
cryptogenic generalized epilepsies   143
cryptogenic localization-related epilepsies   142
cyanotic breath-holding spells   85–86

D
dementia   106
disease normalization   204
disease trivialization   203–204
Doose syndrome *see* myoclonic-astatic seizures
drop attacks *see* atonic seizures; epileptic
    falling seizures
drugs, anti-epileptic   147–156, 188, 216

E
early infantile encephalopathy with
    suppression burst   34
early myoclonus encephalopathy   34
electroencephalography
    epileptic negative myoclonus   *120*
    guidelines for reliable methodology   215
    infantile spasms   77, 215
    juvenile myoclonic epilepsy   *118*
    Lennox–Gastaut syndrome   4
    methodology   65, 67, *67*
    myoclonic absences   *107*
    myoclonic-astatic seizures   103, *104*, 105
    positioning and number of electrodes   69–70
    representation of a startle   *73*
    stereo-electro-encephalography   126, *127*, 128,
        129, 130, *131*, 132, *133*, 134, 169
    technique   69–71
    tonic seizures   4, *98*
    types of patterns   70–71
    use in clinical diagnosis   71, *72–73*, 74
    West syndrome   78, *78*
electromyography
    electrode positioning   67–68, *68*
    guidelines for reliable methodology   215
    representation of a startle   69, *69*, *73*
    running the examination   68
    technique   67–69
    types of EMG manifestations   68–69, *69*
    use in clinical diagnosis   71, *71–73*, 74
epilepsy with continuous spike-waves
    during slow sleep   108–109, *109*
epileptic falling seizures
    classification   96
    clinical and neurophysiological features
        53–61, 168
    control of   177
    cortical origins   60–61
    cortical resection   160, 161–164
    defined   29, 147, 178
    diagnostic issues   60
    'drop attacks'   1, 3, 4, 58
    during adolescence   113–121, 210
    long-term outcomes
        137, *138*, 139, *140–141*, 141–143
    paroxysmal impairment
        of equilibration   125–126, *127*, 128
    paroxysmal kinesigenic choreoathetosis   88–89
    paroxysmal modification of tone and posture
        125, 128, *129*, 130, *131*, 132, *133*
    pathophysiology of   60–61, 178–179
    pharmacological treatment of   147–156, 216
    psychopathological and humanistic aspects
        207–212
    relation to axonal development   25–26
    response to callosotomy   176–177, 185, 188
    risk of injury   193–196
    secondary generalizations   125
    subjects with epileptic frontal focus   5
    types of   1–4, 29–30
    vegetative paroxysmal impairments   125
    see also astatic seizures; atonic seizures;
        infantile spasms; Lennox–Gastaut syndrome;
        myoclonic-astatic seizures; myoclonic
        seizures; non-epileptic falling seizures; poly-
        graphic recording, of falls; social life, of the
        epileptic child; tonic seizures

Index

epileptic negative myoclonus
    age of onset   37
    atonic seizures   4–5
    clinical aspects   54–55
    defined   38, 54
    EEG reading   *54*
    neurophysiological aspects   55–57, *56, 57*
    progressive myoclonus epilepsy   119, *120*, 121
epileptic spasms *see* spasms
ethosuximide   148

F
falling
    'falling sickness'   29, 207–208
    fear of, in religion and mythology   208–211
    symbolism of   210–211
    see also epileptic falling seizures;
        non-epileptic falling seizures
family, of the epileptic child   201–202
FBM *see* felbamate
felbamate   149, 151, 153–156, 216
flexor tonic seizures   29–30
focal epilepsies, of adolescence   121

G
Gastaut, Henri   vii, 1–4, 213, 217
generalized epilepsies   58, 99, 115
GVG *see* vigabatrin

H
head drop, EEG pattern of   *100*
hemispherectomy   169, 178
hereditary startle disease   87–88
hyperrekplexia   87–88
hypertonia   128, 130, 132
hypothalamic hamartoma   168
hypsarrhythmia   77

I
idiopathic generalized epilepsy   142–143, 193–194
idiopathic localization-related epilepsy   141–142
idiopathic partial epilepsy   193–194
infantile epilepsies
    benign myoclonic epilepsy   35, 141–142
    early infantile encephalopathy with
        suppression burst   34
    early myoclonus encephalopathy   34
    infantile spasms   3, 34, 75–79, 81, 215
    myoclonic epilepsies   35–36
    severe myoclonic epilepsy   35–36

West syndrome and related
    conditions   34, 76–78, *78*, 97, 148
injury, risk of in epileptic falls   193–196

J
juvenile myoclonic epilepsy   114–118
    clinical presentation   116–118, *117*
    EEG patterns   *115*, 115–116, *118*
    falling seizures   5
    genetic susceptibility to   116
    onset and symptoms   114–115
    treatment and outcome   37, 116

L
Lafora's disease   109, 119, *120*, 121
lamotrigine   148–149, 151, 154–156, 188, 216
Lennox–Gastaut syndrome   95–102
    aetiology   96–97
    clinical presentation   97–101
    contrasted with myoclonic-astatic epilepsy   36
    defining features   96
    differential diagnosis   101
    drop attacks   147
    EEG patterns   *100*, 100–101, 102
    in adults   118–119
    neurophysiological and psychiatric symptoms
         100–101
    pharmacological treatment of   148–156
    response to callosotomy   177–178, 187
    symptomatic generalized epilepsies   143
    tonic seizures   4, 80
    tonic seizures with spasms   76
    treatment and outcome   101–102
lesionectomy   128, 163, 166
LMT *see* lamotrigine

M
magnetic resonance
    imaging   180–181, 184, 186–187
marginalization, of epileptics   202, 204
medical practitioners, and social issues   203
mental retardation   86, 103, 143
metaphysics, and epilepsy   211–212
modular postural control   13–14
motor programmes, effect of TCS on   49
muscle tone, changes in   5, 12
myoclonic absences   37, 106–108, *107*, 115

myoclonic-astatic seizures	
classification	29, 102
clinical presentation	103, *104*, 105
contrasted with Lennox–Gastaut syndrome	36, 102–103
defining features	102–103
differential diagnosis	105
drop attacks	147
EEG patterns	103, *104*, 105
pharmacological treatment of	149–150, 155–156
treatment and outcome	106
myoclonic-atonic seizures	
drop attacks	148
electroclinical features	58
in Lennox–Gastaut syndrome	98, 101, 118
myoclonia of	4
pathophysiology of	178
pharmacological treatment of	150–156
myoclonic seizures	
classification	1
defined	2
diagnosis of	105
drop attacks	147–148
EEG pattern	73
electroclinical features	58
EMG pattern	69, 73
impairment of postural control	29–30
in Lennox–Gastaut syndrome	98, 101, 118
infancy and early childhood	35–36
late childhood and adolescence	37
pharmacological treatment of	148, 150
relation to cerebral maturation	37
see also juvenile myoclonic epilepsy	

N

narcolepsy	89
neocortex, physiology of	33
neuronal ceroid lipofuscinosis	109
non-epileptic falling seizures	83–90
classification	1, 84
with consciousness loss	84–87
without consciousness loss	87–89
normalization	204

O

ocular tilt reaction	*12*

P

pallid breath-holding spells	85, 86
paroxysmal impairment of equilibration	125–126, *127*, 128
paroxysmal kinesigenic choreoathetosis	88–89
paroxysmal modification of tone	125, 128, *129*, 130, *131*, 132, *133*
partial epilepsies	
benign partial epilepsy	105, 109
classification	1
EEG pattern	70
electroclinical features	60
in Lennox–Gastaut syndrome	99
postoperative	187
postural loss in seizures	37, 137, 148
resective surgery for	168–169
pathological startle	87
phenitoin	148
phenobarbital	148
polygraphic recording, of falls	65–74
clinical diagnosis using	71, *72–73*, 74
drop attacks	148
electroencephalography	69–71
electromyography	67–69
graphic representations of movements	67
guidelines for reliable methodology	215
infantile spasms	76
juvenile myoclonic epilepsy	*117*
picture study	65, 66
video-polygraphic recording	53, 60
West syndrome	78, *78*
posture	
anticipatory postural adjustments	15–17, *16*
cerebral maturation and lapses of	37–39
contrasted with balance	13–14
definition and function	12–13
elements of equilibrium control	*14*, 14–15
loss of	5
modular versus antigravity organization of	13–14
normal development of postural control	30–31, *31*
postural body scheme	14
postural reactions	15
progressive myoclonus epilepsy	109, 119, *120*, 121
psychogenic seizures, with or without loss of consciousness	89

R

Rasmussen's syndrome	164
related epileptic silent period	54
Rett syndrome	86

S

secondary generalizations 125, 148
seizures *see* epileptic falling seizures
severe myoclonic epilepsy 35–36
siblings, of the epileptic child 202
silent periods
    EMG patterns *71*
    following transcranial stimulation 45–50, *46*
social life, of the epileptic child 199–205
    among family members 201–202
    effect of falls on social interaction
        199–201, 204–205
    in school, play and sport 202–203
social rights, of the epileptic child 203–204
sodium valproate 148–151, 153–156, 186, 216
spasms
    infantile spasms 3, 34, 75–79, 81, 215
    pharmacological treatment of 150–156
Spielmeyer–Vogt–Sjogren disease 119
split-brain syndrome 187
startle 87
status epilepticus 4–5
stereo-electro-encephalography
    126, *127*, 128, *129*, 130, *131*, 132, *133*, 134, 169
surgery, for seizures with falls 159–170
    case report 166, *167*, 168
    patients and methods 160–161
    results 161–166
    see also specific procedures
symptomatic generalized epilepsy 143, 193–194
symptomatic localization-related epilepsy 142
symptomatic partial epilepsy 193–194
syncopes 84–85, 121, 148

T

temporal syncope 148
thalamic neurons, maturation of 31–33, *32*
tonic-clonic seizures, generalized 115
tonic seizures
    characteristic muscle contractions 75–76
    classification 1, 81
    contrasted with atonic seizures and spasms 36
    defined 80, 81
    drop attacks 147–148
    EEG patterns 80
    EMG patterns *69*
    epilepsy with continuous spike-waves
        during slow sleep 108–109
    expression of 79–80
    features 2–3, 59–60
    in Lennox–Gastaut syndrome
        97–98, *98*, 101–102, 118
    in myoclonic-astatic epilepsy 103, 105
    pathophysiology of 178–179
    pharmacological treatment of 150–156
    postural loss 29
    relation to cerebral maturation 37
    response to callosotomy 176, 185, 188
transcranial stimulation 45–50
    during epileptic negative myoclonus 56–57, *57*
    inhibitory effects of 48–50, *49*
    muscular silent period following 45–50, *46*
    procedure 45–46
trivialization 203–204
'trunk fits' 128, 134

U

Unverricht–Lundborg's disease 109, 119, 121

V

Valsalva manoeuvre 86
vegetative paroxysmal impairments 125
vertigo 126, 128
vestibular afferents, dysfunctioning of 11–12, *12*
vigabatrin 148, 149, 152–156, 216
visual areas, of the cat 19–20, 23, *23*
VPA *see* sodium valproate

W

West syndrome 34, 76–78, *78*, 97, 148
    see also infantile spasms